Principles of Biomedical Ethics

Principles of Biomedical Ethics

TOM L. BEAUCHAMP   JAMES F. CHILDRESS

New York   Oxford
OXFORD UNIVERSITY PRESS
1979

Library of Congress Cataloging in Publication Data
Beauchamp, Tom L
  Principles of biomedical ethics.

  Bibliography: p.
  Includes index.
  1. Medical ethics.
  I. Childress, James F., joint author.   II. Title.
R724.B36   174'.2   78-15638
ISBN 0-19-502487-7   ISBN 0-19-502488-5 pbk.

Printed in the United States of America

To
Georgia, Ruth, and Don

I can no other answer make but thanks,
And thanks, and ever thanks.

Twelfth Night

Preface

This book offers a systematic analysis of the moral principles that should apply to biomedicine. Many books in the rapidly expanding field of biomedical ethics focus on a series of problems such as abortion, euthanasia, behavior control, research involving human subjects, and the distribution of health care. Rarely do these books concentrate on the principles that should apply to a wide range of biomedical problems—including but not limited to the aforementioned problems. As a result, the moral judgments involved in one dilemma may appear to be unconnected to the moral judgments in others. Such a disjointed approach often relies on the discussion of cases, with little attention to the principles that both create and illuminate the dilemmas. As noted by a character in Tom Stoppard's play, *Professional Foul,* "There would be no moral dilemmas if moral principles worked in straight lines and never crossed each other." Only by examining moral principles and determining how they apply to cases and how they conflict can we bring some order and coherence to the discussion of these problems. Only then can we see that there are procedures and standards for deliberation and justification in biomedical ethics that parallel those in other areas of human activity.

We understand "biomedical ethics" as one type of *applied ethics*—the application of general ethical theories, principles, and rules to problems of therapeutic practice, health care delivery, and medical and biological research. In our discussions of ethical theory per se, we offer analyses of levels of moral deliberation and justification and of the ways two major approaches—utilitarian and deontological theories—interpret principles, rules, and judgments (Chapters 1–2). The systematic core of the book (Chapters 3–6) presents four fundamental moral principles—autonomy, beneficence, nonmaleficence, and justice. Here we analyze the meaning, weight, and implications of these principles, as well as their interrelationships. The next chapter (7) sketches the principles of truthfulness and confidentiality, as well as some of the role responsibilities that frequently come into conflict for health care professionals and researchers. The final chapter (8) examines ideals, virtues, and integrity—other important ingredients of the moral life. We say that Chapters 3–6 constitute the systematic core of the book because these chapters are intended to provide an integrated framework of principles through which diverse moral problems may be handled. If there is either an incompleteness of principles or an ad hoc quality to the selection of these four principles, then we have not fully achieved our goals in this book.

Because biomedical ethics is *applied* ethics, it is essential to examine a wide variety of actual cases involving medical practice, health care delivery, research, and public policy. A systematic analysis of moral principles would otherwise be disembodied and useless. Thus, in our treatment of ethical theories and principles, we also discuss actual cases. Such cases not only illustrate principles and their conflicts, they also provide a way to explicate and to test the principles. And, as we know from the history of law and morals, hard cases sometimes lead to a modification of the principles themselves.

In Appendix I we present twenty-nine detailed cases. At various points in the text we discuss these cases in relation to moral principles. Virtually all these cases are based on actual occurrences, and most were originally reported by medical professionals. They are intended to be as representative of current problems as possible. Several cases are drawn from the law, not because law and morality are coextensive, but because legal decisions commonly appeal to moral principles and rules, or raise issues that must be handled at least in part by moral deliberation. Other cases not presented in the Appendix are used as illustrations in the text. (For teachers of biomedical ethics who wish to supplement these cases, Robert Veatch's *Case Studies in Medical Ethics* offers a number of similarly constructed cases.)

Even a comprehensive treatment of the principles of biomedical ethics cannot indicate all their important applications. We have been selective, and we have tended to concentrate on typical and representative issues and cases. Because of limitations of space, we have not included cases, for example, of transsexual surgery, in vitro fertilization, psychosurgery, or behavior modification. However, we believe that our framework of principles can illuminate such cases.

One major difficulty in a book of this sort is to define and then address the appropriate audience. Our intended audience includes health care professionals such as physicians and nurses, research investigators, policy makers in biomedicine, and students preparing for such roles who are interested in how ethical theories bear on their activities. Our intended audience also includes philosophers, theologians, and students in philosophy and religious studies who are interested in how their reflections on ethical theory relate to biomedicine. For such a mixed audience, it is necessary to eliminate or at least to define technical terms from each specialty. We have tried to presuppose only minimal acquaintance with philosophy, theology, and medicine—merely what the average aware person even on the college level could be expected to possess. Above all we have kept in mind teachers and students who will use this book in the classroom. We have tried to write as clearly and as concisely as possible, with ample cases and examples to clarify the theoretical points. In several cases in Appendix I, we have not, however, eliminated or defined all technical medical terms. In most instances, the gist of the case will be clear, and when we discuss the case in the text, we restate relevant points in nontechnical language.

Although our discussions and cases mainly refer to problems encountered by physicians and researchers, we intend our analyses to be pertinent to other health care professionals and policy makers as well. Consider nursing, for example. Most of the issues that we raise may be redescribed in virtually identical terms for nurses and other members of a health care team. The same moral principles and rules govern nurses as well as physicians. By explicating the presuppositions and implications of such principles and rules, we thus hope to illuminate nursing no less than medicine. What is special about nursing from a moral standpoint is the question of authority and power on the health care team. Special moral dilemmas for nursing may arise from power conflicts. Such conflicts frequently involve disagreements about moral principles and judgments;

but again these disagreements may occur among members of the same profession as well as among members of different professions. In any event, when the nurse has to decide whether to continue to cooperate on a health care team, whether to follow a doctor's instructions, etc., the relevant moral principles and rules for the decision are identical to those for doctors. Similar points could be made about other specialties. Thus, our general analysis of ethical principles is designed to apply to the whole range of biomedicine and health care delivery. (Appendix II is composed of several professional codes, declarations, and regulations derived from ethical and policy reflections within such specialty professions.)

Ethics as the systematic examination of the moral life is designed to illuminate what we ought to do by asking us to consider and reconsider our ordinary actions, judgments, and justifications. While we rarely find knockdown arguments in debates about applied ethics, such debates are subject to rational analysis. However—to paraphrase Aristotle—we can only expect the precision and degree of certainty appropriate to the subject matter. Sometimes the answers cannot be as tidy as we might wish.

T.L.B.
J.F.C.

Washington, D.C.
December 1978

Acknowledgments

Every book has its history, and every author incurs debts of gratitude. In 1976 the authors and Dr. Seymour Perlin, a psychiatrist then at the Kennedy Institute of Ethics and now at the George Washington University School of Medicine, frequently discussed the need for a systematic analysis of the *principles* that should govern a wide range of decisions affecting biomedicine. These discussions led the three of us to embark on the project that eventuated in this book. Our original intention was to produce a jointly authored analysis by a philosopher, a religious ethicist, and a physician. Although Dr. Perlin was prevented from participating in the actual writing because of other commitments, he did complete an anthology with Beauchamp on related matters, and he made important contributions in the early stages of this book. We are grateful to him for his inspiration and enthusiastic support.

Since 1976 the authors have had a range of professional experiences that partially compensate for the absence of a physician on the writing team. In each instance they received assistance that led to changes in this book. First, they assumed primary responsibility for the ethical theory portion of the Kennedy Institute Intensive Bioethics Course, which is held each summer for 50–60 scientists, physicians, nurses, and other health care professionals. In addition, Childress has offered two seminars for physicians and other health care professionals under the auspices of the National Endowment for the Humanities and has taught in several workshops at the Hastings Center. During this same period of time, Beauchamp served as staff philosopher for the National Commission for the Protection of Human Subjects of Biomedical and Behavioral Research (N.I.H.), as a lecturer and consultant to dialysis and transplant societies composed of physicians and nurses, and as a Chautauqua lecturer on these subjects for college teachers under the auspices of the National Science Foundation and the American Association for the Advancement of Science. These experiences, in conjunction with seminars, lectures, and consultations in a variety of clinical and research settings at Georgetown and elsewhere, have made us sensitive to the concrete problems that must be faced by health care professionals. We still have much to learn, but we hope that we have been able to depict realistically and sympathetically many dilemmas faced by these professionals and by their patients and subjects.

This is a jointly authored book in every sense of the term. Although each author initially had primary responsibility for certain chapters, both authors rewrote substantial parts of every chapter and take responsibility for the whole, which at every point bears their dual imprint, whether by conviction or by compromise. The interaction that permitted this collaboration was facilitated by the Kennedy Institute of Ethics, which offers maximal freedom and stimulation to pursue such projects and which brings together medical practitioners and health care professionals, as well as philosophers, theologians, and lawyers. We are grateful to various colleagues—particularly to André Hellegers, Director of the Kennedy Institute, and to LeRoy Walters, Director of the Center for Bioethics at the Institute, for making this setting so attractive. In addition, we are indebted to the Kennedy Foundation for its support of the Kennedy Institute and to Sargent Shriver and Eunice Kennedy Shriver for their personal interest and encouragement.

Writers who influence the authors of books can sometimes go unnoticed because readers customarily look only to chapter and footnote references for such influences. In the present book, however, two hidden sources deserve special mention. First, no footnotes to Gerald Dworkin appear in the first section of Chapter 3 on Autonomy. Nonetheless, one of his unpublished manuscripts heavily influenced some parts of this section. This has since been published as "Moral Autonomy," in H. Tristram Engelhardt, Jr. and Daniel Callahan, eds., *Morals, Science and Sociality*

(The Hastings Center, 1978). Second, the work of the National Commission for the Protection of Human Subjects was carried on almost coextensively with the writing of this book. The deliberations of this body led us to think through old and new problems more carefully. Several commissioners, particularly Donald Seldin, M.D., Al Jonsen, Ph.D., and Patricia King, J.D., influenced the development of the book. Both of us at different times had the good fortune to teach law school seminars with Professor King, and we are also indebted, to her for the perspectives gained from this exposure.

Among the several people who read full drafts of the manuscript, Dr. Joanne Lynn of the George Washington University School of Medicine, Dr. Joan Sieber, a psychologist at the Kennedy Institute and the California State University, Hayward, and Dr. Martin Benjamin of the Philosophy Department at Michigan State deserve special mention for their thorough and valuable commentaries. We are grateful to them and to others who offered criticisms and suggestions.

Several members of the Kennedy Institute staff aided us immeasurably. Our research assistants, James J. McCartney and Dorle Vawter, contributed in numerous ways by checking references, reading proofs, and making helpful suggestions regarding style and substance. In addition, McCartney wrote a number of cases for Appendix I; others who graciously provided cases are identified in footnotes to this Appendix. William Pitt prepared the index with his customary attention to detail. The library staff at the Institute, particularly Doris Goldstein and Betsy Walkup, supplied many references and materials, frequently on short notice. Most importantly, we are grateful to Mary Baker, executive secretary par excellence, who did most of the administrative organization and typing, assisted by Mary Ellen Timbol. We cannot exaggerate our gratitude to Mrs. Baker, whose cheerfulness, friendship, diligence, and remarkable abilities make our various activities easier and more fruitful.

Finally, Beauchamp wishes to express personal debts of gratitude to Ruth Faden of the Johns Hopkins University School of Hygiene and Public Health and the Kennedy Institute and to Don Seldin of the University of Texas Medical School (Southwestern). Sometimes it is impossible to distinguish special friendships from influential professional relationships, and this distinction was never more difficult to make than in the case of his association with these two remarkable individuals. The portion of this book contributed by Beauchamp is dedicated to these cherished friends. Childress expresses his deepest gratitude to his wife, Georgia, to whom he dedicates his portion of this book, and to his sons, Fred and Frank, for contributions that relate to, but also go well beyond, this book. They are an unfailing source of support and joy for him.

Contents

Principles of Biomedical Ethics

1

Morality and Ethical Theory

Moral dilemmas and moral reasoning

People in a variety of roles frequently must make difficult decisions. Consider an example involving two California judges reflecting on a murder (Case #1 in the Appendix). A woman was killed by a man who had previously confided to a psychiatrist his intention to kill her. The psychiatrist attempted to have the man committed, but, because of patient/physician confidentiality, he did not communicate the threat to the woman when the commitment attempt failed. This case eventually reached the California Supreme Court. The judge who wrote the majority opinion in the case held that "When a therapist determines, or pursuant to the standards of his profession should determine, that his patient presents a serious danger of violence to another, he incurs an obligation to use reasonable care to protect the intended victim against such danger," including notification of the police and possibly a direct warning. The judge argued that although the protective privilege of medical confidentiality ought generally to be observed by physicians, it must yield in the present case to the "public interest in safety from violent assault." The judge's position is that rules of professional ethics have a substantial public importance but nonetheless can be overridden by matters of greater importance, such as the protection of persons from violent assault. In the minority opinion in this case, a second judge stated his disagreement. He argued that patient rights are violated when rules of confidentiality are not observed, that patients will lose confidence in psychiatrists and will fail to divulge critical information to them, and that violent assaults will actually increase as a result, because mentally ill persons will not seek psychiatric aid.

This case can be read as a straightforward moral dilemma (and perhaps also as a legal dilemma), because both judges cited strong moral reasons in support of their quite opposite conclusions. But what makes this or any situation a moral dilemma or quandary? In dilemmatic situations the reasons on each side of a problem are weighty ones, and none is in any obvious way the right set of reasons. If one acts on either set of reasons, one's actions will be desirable in some respects but undesirable in other respects. Yet one thinks that ideally one ought to act on all the reasons, for each is, considered by itself, a good reason. If there is a conflict between moral obligation, on the one hand, and self-interest or personal inclination, on the other, we do not usually conceive the situation as presenting a moral dilemma, for *moral* dilemmas arise when one can appeal to moral considerations for taking each of two opposing courses of action. If moral reasons compete with nonmoral reasons, difficult questions can be posed (for example, why be moral?), without creating a *moral* dilemma. Some situations, however, clearly involve moral dilemmas. They take the following forms:[1] (1) Some evidence indicates that act X is morally right, and some evidence indicates that act X is morally wrong, but the evidence on both sides is inconclusive. Abortion, for example, is sometimes said to be "a terrible dilemma" for women who see the evidence in this way. (2) It is clear to the agent that on moral grounds he or she both ought and ought not to perform act X. For example, some have viewed the intentional cessation of lifesaving therapies in the case of comatose patients as dilemmatic in this way.

In this book we examine the reasons that do and should go into moral *deliberation* and into moral *justification* in biomedicine. The reasons that are properly used in justification will also appear in deliberation whenever the agent tries to determine which course of action is right, i.e., morally justified or even obligatory. The reasons present in moral deliberation thus are justifying reasons, because they express the conditions under which a moral action is justified.

Our approach to moral reasoning in deliberation and justification can be diagrammed in the form of hierarchical levels or tiers, which we will call levels of moral justification:

4 *Ethical Theories*
↑
3 *Principles*
↑
2 *Rules*
↑
1 *Judgments and Actions*

According to this diagram, judgments about what ought to be done in particular situations are justified by moral rules, which in turn are grounded in principles and ultimately in ethical theories. For example, a physician who refuses to perform amniocentesis (a process of withdrawing fluid from the amniotic sac of a pregnant woman in order to test for congenital diseases) may hold that it is morally wrong intentionally to kill innocent human beings. When pressed, he may justify the proclaimed moral rule against killing innocent human beings by reference to a principle of the sanctity of human life. Finally, the particular judgment, the rule, and the principle may be grounded in an ethical theory (a theory that for many people may be only implicit and inchoate).

Although our diagram may be oversimplified, it is designed to indicate that in the process of moral reasoning we appeal to different reasons of varying degrees of abstraction and systematization. Let us start with the lowest level and move upwards. A *judgment* is a decision, verdict, or conclusion about a particular action. Although the precise nature of the distinction between rules and principles is somewhat controversial, *rules* state that actions of a certain kind ought (or ought not) to be done because they are right (or wrong). A simple example is, "It is wrong to lie to a patient." *Principles* are more general and fundamental than moral rules and serve as their foundation. The principle of respect for persons, for example, may ground several moral rules of the "it is wrong to lie" sort. Finally, *theories* are bodies of principles and rules, more or less systematically related. They include second-order principles and rules about what to do when there are conflicts. Utilitarian theories, as we shall see, are one important example of ethical theories. Following William Frankena, we will refer to all these levels or tiers, but especially to principles and rules, as "action-guides."

Moral judgments involve applications of action-guides to concrete situations. They also involve factual beliefs about the world. For instance, if we hold that policy X is wrong because it imposes unjustified risks on a group of people, we presuppose certain beliefs about the facts of the situation. Similarly, judgments about the justifiability of abortion may depend not only on rules and principles, but also on factual beliefs about the nature and development of the fetus. As these examples suggest, the conceptualization of the situation in which we act often depends, at least in part, on scientific, metaphysical, or religious beliefs. In addition, such convictions may be invoked to vindicate certain theories and action-guides (as, for example, in the tradition of natural law). As a result, moral debate about a particular course of action may stem not only from disagreement about the relevant action-guides but also about the correct factual description of the situation.

Consider the example of a debate involving diverse moral reasons and complex interplay between action-guides and factual beliefs. In several exchanges, Paul Ramsey and Richard McCormick have urged different policies in the involvement of children in research that does not offer potential medical benefit to the subjects involved in the research, although it may ultimately benefit others. McCormick holds that it is under some conditions morally permissible to use children in such "nontherapeutic" research. His general rule is that this form of research is justified only if it involves minimal or negligible risk and if there is proxy consent—providing, of course, that the research is also scientifically acceptable, etc. His basic principle, which supports this rule, is one of justice: we all ought to bear certain burdens, usually of a minimal sort, for the common good. Such minimal or negligible burdens are not purely charitable, because they are demanded by justice. Thus, in McCormick's view, both adults and children ought to consent to participation in research under some conditions as a matter of justice. He argues that parents (and other proxies) may legitimately consent for children to participate in nontherapeutic research where the child *ought* to consent (if he could consent) because of a moral obligation. A judgment that it is morally acceptable to use children in nontherapeutic research would, for McCormick, depend on factual beliefs about the probable benefit and risks of the research; e.g., if the risks are more than minimal or negligible, the research is never justified. In addition, McCormick's ethical theory, as a version of natural-law thought, depends on certain factual beliefs about human tendencies that allow him to derive principles and rules about what people ought to do. These tendencies, including the human inclination toward community, are grounded in metaphysics and theology: God has created man with tendencies toward certain values.

By contrast, Paul Ramsey holds that we should never use any child in nontherapeutic research. This rule is grounded in a Kantian principle of respect for persons: we should never treat people merely as means to some other end. To use human subjects who cannot consent in nontherapeutic research violates their integrity; it treats them merely as means to the end of scientific knowledge. Because participation in research involves the use of one's body even where the risks are only minimal or negligible, the act of participation is held by Ramsey to be an act of charity, not justice; and we cannot be charitable for other people by enlisting them in an enterprise without their consent. Ramsey's ideal for research is collaboration and coadventure between researcher and subject. Since this ideal presupposes the capacity for consent, it excludes the use of children. One of Ramsey's grounds for the principle of respect for persons and for the ideal of cooperation is a theological belief about covenant that is developed in the Bible. Given Ramsey's principles and rules, as grounded in certain factual beliefs, he does not entertain attempts to determine whether the risks of research are minimal or negligible. If children cannot consent, he thinks it is morally wrong to use them in nontherapeutic research regardless of the risk-benefit ratio. Furthermore, in contrast to McCormick's view that research involving children is of critical importance, and even mandatory, Ramsey views it as entirely optional.[2]

Although several other points in this debate are noteworthy, what has been said is sufficient to illustrate the complex interrelations between tiers of moral justification and between action-guides and factual beliefs. The debate indicates that disputes about particular acts and policies often involve complex disagreements over factual beliefs, as well as over normative rules, principles, and ethical theories.

Ethical theories and biomedical ethics

Which action-guides are worthy of moral acceptance and why? *General normative ethics* is a field of inquiry which attempts to answer this question. It is constituted by what in our levels of justification are called ethical theories. Such theories seek to formulate and defend a system of moral principles and rules that determine which actions are right and which are wrong. These action-guides are presumably valid for everyone. Ideally, any such ethical theory will include a complete set of ethical action-guides and will defend the claim that they are universally valid. While general normative ethics is an attempt to construct an ethical theory, numerous ethical questions would remain even if a fully satisfactory theory were to be developed. For example, what do the various principles and rules imply for concrete decisions that people must make in everyday life? An attempt to apply these action-guides to different problem areas can be labelled *applied normative ethics*. The term "applied" is used because general ethical principles and rules are applied to illuminate and resolve moral problems. For example, one might appeal to principles of justice and utility in order to illuminate and resolve moral dilemmas concerning such issues as the allocation of scarce medical resources or abortion.

In addition to *normative ethics*, either general or applied, there are at least two *nonnormative* approaches to morality. First, there is *descriptive ethics*, the factual investigation of moral behavior and beliefs. Anthropologists, sociologists, and historians determine, for example, whether and in what ways moral attitudes and codes differ from society to society. They study different beliefs about sexual relations, the treatment of the dying, etc. Second, there is the field of *metaethics*. This approach to morality, which has been warmly embraced by numerous philosophers in this century, involves analysis of the meanings of crucial ethical terms such as "right," "obligation," and "responsibility." Students of metaethics also analyze the logic of moral reasoning, including the nature of moral justification.

Descriptive ethics and metaethics can be grouped together because both are nonnormative; that is, they do not attempt to provide prescriptive action-guides. Instead, they attempt to establish what factually or conceptually *is* the case, not what ethically *ought* to be the case.[3] Only in passing do we take positions in this book on problems of descriptive ethics and metaethics. For example, we operate descriptively in trying to determine what professional medical codes say about certain issues. Even so, we are ultimately interested in whether the codes' prescriptions are *defensible*. We also occasionally deal in metaethics—for example, our discussion later in this chapter of the distinction between moral and nonmoral action-guides is metaethical. But both descriptive and metaethical approaches are secondary to the enterprise of normative ethics throughout this book. Accordingly, when we use the term "ethics" without qualification, we shall mean *normative ethics,* either general or applied.

Our focus is *applied normative ethics,* because biomedical ethics is the application of general moral action-guides to biomedicine. Biomedical ethics is thus comparable to political ethics, jurisprudence, and business ethics. The term "bioethics," which is sometimes used to describe the area of our interest, can be misleading. It suggests that we are dealing with an independent field, rather than with the *application* of general moral principles to an area of human activity. It may obscure the continuity between the action-guides in different fields of applied ethics and the way in which general normative ethics is constantly applied to a wide variety of human activities.

As our tiers of justification suggest, attempts to resolve moral dilemmas by applying moral rules and principles ultimately terminate in a general ethical theory. We shall treat issues in general ethical theory that are relevant to biomedical ethics throughout the following chapters. In particular, we shall examine in detail what we take to be the most important moral principles and rules for biomedicine.

Although systematic work in biomedical ethics is fairly recent in origin, many issues in this applied field have been debated for decades and, in some cases, for centuries. While philosophers and theologians have engaged in these debates, the most influential reflection on problems of biomedical ethics has evolved in the form of professional codes of medical ethics and codes of research ethics (for example, see Appendix II). Such codes are sets of highly specific rules which apply to persons in professional roles. These rules specify normative standards for situations likely to arise in the practice of medicine or in research. It is important, then, to distinguish between general moral codes that govern whole societies and apply to everyone alike, and special moral codes that govern special groups such as doctors, nurses, advertising agents, electrical engineers, and lawyers.

A general moral code consists of fundamental moral principles and rules. There should not be so many rules, or rules so heavily qualified, that some members of society cannot remember or grasp them. These rules are usually general statements such as "Whenever you have promised to do something then you ought to do it." By contrast, a special moral code is composed of derivative and very specific moral rules that are justified by reference to more general and fundamental rules and principles (although the justification may only be implicit in the codes themselves). Again, there should not be so many rules that members of the group cannot master them; but some of these rules will be more professional, and technical in detail, than those in the general moral code. Examples of such rules in biomedical practice and research are the following: "Having undertaken the care of a patient, [a physician] may not neglect him; and unless he has been discharged he may discontinue his services only after giving adequate notice" (American Medical Association, Principles of Medical Ethics, Sec. 5); and "Special caution should be exercised by the doctor in performing clinical research in which the personality of the subject is liable to be altered by drugs or experimental procedures" (World Medical Association, Declaration of Helsinki, 1964, I.5).

In order to indicate the advantages and disadvantages of such professional codes, something should first be said about professions themselves. According to Talcott Parsons, a profession is "a cluster of occupational roles, that is, roles in which the incumbents perform certain functions valued in the society in general, and by these activities, typically earn a living at a full-time job."[4] Professions control entry into their occupational roles by certifying that candidates have developed the requisite body of skills and knowledge. Thus, they have some degree of independence and autonomy in performing the functions valued by the society. In addition to attempting to ensure professional competence, professions typically specify and enforce certain responsibilities and obligations, so that those who enter into a relationship with members of the profession can trust them.[5] A professional code represents an articulated statement of role morality *as seen by the members of the profession.* It is distinguished from sets of standards imposed from the outside by other bodies such as governments. Codes also specify responsibilities between members of the profession, e.g., the AMA code instructs physicians not to criticize physicians previously in charge of a case and urges them to offer professional courtesy.

Professional codes are justified if they serve as effective ways to express moral principles and rules in special relationships. Their function is to facilitate relationships of trust and confidence that permit and encourage certain activities to be performed for socially valued ends, such as the promotion of health. No doubt some professional codes oversimplify moral requirements and lead professionals to think that they have met all the relevant moral requirements if they have followed the rules of the code; but such failures may be outweighed by their value in controlling moral conduct. A more serious question concerns the adequacy and comprehensiveness of the specific moral rules found in existing professional codes. In particular, the specific codes for biomedicine do not express all the important principles and rules. For example, most of the medical codes have much to say about some principles, such as nonmaleficence and beneficence, and about some rules, such as confidentiality; but they have little if anything to say about other important principles and rules, such as veracity, autonomy, and justice.[6]

Some neglected principles and rules have been accentuated by two recent developments. First, some groups, including the American Hospital Association, have formulated statements of patients' rights that incorporate such principles as autonomy and veracity. These statements, in effect, are codes of proper professional conduct for a wide range of health professionals, including physicians. They differ from earlier codes by focussing on the rights of those receiving health services, rather than on the obligations of health professionals. Different emphases in content are also important: whereas earlier codes tended to be paternalistic by affirming the professional's judgments about benefits and harms for the patient, these recent statements of rights stress patient autonomy.[7]

Second, in addition to codes formulated by consumer groups, several codes, regulations, and guidelines have been promulgated by governmental agencies. Many past codes of professional and consumer groups have stressed *individual* conduct. Indeed, much work in biomedical ethics has been limited to or primarily focussed on individual conduct—for example, on what a physician should or should not do to a patient. But numerous questions of *public policy* also surround biomedicine. Consider the area of research, for instance. Since the Nuremberg Code of 1947, the United States Department of Health, Education, and Welfare has promulgated several guidelines for research involving human subjects. In 1974 Congress created the National Commission for the Protection of Human Subjects of Biomedical and Behavioral Research to recommend guidelines to the Secretary of the Department of Health, Education, and Welfare.[8] Their conclusions and lengthy recommendations, along with other governmental policies in biomedicine, raise questions about the proper relation between the government and professional groups in formulating standards and controlling conduct. Many of these questions are, at least in part, moral in nature.

But what is meant by "public policy," and how is it connected to ethics? According to one recent author, "Public policy is whatever governments choose to do or not to do."[9] More adequately, public policy is purposive action or inaction by government officials in such a way as to display a course or pattern. As such, public policies typically involve one or more of the following actions: regulation (e.g., prohibition of an activity) and allocation and distribution of both social benefits (e.g., services and goods) and social burdens (e.g., taxation). In this book we will deal briefly with selected problems of public policy; for instance, we will consider whether the government should prohibit active euthanasia, regardless of the conclusions individuals and health professionals reach, and we will inquire whether one pattern of allocating health resources is more just than another.

The same principles and rules that apply to ethical issues in biomedicine also apply to public policies regarding biomedicine. However, it is rarely possible to move assuredly from a judgment that *act* X is morally right (or wrong) to a judgment that *policy* X is morally right (or wrong), because of numerous factors such as the symbolic value of law and the cost of enforcement. Thus, the judgment that an act is morally wrong does not necessarily lead to the judgment that the government should prohibit it or even refuse to allocate funds for it. For example, it is possible to hold that sterilization or abortion is morally wrong without simultaneously holding that the law should prohibit it or deny funds to poor women who without government support could not have a sterilization or an abortion. Nor does the judgment that an act is morally acceptable in some circumstances imply that the law should permit it. An example may be found in debates about active euthanasia. It is possible to hold that some *acts* of active euthanasia where patients face uncontrollable pain and suffering are morally justified, and yet to hold simultaneously that the government should prohibit active euthanasia because it is not possible to design a *law* that would prevent abuses.

Tests of ethical theories

Several general tests can be used to determine the adequacy of ethical theories. Although it is possible that no ethical theory will satisfactorily meet all the tests, we do and should appeal to them in trying to determine which elements in a theory are acceptable.

First, an ethical theory should be internally consistent and coherent. Ralph Waldo Emerson dismissed a foolish consistency as "the hobgoblin of little minds," but a theory that is not internally consistent and coherent is to that extent unacceptable. Indeed, it is questionable that such a "theory" could really count as a theory, because it would not yield similar results when used by different people or even by the same persons in different but relevantly similar circumstances. Second, a theory should be complete and comprehensive. There should be no major gaps or holes in the theory. A theory that is more complete and comprehensive is, *ceteris paribus,* preferable to less complete and comprehensive theories. Third, simplicity is a virtue of theories. For example, a theory should have no more rules, principles, and concepts than are necessary, and certainly no more than people are able to remember and able to apply without confusion.

Fourth, a theory must be complex enough to account for the whole range of moral experience, including our ordinary judgments. We daily participate in morality as we make decisions, reach judgments, and offer reasons in the name of morality. Ethical theories must account for what we already do. Indeed, they build on, systematize, and criticize our ordinary notions. Our moral experience and our moral theories are also dialectically related. We develop theories to illuminate experience and to determine what we ought to do, but we also use experience to test, corroborate, and criticize theories. If a theory yields conclusions that are totally incompatible with our ordinary judgments—for example, if it allows human subjects to be used purely as means to the ends of scientific research—we have reason to be suspicious of that theory and to look for another. But in many matters of morality, we may be uncertain whether the theory is in error and needs to be modified, whether the theory should be rejected, or whether our ordinary judgments are mistaken. As Joel Feinberg suggests, our procedure is similar to the dialectical reasoning which occurs in courts of law:

If a principle commits one to an antecedently unacceptable judgment, then one has to modify or supplement the principle in a way that does the least damage to the harmony of one's particular and general opinions taken as a group. On the other hand, when a solid well-entrenched principle entails a change in a particular judgment, the overriding claims of consistency may require that the judgment be adjusted.[10]

The relations between the different tiers of justification follow a similar dialectical pattern.

Although other tests could be formulated, these are among the most important ones that we will use in analyzing and appraising various theories in subsequent chapters. A theory may receive a high score on the basis of one test, but a low score on the basis of another test. As we shall see in Chapter 2, utilitarianism is relatively consistent, coherent, simple, and comprehensive, but its critics claim that it is in tension with our ordinary judgments, especially our judgments about just actions and policies. By contrast, critics of some deontological theories may agree that such theories appear to be fairly consistent with our ordinary judgments, but they insist that these ordinary judgments should at least occasionally be modified by a more consistent, coherent, simple, and comprehensive theory.

Moral and nonmoral action-guides

What makes some dilemmas and judgments—and not others—moral? That is, by what criteria can we say that any given normative standard is properly moral rather than religious, legal, political, or whatever? This question is not merely theoretical; it has practical significance. For instance, in 1974, Congress charged the National Commission for the Protection of Human Subjects of Biomedical and Behavioral Research to "conduct a comprehensive investigation and study to identify the *basic ethical principles* which should underlie the conduct of biomedical and behavioral research involving human subjects."[11] The National Commission then attempted to determine during its deliberations whether and how ethical principles can be distinguished from, for example, legal principles.

Although many believe they can recognize moral action-guides when they see them, there is pronounced disagreement about the criteria that make them moral. We shall indicate some of the main criteria for distinguishing moral and nonmoral action-guides. However, it should be noted from the outset that some action-guides involve both moral and nonmoral elements, and that several diverse action-guides thus may be employed in judgments about a single act.

Consider six very different reasons that might be given for holding that we should not allow Baby X, a genetically defective newborn, to die.

Some of the reasons are moral; others are nonmoral. We are not now interested in determining how much *weight* these reasons should have in our deliberations, but whether they are *moral* reasons. The question is *whether* they should count as moral reasons, not *how much* they should count in our deliberations.

(1) We should not allow Baby X to die because we have provided treatment for similar babies in the past, and it is therefore arbitrary and capricious to deny treatment to Baby X. This argument from fairness or justice could also be stated in broader terms: the defect is a morally irrelevant dissimilarity between Baby X and babies that have been previously treated.

(2) We should not allow Baby X to die because death is not in his best interest. Since he has a good probability of a reasonably good quality of life, his interests would be better served by continued treatment.

(3) We should not allow Baby X to die because this action might become publicly known, and, given the attitudes in this community, we might not be able to raise money for a needed addition to the hospital.

(4) Our institution is committed by its own public statements to maximal treatment for all who need it.

(5) Allowing Baby X to die is against the law.

(6) In the light of what the *Bible* says about children and human life, Baby X should not be allowed to die.

Reasons (1) and (2) are clearly moral reasons. Whether they should prevail in this situation would depend on further facts of the case and on whether there are competing and stronger moral claims. Reasons (3–6), as stated, are nonmoral, although all of them could be stated in ways that would render them moral. For example, reason (5), which holds that the act is illegal, could be offered as a moral reason if it were connected with some other convictions, such as that one has a fundamental moral obligation to obey the law.

Contemporary philosophers have delineated three main conditions of moral action-guides (in contrast to nonmoral ones). The first two conditions are formal. They refer to the form, not the content, of moral judgments, rules, and principles. Because they do not pertain to content, they would (if used alone) allow more action-guides to be counted as moral than the third condition would allow. According to the first condition, moral action-guides are whatever a person or, alternatively, a society accepts as *supreme, final,* or *overriding* in judgments about actions. Unless this condition of overridingness is combined with other conditions, it permits almost anything to count as moral if a person, or a society, is committed to its overriding pursuit. For example, a person's primary commitment to scientific knowledge could be taken as that person's morality. True, we often do say that a person or a society has a morality even when we think that it is an unacceptable morality. It is difficult, however, to hold that supremacy is either necessary or sufficient for morality. Because other conditions such as the second one to be mentioned (universalizability) appear to be indispensable, we cannot say that *every* overriding action-guide counts as moral. Furthermore, to hold that supremacy is a necessary condition of morality is to prejudge the weight that moral action-guides should have in our deliberations when they conflict with political, legal, and religious action-guides. We cannot with certainty say that moral considerations, by definition, must outweigh or override all other considerations in competition with them.

A second and widely accepted condition for moral action-guides is *universalizability*, which requires that all relevantly similar cases be treated in a similar way. This formal condition may be a necessary condition of moral thinking, but it is insufficient to distinguish moral judgments from other judgments which also meet this requirement. A judgment that an act is right (or wrong) commits one to judging relevantly similar acts right (or wrong); and if a person holds that act X is right and act Y is wrong but cannot point to any significant differences between them, the person is not making a moral judgment. But clearly many universalizable action-guiding propositions are not moral—e.g., "Always train your dogs before they are one month old."

The practical significance and the limits of the principle of universalizability (which, as we shall see in Chapter 6, can also be formulated as the principle of formal justice) can be seen in the deliberations and recommendations regarding fetal research of the aforementioned National Commission for the Protection of Human Subjects of Biomedical and Behavioral Research. (1) The Commission affirmed the equality of the fetus to be aborted and the fetus to be brought to term in cases of experimentation *in utero*. It affirmed "that the woman's decision for abortion does not, in itself, change the status of the fetus for purposes of protection. Thus, the same principles apply whether or not abortion is contemplated; in both cases, only minimal risk is acceptable."[12] (2) The Commission was otherwise divided, however, because similar treatment is not identical treatment. "Minimal risk" for a fetus intended to be brought to term is different from "minimal risk" for a fetus intended to be aborted, if we assume that the woman will not change her mind. For example, the injection of a drug that crosses the placenta might not injure a fetus aborted within two weeks after the injection, but it might injure the fetus two months after the injection. Thus, the Commission agreed that the principle of universalizability (in this case, a principle of equal treatment) is applicable to fetal research, yet they disagreed about what this principle implies for research involving differently situated fetuses.

Some philosophers have also proposed a third criterion of morality, one which has moral content. They argue that it is necessary for a moral action-guide to have some direct reference to the *welfare of others*. This condition of other-regardingness excludes egoistic principles, for example, from the realm of moral action-guides; and it would exclude certain religious action-guides. But clearly most principles and rules of interest in biomedicine, whether moral or not, involve some direct reference to human welfare. Also, the contention that moral action-guides must have some reference to the welfare of others does not indicate that the welfare of *all* parties must receive the same weight. For example, if someone argued for a policy of massive, high-risk, nontherapeutic research on prisoners for the benefit of the society, we could not count that recommendation as *nonmoral* merely because it sacrifices some individuals for the sake of others. It would, however, be *immoral* according to most ethical theories.

In order to determine the grounds on which such a policy could be held to be immoral, we shall now turn to an examination of major ethical theories and their moral principles, rules, and judgments.

Notes

1. See John Lemmon, "Moral Dilemmas," *Philosophical Review* 71 (1962): 139–58.
2. Paul Ramsey, *The Patient as Person* (New Haven: Yale University Press, 1970), pp. 1–58; "The Enforcement of Morals: Nontherapeutic Research on Children," *The Hastings Center Report* 6 (August 1976): 21–39; "Children as Research Subjects: A Reply," *The Hastings Center Report* 7 (April 1977): 40–42; and Richard McCormick, S.J., "Proxy Consent in the Experimental Situation," *Perspectives in Biology and Medicine* 18 (Autumn 1974): 2–20; "Experimentation in Children: Sharing in Sociality," *The Hastings Center*

Report 6 (December 1976): 41–46. See also William E. May, "Experimenting on Human Subjects," *Linacre Quarterly* 41 (November 1974): 238–52; and the National Commission for the Protection of Human Subjects of Biomedical and Behavioral Research, *Report and Recommendations: Research Involving Children* (Washington, D.C.: U.S. Department of Health, Education, and Welfare, 1977).

3. For various reasons it is controversial whether such a sharp distinction can be drawn between metaethics and normative ethics. See for example Philippa Foot, "Goodness and Choice" and J. R. Searle, "How to Derive 'Ought' from 'Is'," in W. D. Hudson, ed., *The Is/Ought Question* (London: Macmillan, 1969).

4. Talcott Parsons, *Essays in Sociological Theory,* rev. ed. (Glencoe, Ill.: The Free Press, 1954), p. 372.

5. *The American Medical Association Code of Ethics* of 1847, largely adapted from Percival's *Medical Ethics* (1803), was to a great extent a response to a crisis in public confidence. See Donald E. Konold, "History of the Codes of Medical Ethics," *Encyclopedia of Bioethics,* ed. Warren T. Reich (New York: The Free Press, 1978). Professional ethics may be formal or informal and may or may not be backed by sanctions held by a disciplinary body. Medicine is characterized by formal codes and disciplinary bodies, but some other health professions are less formal and lack the disciplinary structure and sanctions (e.g., social workers).

6. See Sissela Bok, "The Tools of Bioethics," in Stanley Joel Reiser, Arthur J. Dyck, and William J. Curran, eds., *Ethics in Medicine: Historical Perspectives and Contemporary Concerns* (Cambridge, Mass.: MIT Press, 1977), pp. 137–41.

7. See George J. Annas, *The Rights of Hospital Patients: The Basic ACLU Guide to a Hospital Patient's Rights* (New York: Avon Books, 1975). For a discussion of the evolution of medical codes, see *Encyclopedia of Bioethics,* "History of the Codes of Medical Ethics."

8. See Public Law 93–348 and the listing of the publications of this Commission in the Bibliography in the present volume, under "Government Documents."

9. Thomas R. Dye, *Understanding Public Policy,* 2nd ed. (Englewood Cliffs, N.J.: Prentice-Hall, 1975), p. 1.

10. Joel Feinberg, *Social Philosophy* (Englewood Cliffs, N.J.: Prentice-Hall, 1973), p. 34.

11. Public Law 93–348, emphasis added. See footnote # 8 above. For a discussion of some of the issues and major positions, see James F. Childress, "The Identification of Ethical Principles," *Journal of Religious Ethics* 5 (Spring 1977): 39–68. We will often use the term "moral" and "ethical" interchangeably, although some distinctions can be drawn between them. Cicero apparently formed the Latin word *moralis* (from *mores*) to translate the Greek term *ethikos.* Etymologically their meanings are similar and stress manners, character, and customs. Contemporary usage suggests some rough but not

very precise distinctions between them. "Ethics" often refers to reflective and theoretical perspectives, while "morality" often refers more clearly to actual conduct and practice. Our use of the terms "ethics" and "morality" in this book respects this rough distinction, although we use the adjectives "moral" and "ethical" less precisely.

12. The National Commission for the Protection of Human Subjects of Biomedical and Behavioral Research, *Report and Recommendations: Research on the Fetus* (Washington, D.C.: U.S. Department of Health, Education, and Welfare, 1975), p. 66.

2

Utilitarian and Deontological Theories

A developed ethical theory, as we saw in the previous chapter, provides a framework within which an agent can determine morally appropriate actions. But, in the light of the tests we developed, which ethical theory is the most satisfactory? In this chapter, we shall concentrate on two types of ethical theories that have received the most attention in recent years: utilitarian and deontological theories.

The classical origins of utilitarianism are found in the writings of David Hume (1711–76), Jeremy Bentham (1748–1832), and John Stuart Mill (1806–73). Utilitarianism is only one of several ethical theories that gauge the worth of actions by their ends and consequences. These theories are sometimes said to be consequentialist or teleological (derived from the Greek term *telos,* meaning "end"). They hold that morally right actions are determined by the nonmoral value (e.g., pleasure, friendship, knowledge, or health) produced by their performance. The value is said to be *nonmoral* because it is the general goal of human strivings (e.g., in art, athletics, and academics), and thus is not a distinctly moral value as is, for example, fulfilling a moral obligation. A common feature of these theories is that duty and right conduct are subordinated to what is good, for right and duty are defined in terms of goods or that which produces goods.

By contrast, deontological theories (derived from the Greek term *deon,* meaning "duty") deny precisely what teleological theories affirm. Their classical origins are more diverse and include, for example, some religious ethics that concentrate on divine commands; but the ethical theory of Immanuel Kant (1734–1804) is generally regarded as the first unambiguous formulation. Deontologists maintain that the concept of duty is independent of the concept of good and that right actions are not determined exclusively by the production of nonmoral goods. The basic difference between these two general approaches may be briefly expressed as follows: the teleologist (and thus the utilitarian) holds that actions are determined to be right or wrong by only one of their features, viz., their consequences, while the deontologist contends that even if this feature sometimes determines the rightness and wrongness of acts, it does not always do so. Other features are also relevant, e.g., the fact that an act involves telling a lie or breaking a promise. In this chapter we consider these two general approaches to ethics as ways to account for rightness and wrongness in biomedical ethics. Rather than considering the many different versions of teleological theories, we focus on the most prominent version, utilitarianism.

Utilitarianism

While the term "utilitarianism" is familiar to most of us, its popular usage can be confusing and misleading. It is said, for example, to be the theory that "the end justifies the means." It is also said to be the view that "we ought to promote the greatest good of the greatest number." Since "utility" is commonly translated as "usefulness," this theory is also said to be the view that what is right is that which is most useful. In some respects each of these popular characterizations is accurate, but utilitarianism is considerably more sophisticated and refined than such characterizations indicate. In this book the term "utilitarianism" refers to the moral theory that there is one and only one basic principle in ethics, the principle of utility. This principle asserts that we ought in all circumstances to produce the greatest possible balance of value over disvalue for all persons affected (or the least possible balance of disvalue if only evil results can be brought about).

An example of utilitarian thinking is the following: It is universally agreed that physicians should minimize the cost to and suffering of patients. This obviously does not mean that physicians should never charge patients for their work or should never allow any suffering or risk of harm whatsoever. But it does mean that whenever there is a choice between different but equally efficacious methods of treatment, patients' benefits should be maximized and the costs and risks minimized. Any other approach would rightly be regarded as an unethical practice. While this example does reflect elementary utilitarian thinking, there are disputes among utilitarians concerning how the theory may be best characterized, as well as disputes over which values are most important. Some grasp of these internal disputes is required if we are to understand utilitarian ethics.

The concept of utility

We have seen that all utilitarians share the conviction that human actions are to be morally assessed in terms of their production of maximal nonmoral value. But how are we to determine, it may be asked, what value could and should be produced in any given circumstance? Utilitarians agree that ultimately we ought to look to the production of what is intrinsically valuable rather than extrinsically valuable. That is, what is good in itself and not merely what is good as a means to something else ought to be produced. For example, neither undergoing nor performing an abortion is considered by anyone to be an intrinsically good event. However, many people would sometimes consider it extrinsically good as a means to another end, such as the restoration of an ill woman to a state of health. Utilitarians believe that we really ought to seek certain experiences and conditions in life that are good in themselves without reference to their further consequences, and that all values are ultimately to be gauged in terms of these intrinsic goods. Health and freedom from pain would be included among such values by most utilitarians.

An intrinsic value, then, is a value in life that we wish to possess and enjoy just for its own sake and not for something else which it produces. Without such values, the things we pursue as means to other things would probably lose their value. If, for example, a surgical procedure is employed to restore a person to a state of health, but the health is not itself valued, then it is hard to understand what the value of the surgical procedure could be for that person. The value of most procedures in medical practice and research is derivative from some other nonderivative value, such as health. Sometimes, of course, a single thing can possess both intrinsic and extrinsic value. For example, new knowledge about nuclear-powered, artificial hearts may be intrinsically valuable to scientific investigators, but it may also be extrinsically valuable for thousands of (future) patients. Health also can be extrinsically good, as a means to the end of an enjoyable and productive life. Still, the main task for utilitarians is to provide an acceptable theory that explains why things are intrinsically good and that develops lists and categories of such goods.

A major distinction within utilitarian theories of intrinsic value is drawn between hedonistic utilitarians and pluralistic utilitarians. Bentham and Mill are referred to as hedonistic utilitarians because they conceived utility entirely in terms of happiness or pleasure—two terms that may here be taken as synonymous and as very broad in scope. Bentham, for example, viewed utility as that aspect of any object or event whereby it tends to produce different pleasures in the form of benefit, advantage, good, the prevention of pain, etc.[1] Mill went to considerable lengths not to be misunderstood on the matter of what "happiness" means. He insisted that happiness does not refer to "a continuity of highly pleasurable excitement," but rather encompasses a realistic appraisal of the pleasurable moments afforded in life, whether they take the form of tranquillity or passionate excitement.[2]

The principle of utility for Bentham and Mill thus demands courses of action which produce the maximum possible happiness in the broad sense of the term employed by these philosophers. That is, an action ought to be performed if the sum of the happiness interests of all affected individuals would be maximized by the performance of that action. If Mill and Bentham had believed other things in life besides happiness were desirable as ends in themselves, they no doubt would have held a different view. But both believed that pleasure and freedom from pain are the only things desirable as ends, and therefore that all desirable things (which are numerous) are desirable because they either produce pleasure or prevent pain.

Mill and Bentham knew, of course, that many human actions do not appear to be performed merely for the sake of happiness. For example, they were aware that highly motivated professionals—such as research scientists—can work themselves to the point of exhaustion for the sake of knowledge they hope to gain, even though they might have chosen different and more pleasurable pursuits. Mill's explanation of this phenomenon is that such persons are initially motivated by pleasure. They are at that time interested either in prestige or in the prospect of money, both of which promise pleasure. Along the way, however, either the pursuit of knowledge becomes itself productive of happiness or else such persons never stop associating the money or prestige they hope to gain with an ultimate goal of pleasure (despite their not actually deriving much, if any, pleasure). Mill also believed that there are qualitatively different kinds of pleasure, some worth cultivating more than others because intrinsically more valuable. This claim proved difficult to sustain, but Mill's problems with it cannot be considered here. The main point is that for some utilitarians, including two of its leading proponents, happiness or pleasure is the single form of intrinsic value, even though it may be analyzed into many different subtypes.

Later utilitarian philosophers have not looked kindly on this monistic conception of intrinsic value. They have argued that other values besides happiness possess intrinsic worth—e.g., values such as friendship, knowledge, courage, health, beauty, and perhaps even certain moral qualities. According to one defender of this view, G. E. Moore, even some states of consciousness can be valuable apart from their pleasantness.[3] The idea that there are many kinds of intrinsic value eventually received widespread acceptance among utilitarians. Its proponents held that the rightness or wrongness of an action is to be assessed in terms of the total range of intrinsic value ultimately produced by the action.

In recent philosophy, economics, and psychology, neither the approach of the hedonists nor that of the pluralists has prevailed. Both approaches have seemed relatively useless for purposes of objectively aggregating widely different interests in order to determine where maximal value and, therefore, right action, lies. The major alternative approach is to appeal to the language of individual *preferences*. For this approach, the concept of utility refers not to experiences or states of affairs, but rather to an individual's actual preferences, as determined by his behavior. To maximize a single person's utility is to provide what he has chosen or would choose from among the available alternatives that might be produced. To maximize the utility of all persons affected by an action or policy is to maximize the utility of the aggregate group. This approach is indifferent as regards hedonistic or pluralistic views of intrinsic value. What is intrinsically valuable is what individuals prefer to obtain, and utility is thus translated into the satisfaction of those needs and desires that individuals choose to satisfy.

This modern approach to value is preferable to its predecessors for two main reasons. First, recent disputes about hedonism and pluralism have proved interminable, sometimes ideological, and in the view of many, irresolvable. One's choice of a range of these values seems deeply affected by personal experiences—a problem the concept of preference seems to provide a way of avoiding. Second, to make utilitarian calculations it is necessary in some way to measure values. In the monistic theory espoused by Bentham and Mill, for example, we must be able to measure pleasurable and painful states and then compare one person's pleasures with another's in order to decide which are quantitatively greater. Yet, it is uncertain what it means to measure and then compare the values of pleasure, health, and knowledge—or any value at all, for that matter. It does make sense, however, to measure preferences by devising a utility scale that measures strengths of individual and group preferences numerically. This approach has proved fruitful in recent discussions of health economics, to take just one of many examples.

The preference approach nonetheless is not trouble-free. A major theoretical problem for utilitarianism arises when individuals have what are, according to ordinary views about morality, immoral or at least morally unacceptable preferences. For example, if a skillful researcher derived supreme satisfaction from inflicting pain on animals or human subjects in experiments, we would condemn and discount this person's preference and would seek to prevent it from being actualized. Utilitarianism based on subjective preferences is satisfactory only if a range of acceptable values can be formulated. This task has proved difficult, however, and may even be inconsistent with the preference approach. This problem cannot be ignored, but since most people are not deviant in the manner envisioned and do have acceptable (even if we may think odd) values, we shall proceed here under the assumption that the utilitarian approach makes sense and is not wildly implausible if a theory of appropriate (nonmoral) values could be provided to buttress its moral perspective.

If utilitarianism could be fully worked out along the lines we have envisioned, it would give us a definite procedure for making ethical choices. We would first calculate to the best of our knowledge the consequences that would result from our performance of the various options open to us. In making this calculation we would ask how much value and how much disvalue—as gauged by the preferences of those affected by our actions—would result in the lives of all affected, including ourselves. Once we have completed all these calculations for all relevant courses of action, we are morally obliged to choose that action which maximizes intrinsic value (or minimizes intrinsic disvalue). Knowingly to perform any other action is to take a morally wrong course.

It would be easy to overestimate the demands of this moral theory. While we must always attempt to make accurate measurements of the preferences of others, this seldom can be done because of our limited knowledge and time. Often in everyday affairs we must act on severely limited knowledge of the consequences of our action. The utilitarian does not condemn any sincere attempt to maximize value merely because the consequences of the attempt turn out to be less than ideal. What is important, morally speaking, is that one conscientiously attempts to determine the most favorable action, and then with equal seriousness attempts to perform this action. Since common sense and fair-minded deliberation will ordinarily suffice for these calculations, utilitarians cannot be accused of presenting overly demanding moral requirements, as some critics have alleged.

Act and rule utilitarianism

The next and most important distinction to be considered is that between act and rule utilitarians. For all utilitarians the principle of utility is the ultimate source of appeal for the determination of morally right and wrong actions. Controversy has arisen, however, over whether this principle is to be applied to particular *acts* in particular circumstances in order to determine which act is right *or* whether it is to be applied instead to *rules* of conduct which themselves determine the acts that are right and wrong. Using the scheme of ascending levels of justification introduced in Chapter 1, we may outline how utilitarians attempt to justify moral actions and, at the same time, illustrate how act and rule utilitarians differ:

Rule Utilitarianism	Act Utilitarianism
Principle of Utility	Principle of Utility
↑	↑
Moral Rules	Individual Actions
↑	
Individual Actions	

According to the schema on the left, actions are justified by appeal to rules, which in turn are justified by appeal to utility. An act utilitarian simply skips the level of rules and justifies actions directly by appeal to the principle of utility.

The act utilitarian considers the consequences of each particular act, while the rule utilitarian considers the consequences of generally observing a rule. Accordingly, the act utilitarian asks, "What good and evil consequences will result from this action in this circumstance?" and not "What good and evil consequences will result from this sort of action in general in these sorts of circumstances?" The act utilitarian sees rules such as "You ought to tell the truth" as useful rules of thumb in guiding human actions, but not as unbreakable prescriptions. According to this species of utilitarian the question is always, "What should I do now?" and not "What has proved generally valuable in the past?" Act utilitarians take this position because they think observance of a general rule (of truth-telling in this case) would not on some occasions be for the general good.

For roughly this latter reason, act utilitarians regard rule utilitarians as unfaithful to the demands of the principle of utility. This principle requires that we maximize happiness, or at least that we maximize intrinsic value. But there are individual cases in which abiding by a generally beneficial rule will not prove most beneficial to the persons involved, even in the long run. So, why then ought the rule to be obeyed in individual cases when obedience does not maximize value? The contemporary utilitarian, J. J. C. Smart, has argued that the rule utilitarian cannot reply to this criticism that it would be better that everybody should obey the rule than that nobody should. This objection fails, according to Smart, because there is a third possibility between never obeying a rule and always obeying it—viz., that it should *sometimes* be obeyed.[4] For example, physicians do not always tell the truth to patients. They withhold information and even lie. Perhaps they invoke the legal doctrine of therapeutic privilege as a justification for their action, but they nonetheless violate general moral rules of truth-telling. They do so because they think it is better for the patient and for all concerned, and they do not think their act really undermines morality. Smart's objection seems in the end reducible to the empirical prediction that we will be better off in the moral life if we sometimes obey and sometimes disobey rules, because this selective obedience will not erode either moral rules or our general respect for morality. The rule utilitarian would, of course, challenge Smart's apparent empirical prediction that less rather than more damage will be done to the institution of morality by adopting an act-utilitarian position.

An intriguing example of act-utilitarian thinking emerged in a recent case of research in the social sciences (included in the Appendix as Case #4). In this case, a sociologist posed as a lookout for male homosexuals using such public facilities as isolated bathrooms on highways (so-called "tearooms") in order to observe homosexual behavior. His desire to provide a thorough study of this form of life-style led him to record the automobile license plate numbers of the participants so that he could subsequently locate their residences. He then gained entrance to their homes by falsely posing as a researcher pursuing a different and innocuous kind of study, rather than his actual study, in order to obtain data on family background, marital status, etc. This research methodology has been heavily criticized not only because it put the subjects studied at risk (since the police might have obtained damaging data, including the license plate numbers) but also because it involved outright deception, including a set of lies to gain entrance to private homes. In other words, it violated a number of standard moral rules about deception, lying, invading privacy, and placing other persons at risk.

The sociologist involved defended his work on act-utilitarian grounds. He argued that his study would provide a valuable understanding of the motives and general behavioral patterns of those who perform homosexual acts—and also that it would help others appreciate the social pressures that lead to homosexual activity. In short, he attempted to justify the violation of standard moral rules by appeal to the valuable and otherwise unattainable goals of his research.

Act utilitarianism has been subjected to sharp criticism in recent moral philosophy—justifiably, in our view. One major theoretical reason for its rejection relies on examples of obviously wrong actions which are un-detectable by others. For example, suppose a physician treating an end-stage dialysis patient who will die in two to three months kills the patient by an undetectable means on grounds that the patient's death would maximize utility in the circumstances, all things considered. A case of this sort, minus the actual killing, is found in Case #13 in the Appendix. Now imagine a second physician who performs the identical action under the identical circumstances, except that his action is detectable, and is detected. It would seem that, according to act utilitarianism, the second action is morally worse than the first. The first action plausibly does maximize utility in the circumstances. After all, the dialysis patient has little life left and is a severe financial and psychological burden to his family. Additionally, the first doctor does not suffer the consequences of public criticism or even imprisonment. In the second case, however, the doctor does suffer imprisonment, and the family suffers the embarrassment, guilt, and anguish which invariably accompany such events.

This conclusion of act utilitarianism strikes many as odd and unacceptable, for at least two reasons. First, the crime of murder is equally wrong in both cases on the same moral grounds; the first action does not appear less blameworthy simply because of the absence of a chain of unpleasant consequences. Second, we are inclined to say that the consequences of the physician's action, apart from the immediate consequence for the victim, are disconnected from our *moral* assessment of the action as wrong. Act utilitarianism seems to make this extraneous set of consequences, e.g., imprisonment, not only relevant when it is irrelevant, but relevant in such a way that it should change our assessment of the moral value of the action.

A similar and by now standard form of counterexample to act utilitarianism is captured in the following imagined sequence of events: Suppose that you are mountain climbing with your closest friend, a person whom you admire and respect, and from whom you have received many favors. Now suppose you lose your grip on a rope while he is descending a sheer cliff. He falls. By the time you reach him he is dying. In these dying moments he asks that you make a promise to him, and you agree. He reveals a great financial secret he has been harboring. Through years of hard work and careful investments he has hoarded a million dollars. He asks you to deliver this money to an uncle who has helped him in the past. But you know that this uncle is very rich and will eventually squander this money. No one else knows about either the promise or the secret cash. On act-utilitarian principles, it would appear that you should not carry out your promise to your dying friend. You can surely put the money to much better use by giving it to charitable institutions. In this way you would do a lot of good and virtually no harm. You do not disappoint the man to whom you made the promise, because he is dead. Nor by breaking the promise do you do indirect harm by weakening faith in the socially useful institutions of promise-making and promise-keeping.

The point of this counterexample is to show that act utilitarianism is inconsistent with our common convictions about moral rightness, or what might be called the common moral consciousness. We saw in Chapter 1 that one test of an ethical theory is its congruence with these common, but considered, ethical convictions. The rule utilitarian would agree with this objection from common morality because of the utility of the rule of promise-keeping in general. The act utilitarian would reply that although promises usually should be kept in order to maintain a climate of trust, this consideration fails to apply in the present case, because more good is produced by breaking the promise, which, in any event, is not public. The act utilitarian willingly admits that his system is inconsistent with ordinary moral convictions in cases like this one, but will respond that we need to revise our ordinary convictions, not to scrap act utilitarianism.

The objections thus far considered are exclusively directed to act utilitarianism and cannot without modification be used to refute the rule utilitarian. According to rule utilitarians, rules themselves have a central position in morality and cannot be disregarded because of the exigencies of particular situations. Because rules maximize utility, the act of a physician who withheld information from a patient would be immoral unless he were able to justify it by appeal to a moral rule strong enough to override the rule requiring that the truth be told. Because of the substantial contributions made to society by the general observance of rules of truth-telling, the rule utilitarian would not compromise them for a particular situation. Such compromise would threaten the integrity and existence of the rule itself, and a rule is selected in the first instance because its general observance would maximize social utility better than would any alternative rule, or no rule. For the rule utilitarian, then, the conformity of an act to a valuable rule makes the act right, whereas for the act utilitarian the beneficial consequences of the act alone make it right.

A relevant example of rule-utilitarian thinking is found in Case #1 in the Appendix. In this case, which we discussed in Chapter 1, a woman was killed by a man who had previously confided to a psychiatrist his intention to kill her. The psychiatrist did attempt to have the man committed but did not communicate the threat to the woman when the commitment attempt failed, on grounds of patient/physician confidentiality. The majority opinion in the case holds that the danger of violence a patient presents to another person generates a psychiatric obligation to use reasonable care in protecting the intended victim, possibly by a direct warning. Justice Tobriner goes on to argue that "public policy" in such matters turns on the importance of rules—in this case the rules of protecting confidentiality and of protecting persons from violent assault. The judge is not only appealing to the public importance of observing rules but appears on utilitarian grounds to be judging the rule of confidentiality to be less important than rules protecting persons from violent assault.

The opinion of the dissenting judge in this case—Justice Clark—is even more directly rooted in rule-utilitarian thinking. Justice Clark reasons as follows:

Policy generally determines duty. . . . Overwhelming policy considerations weigh against imposing a duty on psychotherapists to warn a potential victim against harm. While offering virtually no benefit to society, such a duty will frustrate psychiatric treatment, invade fundamental patient rights, and increase violence.

Following this paragraph the judge lists a series of consequence-regarding reasons in support of a firm rule protecting the confidentiality of information transmitted to psychiatrists. Not observing such a rule would cause irreparable harm to "the very practice of psychiatry" and would deter people from seeing psychiatrists. Even though the judge does not expressly invoke utilitarian ethical theory in support of his views, his opinion is a fine example of rule-utilitarian reasoning.

Although many rule utilitarians justify various rules by their consequences, some rule utilitarians propose that we consider the utility of *whole codes or systems of rules* rather than *independent* rules. Among the defenders of different versions of this position are David Hume, the eighteenth-century Scottish philosopher, and R. B. Brandt, a contemporary American philosopher.[5] According to this approach, the rightness or wrongness of individual acts is determined by reference to moral rules that have a place in a code or system of rules. The system is assessed as a whole in terms of its overall consequences. It is necessary to consider the consequences of moral rules not as independent rules, then, but as parts of a whole code of rules. By again using the scheme of ascending levels of justification introduced in Chapter 1, we may illustrate this version of rule utilitarianism:

Principle of Utility	[Supreme Principle]
↑	
Moral Code	[Whole Scheme of Rules]
↑	
Moral Rules	[Single Rules]
↑	
Individual Actions	[Judgments and Actions]

While this whole code approach bears a resemblance to simple rule utilitarianism, it allegedly has additional advantages. Most importantly, proponents claim that we are more likely to be able to maximize utility across a society by the advocacy of a whole system of rules than merely by testing and attempting to gain adherence to single rules, each isolated from the consequences of other rules in the system. It would be difficult to motivate individuals in society to conform to rules if they were individually tested for their consequences, and we rarely think of morality in this way. Most of us are motivated to the acceptance of a whole way of life that is moral, and we generally think of morality as a system of integrated principles and rules, none of which stands in isolation.[6]

It is important to note, in concluding this section, that from the rule utilitarian's perspective no rule (and hence no moral action) is ever absolutely wrong in itself, and no rule in the system of rules is absolute and unrevisable. A rule's acceptability in the system of rules depends strictly on its consequences. Even rules against killing may be revised or substantially overturned. There has, for example, been considerable discussion in recent biomedical ethics of the possibility that seriously defective newborn infants should be killed rather than merely "allowed to die," as is now the practice in some cases. (See Case #17 in the Appendix.) The rule utilitarian would argue that we should support rules permitting such killing if the rules would maximize intrinsic value; but the rule utilitarian also insists that there should be rules *against* such killing if those rules would maximize intrinsic value. To some this utilitarian approach seems shocking and outrageous, because in theory it would permit radical shifts in our present system of moral rules. But utilitarians are not impressed by this objection. They point to the reason why we now have the rules we do have. Specifically, we presently do not permit the killing of newborn infants because of the deprivation of happiness, and even the outright anguish, that would be produced for many affected by such actions. But if this unhappy series of consequences did not generally occur, then the utilitarian would see no reason *in principle* why there should not be such killing. Such cases indicate why utilitarianism is strictly a consequentialist theory.

Deontological theories

We have seen that a teleological or consequentialist theory holds that the right is a function of the good, specifically of intrinsically valuable ends or consequences. Within such a theory one would determine what is right or wrong by asking whether an act or class of acts would probably produce the greatest possible balance of good over evil in the world. By contrast, deontological theories (sometimes called formalist theories) hold that features of some acts other than their consequences make them right or wrong. In Case #5, where a therapist deceives a patient by substituting a placebo, a deontologist would consider both the feature of deception in and of itself (not merely the effects of the deception) and the therapist's motives. For many deontologists deception is a wrong-making characteristic regardless of its consequences. As we shall see, a deontologist need not hold that deception is absolutely wrong and never justifiable. However, to be a deontologist, one must hold that at least some acts are wrong and others are right independent of their consequences. Examples of right-making characteristics in deontological systems include fidelity to promises and contracts, gratitude for benefits received, truthfulness, and justice.

Versions of deontology

Different deontological theories compete with each other, as well as against teleological theories. It is possible to analyze these theories from several perspectives. First, we could explore the different ways deontologists try to vindicate their judgments that certain acts are right or wrong. Some moralists in religious traditions appeal to divine revelation (e.g., to God's promulgation of the Ten Commandments), while others appeal to natural law, which they contend can be known by human reason. Some philosophers, including W. D. Ross, find intuition and common sense sufficient, while others, such as John Rawls, derive their principles from the notion of a hypothetical social contract.[7] To analyze and assess these and other warrants for judgments about moral acts would lead us into the thickets of metaethics (theories of the meaning and justification of ethical terms), and this pursuit would consume too much space. Most of the principles and rules that we will consider are accepted by most deontological theories and can also be discovered in the "common morality."[8] Thus, for our purposes it is not necessary to examine different metaethical theories.

Second, like utilitarian theories, deontological theories may be *monistic* or *pluralistic*. A *monistic* deontological theory holds that there is one single rule or principle from which one can derive all other rules or judgments about right and wrong. Thus, one could affirm basic principles such as love and respect for persons and derive other rules such as truth-telling and fidelity from them. In his classic attempt, Immanuel Kant proposed a single "categorical imperative" through which he tested all maxims of action. As an example, consider a person who desperately needs money and knows that he will not be able to borrow it unless he promises to repay it in a definite time, although he also knows that he will not be able to repay it within this time period. He decides to make a promise that he knows he will break. According to Kant, when we examine the maxim of his action—"When I think myself in want of money, I will borrow money and promise to pay it, although I know that I never can do so"—we discover that it cannot pass the basic test of what Kant calls the categorical imperative, according to which maxims must be *universalizable*. To be universalizable, the maxim must be capable of being conceived and willed without contradiction as a universal law. The above maxim about misleading promises cannot be *conceived* as a universal law, for it would contradict itself. As Kant writes,

"How would things stand if my maxim became a universal law?" I then see straight away that this maxim can never rank as a universal law of nature and be self-consistent, but must necessarily contradict itself. For the universality of a law that everyone believing himself to be in need can make any promise he pleases with the intention not to keep it would make promising, and the very purpose of promising, itself impossible, since no one would believe he was being promised anything, but would laugh at utterances of this kind as empty shams.[9]

Some maxims which can be *conceived* as universal nonetheless cannot be *willed* without contradiction. Consider the maxim of a person who is well-off but refuses to help those who are struggling. According to Kant, an agent cannot, without contradiction, will that his maxim of refusing help become universal law, for he might be in need of others at some point in time, and he would certainly want their help.

Although few philosophers would hold, as Kant appears to, that the universalizability of a maxim is both necessary and sufficient for determining its acceptability, most concur that it is a necessary condition of the validity of ethical judgments, rules, and principles. Kant may actually have had more than one basic principle, since the several formulations he offers of the categorical imperative are not clearly equivalent. In any case, neither Kant nor others who have proposed monistic theories have carried the day.

Pluralistic deontologists, by contrast, affirm more than one basic rule or principle. For example, W. D. Ross, a prominent twentieth-century deontologist, held that there are several basic and irreducible moral principles, such as fidelity, beneficence, and justice. While this pluralistic approach may at first glance appear more plausible than monistic approaches because it is closer to our ordinary judgments, it quickly encounters the difficulty—as Ross recognized—of what to do when these principles or rules come into conflict. Case #3 provides an example of this problem. A physician has to determine whether to tell the truth or to break a confidence. He cannot do both, yet each of the two principles or rules commands his allegiance. The pluralistic deontologist may give us little guidance about which rules or principles take priority in such cases of conflict. For example, Ross held that the principle of nonmaleficence (noninfliction of harm) takes precedence over the principle of beneficence (production of benefit) when they come into conflict, but he gave no answer about the priorities among the other principles except to say that several duties (such as keeping promises) have "a great deal of stringency." Finally, he quoted Aristotle: "The decision rests with perception."[10] While we intuit the principles, according to Ross, we do not intuit what is right in the situation; rather we have to find "the greatest balance" of right over wrong. If a pluralistic deontological theory does not provide some ordering or ranking of its principles and rules, it offers little guidance in the moment of decision making.

One major recent attempt to overcome the difficulties of pluralistic theories is John Rawls's *A Theory of Justice,* which provides a serial or lexical ordering of quite general principles of justice (but not the whole of morality). Rawls's lexical order avoids the need to balance principles, since we have to satisfy the first principle before we consider the second; the prior principle has absolute weight relative to the later ones. Using this approach he argues that the principle of equal liberty is prior to the principle of distributing social and economic benefits. Rawls does not, however, propose this sort of ordering for all moral principles.[11]

Finally, just as there can be act and rule utilitarians, deontologists may focus on *acts* or *rules* that cover classes of acts. Few philosophers or theologians have tried to defend act deontology, though traces of it can be seen here and there. It has been held, for example, that an individual by intuition, or conscience, or faith in God's revelation and grace, can immediately and directly perceive what he or she ought to do. But act deontology is problematic for several reasons. We do not have firm grounds for confidence in our own or others' intuition, conscience, or faith to perceive right and wrong in the situation—particularly in the light of immediate pressures, lack of time for deliberation, and the power self-interest has to distort perception. Rules appear to be an important stabilizing influence in the moral life. Furthermore, to judge that a particular act is wrong in the situation is implicitly to appeal to a rule. *If* we are making a moral judgment when we say that act X is wrong, we are saying that all relevantly similar acts in similar circumstances are wrong. To say it is wrong to tell a lie to a patient who asks a direct question about his prognosis is to say that it is wrong to tell such a lie in similar circumstances. Such a statement is at least an incipient rule.

For *rule deontologists,* the heart of morality is a set of principles and rules that identify classes of acts that are right or wrong and obligatory or prohibited. Kant, for example, held that several rules could be derived from the basic categorical imperative. According to Ross, there are several independent duties that can be stated as rules or principles. Some of these duties rest on one's own previous acts. For example, promises and implicit promises give rise to *duties of fidelity.* And one's previous wrongful acts engender *duties of reparation.* Some other duties rest on the previous acts of other persons. When they render services to us, we have *duties of gratitude.* Ross goes on to develop duties of *self-improvement, nonmaleficence, beneficence,* and *justice.* Several of these duties will be central in later chapters. At the moment we only want to indicate how one version of rule deontology regards some classes of acts as right or wrong independent of their consequences.[12]

Deontology as an ethical theory

What are some of the major characteristics, as well as the strengths and weaknesses, of deontological theories as compared to utilitarian theories? First, utilitarians hold that ultimately there is only one significant moral relationship between persons: the relationship of benefactor and beneficiary. Deontologists, however, take seriously various relationships between people. For them it is not sufficient to say, as utilitarians do, that we should maximize the good and that each person counts as one and only one. They claim that we do not encounter other people merely as depositories of good, as beneficiaries, each one counting as one and only one; rather, we are related to them in various ways by their and our own previous acts. For example, the physician does not confront each sick person merely as someone needing his attention and care. If he has already been treating a patient, his relationship to that person is different from his relationship to another who appears at the office door at the same time with the same ailment. The physician who makes an implicit commitment to a patient by taking the patient into his care generally does not have the right to abrogate that relationship merely because he thinks that he can do more good for others. The texture of the moral life thus seems richer and more complicated than any simple utilitarian model suggests, for numerous relationships with others have special moral significance: parent and child, friend and friend, promisor and promisee, as well as physician and patient. Parents assume certain obligations to their children, and the children incur certain obligations to their parents.

A second and closely connected point concerns the role of past actions in our moral assessments. Utilitarianism seems to have little room for the past in moral judgments, because of its orientation toward the present and future. If utilitarianism considers the past from a moral standpoint, it is only because paying attention to the past appears to be important for future consequences. For example, to reward people for what they have done may encourage them to act in similar ways in the present and the future. But for a rule deontologist like Ross, the fact that one has performed certain acts in the past by itself creates certain obligations. If I have made a promise, I am bound in certain ways to the promisee, independent of the consequences of keeping or not keeping the promise.

Both of these points about morally significant relations with others and about the role of past actions can be illustrated by the debates a few years ago about kidney dialysis as a scarce lifesaving medical technology that could not be provided to everyone who needed it for survival. Some utilitarians held that we should distribute this resource by considering (after the appropriate medical and psychiatric judgments) which patients would probably be the most productive for the society; but these utilitarians usually applied this standard only to *admission* to dialysis. With a few exceptions, they held that once a commitment had been made to a patient, it would be morally improper to remove that patient from the machine to make room for a more qualified patient, i.e., one who would probably contribute more to society. Utilitarians were not willing to say that every few weeks or months we ought to reassess all the patients on, and candidates for, dialysis to determine which ones were worth more to the society. Of course, the utilitarian would probably hold that a rule calling for faithfulness to those to whom we have made implicit if not explicit commitments will ultimately maximize good, in part because frequently reassessing patients and breaking commitments would probably destroy the morale of the patients and undermine productivity. The deontologist, however, would concentrate on the commitment itself, apart from the consequences of respecting that commitment. Here, as well as elsewhere, the rule utilitarian and the rule deontologist may wind up holding similar positions but for apparently different reasons.

Third, utilitarianism conceives the moral life in terms of means to ends reasoning. It asks: "What is our objective?" and "How can we most effectively and efficiently realize our objective (e.g., the production of the greatest possible good)?" This conception of the moral life in terms of means to ends makes it congenial to empirical science. Deontologists, by contrast, hold not only that there are standards independent of the ends for judging the means, but that it is a mistake to conceive the moral life in terms of means and ends. Why? In part, because it seems to presuppose a greater capacity to predict and control than we actually have. We lack the level of capacity to predict and control the future that act utilitarians and some rule utilitarians seem to presuppose. Deontologists also insist that the utilitarian model of choosing effective and efficient means to good ends distorts the moral life in fundamental ways. As Antony Flew argues, "to do one's duty, or to discover what it is, is rarely if ever to achieve, or to find a way to achieve, an objective. Rather and typically, it is to meet, or to find a way to meet, claims; and also, of course, to eschew misdemeanors. Promises must be kept, debts must be paid, dependents must be looked after; and stealing, lying, and cruelty must be avoided."[13] From this view we are not merely agents who initiate acts for good ends; we are also responders who encounter the claims of others. Our responsibilities to others are more varied and more specific than the responsibility to promote good.

Fourth, the deontologist's standard and perhaps most attractive objection is that utilitarianism can lead to morally unacceptable conclusions. One test of moral theories, as we saw earlier, is their congruence with our ordinary moral convictions. Deontologists pose this situation against act utilitarians: suppose that we have two acts, A and B, which appear to yield the same score when we balance their respective good and evil results. The scales appear to be perfectly balanced. But suppose that A involves lying to a patient, while B does not. In the end, the result is the same: the patient can be expected to get well. The consistent act utilitarian must say that the acts are equally right. Now suppose that act A, which involves lying to a patient about his or her condition, is preferable on utilitarian grounds because it offers a greater chance of success in restoring the patient's health, while act B, which does not involve lying, has a slightly lesser chance of success. According to act utilitarianism, A is right and obligatory and the physician should therefore lie to the patient. The deontologist claims that in both cases act utilitarianism leads to judgments that are morally unacceptable.[14]

The rule utilitarian perhaps can avoid these difficulties by holding that a fuller analysis of the consequences, including the remote or long-term consequences, leads us to assign greater weight to the rule of truth-telling. But while rule utilitarianism thus appears to be more congruent with our ordinary judgments, it does not, according to many critics, adequately account for rules of justice, which we find valid apart from the consequences of those rules or principles. For example, consider fairness in bearing the burdens of some common enterprise such as conserving water in a crisis. According to one utilitarian, "if a person happened to know that nearly everybody else was in fact going to make a sacrifice that no one wants to make, and if he knew that, as a result, a similar sacrifice by him was not really essential for the public welfare, then he need not make it."[15] If he has good grounds for thinking that his act will not be known (and emulated) by others and that the enterprise will in no way suffer from his using water, he appears to have no obligation to conserve water on either act- or rule-utilitarian grounds. Nevertheless, according to some interpretations of our ordinary judgments about fairness, we would insist that the person acts unfairly and wrongly, regardless of the consequences. Such a case indicates that our sense of fairness or justice may not be reducible to utility.[16]

On balance, which ethical theory is to be preferred? For one author of this volume rule utilitarianism is preferable to any deontological theory presently available, while for the other, rule deontology is more acceptable than utilitarianism. We come to these different conclusions after testing the various theories for their consistency and coherence, their simplicity, their completeness and comprehensiveness, and their capacity to take account of and to account for our moral experience, including our ordinary judgments. Still, for each of us, the theory that we find more satisfactory is only slightly preferable, and no theory is fully satisfactory on all the tests. Whether one takes the utilitarian or deontological standpoint no doubt makes a great deal of difference at many points in the moral life and in moral reflection and justification. Nevertheless, the differences can easily be overemphasized. In fact, we find that many forms of rule utilitarianism and rule deontology lead to identical rules and actions. It is possible from both utilitarian and deontological standpoints to defend the *same rules* (such as truth-telling and confidentiality) and to assign them roughly the same weight. These standpoints draw even closer if utilitarians take a broad view of the values that support the rules and consider a wide range of direct and indirect, immediate and remote consequences of classes of acts, while deontologists admit that moral principles or rules such as beneficence and nonmaleficence require us to maximize good and minimize evil outcomes.

An indication that rule utilitarianism and rule deontology lead to similar or identical rules, and therefore to a similar conception of the moral life as rule-governed, is found in the writings of the utilitarian philosopher R. B. Brandt. As we have seen, he argues that morality should be conceived as an ideal code consisting of a set of rules that guides the members of a society to maximize intrinsic value. While Brandt appeals to utilitarian reasoning to justify the rules in the code, the following statement is a revealing one:

[The best set of rules] would contain rules giving directions for recurrent situations which involve conflicts of human interests. Presumably, then, it would contain rules rather similar to W. D. Ross's list of prima facie obligations: rules about the keeping of promises and contracts, rules about debts of gratitude such as we may owe to our parents, and, of course, rules about not injuring other persons and about promoting the welfare of others where this does not work a comparable hardship on us.[17]

That Brandt appeals to utility and that Ross appeals to intuition to ground an identical set of rules is a significant difference on the level of ethical theory, but it is a trivial difference when it comes to what we ought to do as a matter of moral rightness and how we should judge the actions of others.

Moreover, within what we would consider the most adequate rule-utilitarian theory and the most adequate rule deontology, moral agents have to face some of the same issues. What should we do when rules come into conflict? What should we do when we cannot realize all the claims upon us or all the goods that we seek? How can we resolve these competing demands? The fact that no presently available rule utilitarianism or rule deontology adequately resolves all moral conflicts perhaps points to their incompleteness. But this incompleteness may reflect more the complexity and tragedy of the moral life than any failures of the theories.

The place of rules

Many utilitarians and deontologists, as we have seen, find that the moral life requires various rules. They reject "situation ethics," which may take either act-deontological or act-utilitarian forms. Although there are several versions of situation ethics, many of its proponents hold that there is a single fundamental principle such as utility, love, or obedience to the divine command, and that all the moral agent has to do is discern the meaning of that principle in the situation. Thus, the agent asks what would serve the greatest good for the greatest number, what would be the most loving deed, or what God commands at the moment, without relying on intermediate rules, i.e., rules connecting the basic principle and the situation. In defending both rule deontology and rule utilitarianism, we have rejected situation ethics. Such a rejection does not, of course, deny the importance of factual considerations, empirical data, and the like, in moral decision making and justification; it only contends that some rules and derivative principles are also required in the situation.

Along the way, we have given several reasons for favoring either rule utilitarianism or rule deontology over their act competitors. Some of those reasons are general; e.g., rules are essential in decision making, since agents frequently do not have the time to recapitulate all the steps from basic principles to conclusions. Other reasons may hold against act utilitarianism, but not against act deontology, and vice versa. Any form of situation ethics, however, appears to run into serious problems of co-ordination, cooperation, and trust. The following encounter between act utilitarians in a medical setting, as envisioned by G. J. Warnock, is instructive:

Suppose that I, a simple Utilitarian, entrust the care of my health to a simple Utilitarian doctor. Now I know, of course, that his intentions are generally beneficent, but equally that they are not *uniquely* beneficent towards me. Thus, while he will not malevolently kill me off, I cannot be sure that he will always try to cure me of my afflictions; I can be sure only that he will do so, *unless* his assessment of the 'general happiness' leads him to do otherwise. I cannot of course condemn this attitude, since it is the same as my own; but it is more than possible that I might not much like it, and might find myself put to much anxiety and fuss in trying to detect, at successive consultations, what his intentions actually were. But conspicuously, there are two things that I could not do to diminish my anxieties: I could not get him to promise, in the style of the Hippocratic Oath, always and only to deploy his skills to my advantage; nor could I usefully ask him to disclose his intentions. The reason is essentially the same in each case. Though he might, if I asked him to, promise not to kill me off, he would of course keep this promise only if he judged it best on the whole to do so; knowing that, I could not unquestioningly rely on his keeping it; and knowing *that*, he would realize that, since I would not do so, it would matter that much less if he did not keep it. And so on, until his 'promise' becomes perfectly idle. Similarly, if I ask him what his intentions are, he will answer truthfully only if he judges it best on the whole to do so; knowing that, I will not unqualifiedly believe him; and knowing *that*, he will realize that, since I will not do so, it will matter that much less if he professes intentions that he does not actually have. And so on, until my asking and his answering become a pure waste of breath. And this is quite general; if general felicific beneficence were the only criterion, then promising and talking alike would become wholly idle pursuits. At best, as perhaps in diplomacy, what people said would become merely a part of the evidence on the basis of which one might try to decide what they really believed, or intended, or were likely to do; and it is not always obvious that there is much point in diplomacy.[18]

Situation ethics, of course, can recognize rules, but it treats them as *summary rules* or *rules of thumb* that are expendable in decision making, since they only summarize the wisdom of the past. Such rules illuminate but do not prescribe what we ought to do. A rule of thumb in baseball is "Don't bunt on third strike," but in some situations it would be advisable for the batter to bunt despite having two strikes. For act deontology or act utilitarianism, all moral rules are like this rule of thumb in baseball. We have argued against this view of moral rules. Although some moral rules may resemble rules of thumb, others are more binding, e.g., the rules that prohibit murder, rape, and cruelty. It is, therefore, important to consider whether some rules are *absolute*.

If moral rules are conceived as absolute, they cannot be overridden under any circumstances. Obviously, there are good reasons for being suspicious of such a view of moral rules. It undermines the freedom and discretion of moral agents, and it sometimes results in moral victims who suffer the consequences of overly rigid adherence to rules. Even if it is not true that everything depends on the consequences, it may be true that in some cases, such as emergencies, the consequences of following some rules would be so terrible that those rules should be overridden.

Nevertheless, we have to face the possibility that some moral rules are virtually exceptionless or absolute: (a) Some rules that refer to traits of character whose development and expression are always good may be absolute. To exhort a physician colleague to "Be caring" or "Be a loving physician" or "Be conscientious" is to call for the development and expression of traits of character that are good. Of course, one may be too loving or too conscientious and thereby obscure important aspects of one's responsibilities. (In the final chapter we will examine traits of character and virtues.) (b) We might also state some rules of action so as to include all exceptions. These rules, with all exceptions built into them, would be absolute. An example might be, "Always obtain the informed consent of your competent patients except in emergency or low-risk situations." There might still be considerable debate about what constitutes an "emergency" or a "low risk," but the rule would be absolute. (c) Finally, some rules that do not specify exceptions may also be virtually absolute. If "murder" is taken to mean "unjustified killing," then its prohibition would be absolute; and the prohibition of cruelty can be considered absolute if the term means "do not inflict suffering for the sake of suffering." In medical contexts, especially some therapeutic settings, there might appear to be exceptions to this second prohibition; but if the therapist intentionally makes a patient suffer so that the patient will become angry and assume responsibility for his decisions, this act does not fall under the prohibition of cruelty, since the infliction of suffering is strictly a means to the valuable end of assuming responsibility.

These examples indicate that the debate about whether some rules can be defended as absolute hinges in part on the definition of moral terms such as "murder," "cruelty," and "lying." Suppose Nazi soldiers had come to a hospital in Germany in the late 1930s and asked the administrator whether there were any Jewish patients in the hospital. If the administrator insisted that the hospital had no Jewish patients, although he knew there were in fact several, how should we describe this exchange and, in particular, the administrator's statement? Consider two possibilities: (1) The administrator's statement is a *lie,* but the lie is justified because it is intended to save the lives of several innocent patients. (2) The administrator's statement is not a lie because his questioners have no right to the truth. In (1), "lying" may be defined as intentionally telling a person what one believes to be untrue in order to deceive him. In (2), "lying" may be defined as not giving the truth to a person to whom it is due. The first involves a "neutral and relatively definite description" of lying, while the second involves a "nonneutral and relatively indefinite description."[19] The first definition indicates what counts as lying or truth-telling, but not how much moral weight lying or truth-telling has. The second definition, however, indicates how much lying or truth-telling counts, but not what is to count as lying or truth-telling. Although the second approach holds that lying is always wrong, it leaves open the question when the truth is *due* someone. If one takes the first approach, one could stress the reality that the moral life often involves doing the "lesser of two evils." For one taking the second approach, harmony between moral principles and rules is more evident than conflict, once their range of applicability is understood. Often this view of harmony is joined with the conviction that one should never do evil that good might result.

The importance of our understanding of central moral terms may be illustrated as follows: In Case #3, a father decided that he did not want to donate a kidney to his five-year-old daughter. His reasons are complex, but they include the uncertain prognosis for his daughter who had been on chronic renal dialysis for three years. He asked the physician to tell the other family members that he was not histocompatible, because he feared that the truth would lead to recriminations against him and would wreck the family. The physician told the family that "medical reasons" prevented the father from being a donor. One could hold that the physician told a lie by intentionally deceiving the wife, but that it was justified because of the evil it prevented. Or one could hold that it was justified because, in a conflict of duties, the protection of confidentiality takes precedence over telling the truth to another "patient," and the father had entered into a relationship of confidentiality with the physician. Or one could hold that the "lie" was justified not because there was another stronger duty but because the physician had no duty to tell the wife the truth. Because what transpired between the father and the physician was confidential, the wife had no right to that information; hence, deceiving her was not even an act of lying. In this analysis, we have not eliminated the possibility of holding that the statement to the wife was an unjustified lie. The present point is merely that different approaches to moral dilemmas and rules may hinge on different understandings of the relevant moral terms, such as lying, as well as on their weight and stringency.

In addition to conceiving of moral rules as rules of thumb and absolute rules, a third possibility is to conceive them as prima facie binding. W. D. Ross has usefully distinguished *prima facie* duties from *actual* duties. He uses the phrase "prima facie duty" to indicate that duties of certain kinds are on all occasions binding *unless* they are in conflict with stronger duties. One's *actual duty* in the situation is determined by an examination of the weight of all the competing prima facie duties. Prima facie duties such as beneficence and promise-keeping are not absolute, since they can be overridden under some conditions. Yet they are more than rules of thumb. Because they are always morally relevant, they constitute strong moral reasons for performing the acts in question, although they may not always prevail over all other prima facie duties. One might say that they count even when they do not win.

For example, Ross considers nonmaleficence—noninfliction of harm—as a prima facie duty. (Indeed all the moral principles taken as primary in this book state prima facie duties in Ross's scheme.) While it may make sense, as we have seen, to say that murder is absolutely prohibited because of what "murder" means, it does not make sense for most moral theories to say that killing is absolutely prohibited. Even the prohibition against killing in the Ten Commandments is more accurately translated as the prohibition of "murder" or "unjustified killing," since the Hebrew people recognized justified killing in self-defense, in war, and as a form of punishment. But "killing" nonetheless is prima facie wrong, because it is an act of maleficence. To call "killing" prima facie wrong, then, is to say that insofar as an act involves killing, it is wrong. But since acts have many features, these features may lead to moral conflicts. For example, the duty not to kill someone may come into conflict with the duty of justice, which includes protecting innocent persons from aggression. But it may also come into conflict with the duty of beneficence, the duty to benefit others. Mercy killing provides an example. Imagine a patient suffering from what appears to be uncontrollable and unmanageable pain. Ross holds that the duty of nonmaleficence takes precedence over the duty of beneficence, but he apparently thought about these duties in relation to different individuals; thus, it would not be right to injure A in order to benefit B (although it might be right to injure A in order to prevent A from injuring B). But suppose the duties of nonmaleficence and beneficence come into conflict in the case of the same suffering patient. It is not clear that killing a person in order to alleviate that person's pain would always be wrong. A person trapped in a burning wreck provides such a case. The point of the notion of prima facie duties, however, is that insofar as the act involves killing, it is wrong. Yet killing may be the only way to satisfy some other prima facie duties. *If so,* then killing can become an actual duty.

To choose a different example, if lying is prima facie wrong, the fact that a physician deceives a patient by giving a placebo (see Case #5) is a moral reason against the action. One traditional formulation of the rule for truth-speaking in medical matters is, "When you are thinking of telling a lie, ask yourself whether it is simply and solely for the patient's benefit that you are going to tell it. If you are sure that you are acting for his good and not for your own profit, you can go ahead with a clear conscience."[20] From the Kantian perspective it would be impossible to *universalize* this rule without contradiction. Another difficulty is that this rule always gives beneficence priority over both truth-telling and autonomy when there is a conflict. It also fails to recognize the weight of the duty not to lie in the medical context, for it would authorize any lie for benevolent motives. But if the duties of veracity and respecting autonomy are strong ones, as we think they are, then at the very least there must be no other acceptable and effective alternative to lying in the situation in order to justify lying.

Furthermore, when a prima facie duty, such as veracity, is outweighed or overridden, it does not simply disappear or evaporate. It leaves what Nozick calls "moral traces."[21] The agent should not only approach his decision conscientiously, but he should also experience regret and, perhaps, even remorse at having to neglect or violate this duty. The duty's "moral traces" should also lead the agent to minimize the effects of the violation. For example, in the case (#5 in Appendix I) in which a therapist deceives a patient by giving a placebo, there is a danger that the deception, which in this case has to become known, will affect the patient's self-conception and his confidence in and reliance upon the therapists. Other moral rules and principles require conscientious efforts to minimize these risks. At the very least, the overridden duties of veracity and respect for autonomy should require that an explanation and apology be given the patient.

Rights

Throughout our discussion we have used terms like "right," "wrong," "obligatory," "obligation," and "duty." We have stressed rightness and duty with some attention to goodness. And we have examined how principles and rules in both deontological and utilitarian theories establish our duties and obligations, as well as the rightness and wrongness of our acts. It may seem odd that we have not employed the language of *rights,* since so many moral controversies in biomedicine and public policy seem to be debates about rights. Controversies about abortion often pit the woman's right of privacy or right to determine the use of her body against the right of the fetus to life. In discussions of health care delivery, proponents of a broad extension of medical services often appeal to the "right to health care," while some of their opponents appeal to the "rights of the medical profession." We have witnessed an explosion of rights language in numerous contexts, from biomedicine to foreign policy—e.g., the debates about "human rights" on the international level. It has been asserted that we have a right to die, a right to treatment, and a right to privacy. Indeed, our moral, political, and legal debates often appear to presuppose that no arguments or reasons can be persuasive unless they can be couched in the language of rights.

Rights language is especially congenial to the liberal individualism that is pervasive in our society. From Thomas Hobbes and John Locke to the present, liberal individualists have employed the language of rights to make their moral, social, and political arguments. Our Anglo-American legal tradition has broadly incorporated this language. In the tradition of liberal individualism, the language of rights has often served such functions as opposing the status quo and forcing social reforms. Historically it was instrumental in securing certain freedoms from established orders of religion, society, and state, e.g., freedom of conscience and freedom of the press. Although statements of important rights are shared across many societies, such statements are not universal. As has often been pointed out, many languages, such as ancient Hebrew and Greek, do not have equivalent expressions for our terms "a right" or "rights." Nevertheless, rights language is very important, not only because of its symbolic significance in our society but also because it plays a legitimate role in ethical theory. It is difficult, however, to determine the status and content of those rights that deserve recognition.

Most recent writers in ethics recognize that "rights" should be defined in terms of claims. In our framework, rights are best seen as justified claims that individuals and groups can make upon others or upon society. Just as legal rights are claims that are justified by existing legal principles and rules, so moral rights are claims that are justified by moral principles and rules. A moral right, then, is a morally justified claim—i.e., a claim validated in terms of moral principles and rules.[22] Just as obligations and duties may take many different forms (religious, legal, moral, etc.), rights may be justified by different forms of principles and rules. In dealing with the abortion issue, the Supreme Court had to determine whether the Constitution and the law embodies rights relevant to this issue. It did not confront the question of moral rights (except by implication), but moral rights and legal rights often are similar and sometimes even identical.

We have concentrated on moral principles and rules, some of which establish duties and obligations, as well as on the rightness and wrongness of acts. In this context we use "duty" and "obligation" interchangeably, though it is important in some other contexts to distinguish them. From our standpoint, there exists what David Braybrooke calls "a firm but untidy correlativity" between obligations and rights, and both obligations and rights can be analyzed in terms of principles and rules.[23] According to the doctrine of the "logical correlativity" of obligations and rights, a right implies that someone else has an obligation to act in certain ways.[24] Rights thus imply obligations. For example, if a physician agrees to take John Doe as a patient and commences treatment, he incurs an obligation to Doe which he does not have toward strangers, and Doe has certain rights against the physician. There are rights to a certain standard of care and rights in care, e.g., the right to the truth. We thus could analyze the moral issues in the relationship between the physician and Doe either by examining the physician's duties or by examining the patient's rights, because the doctrine of the logical correlativity of rights and obligations holds that it is possible to start from a right and infer a correlative obligation, and vice versa. It indicates that we can secure the same moral content from either standpoint, that of the right or of the obligation. However, the doctrine does not tell us whether obligations are grounded in rights or vice versa, and we take no stand on this issue here.

While the doctrine of the logical correlativity of rights and duties is for the most part sound, there is a generalized use of "requirement," "obligation," and "duty" which sometimes appears not to imply correlative rights. For example, we sometimes refer to "duties" or "requirements" of love, charity, and self-sacrifice that do not seem to be restatable in terms of rights. It seems awkward in most instances to hold that one person can claim another person's love or charity as a matter of right. The problem is that some so-called duties and obligations express what we ought to do in the light of ideals and supererogatory actions, such as those of heroes and saints, that may not be appropriately labelled *moral* requirements. Often they express self-imposed requirements, as when we believe that we ought to contribute substantially to charity, even though morality does not require it. We will discuss such ideals and self-imposed requirements in the final chapter.

John Stuart Mill usefully approached this problem by employing the distinction between duties of perfect obligation and duties of imperfect obligation: "duties of perfect obligation are those duties in virtue of which a correlative *right* resides in some person or persons; duties of imperfect obligation are those moral obligations which do not give birth to any right."[25] Mill goes on to indicate that duties of perfect obligation are duties of justice, while duties of imperfect obligation belong to other spheres of morality: "Justice implies something which is not only right to do, and wrong not to do, but which some individual person can claim from us as his moral right. No one has a moral right to our generosity or beneficence, because we are not morally bound to practice those virtues towards any given individual."[26]

Either rule utilitarianism or rule deontology, as obligation-oriented theories, can incorporate the language and substance of rights. This claim may appear to be somewhat surprising, since some utilitarians have vigorously opposed certain conceptions of rights, and many of the strongest supporters and theoreticians of rights have operated within deontological frameworks, emphasizing particularly respect for persons. Indeed, in our ordinary moral discourse, we frequently set the rights of individuals and groups in opposition to social utility. Nevertheless, it follows from the doctrine of the logical correlativity of rights and obligations that rule utilitarianism as well as rule deontology can provide a foundation for both rights and obligations.[27]

Ronald Dworkin's argument about the possibility of rights within a rule-utilitarian political theory also holds for moral theory:

> a political theory might provide for a right to free speech, for example, on the hypothesis that the general acceptance of that right by courts and other political institutions would promote the highest average utility of the community in the long run. . . . If the theory provides that an official of a particular institution is justified in making a political decision, and not justified in refusing to make it, whenever that decision is necessary to protect the freedom to speak of any individual, without regard to the impact of the decision on collective goals, the theory provides free speech as a right.[28]

Rights, according to this view, may serve as constraints or "political trumps" within either rule utilitarianism or rule deontology. In rule utilitarianism, they are justified by their likely contributions to utility, and Mill defended rights of autonomy and liberty in these terms (as we will see in subsequent chapters). In a deontological framework, on the other hand, rights are likely to be based on respect for persons, autonomy, and similar nonutilitarian principles; rights express and embody those principles and are not merely instrumental to the maximization of good consequences. Of course, there will be disputes about whether certain claims are "rights," about their relative weight, etc., but these disputes will probably be no more frequent or intractable *between* rule utilitarians and rule deontologists than within these two approaches to ethical theory.

An important distinction is that between positive rights and negative rights. As Joel Feinberg writes, "A *positive* right is a right to other persons' positive actions; a *negative* right is a right to other persons' omissions or forebearances. For every positive right I have, someone else has a duty to *do* something; for every negative right I have, someone else has a duty to *refrain* from doing something."[29] Examples of both sorts of rights can be found in biomedical practice and research. If there is a right to health care, it is obviously a positive right to goods and services, while the right not to be operated on without one's consent is a negative right, grounded in the principle of autonomy. The liberal tradition has generally found it easier to justify negative rights, especially those that call for noninterference with liberty, than positive rights; but the recognition of welfare rights has extended the range and power of positive rights.

Much confusion in moral discourse about public policies governing biomedicine can be traced to a failure to distinguish positive rights from negative rights. One example comes from the controversy surrounding the Supreme Court decisions on abortion.[30] Some who contend that the abortion decisions are contradictory fail to see that the Court recognized a negative right in 1973 and refused to recognize a positive right in 1977. In *Roe v. Wade* and *Doe v. Bolton* in 1973, the Court ruled that a woman's right to privacy, especially in relation to her physician, gives her a right to abort her fetus within certain limits. If the decision is made within the first trimester of the pregnancy, the state may not interfere with it. The state may, however, regulate abortions for the protection of maternal health in the second trimester; and in the third trimester it may even prohibit abortions, except in cases where there is a threat to the mother's life or health. The constitutionally protected right of privacy is here construed as a negative right. It identifies a sphere of general noninterference and limits state interference to certain specified circumstances. This right was interpreted in the *Danforth* decision (1976) to exclude a husband's veto of his wife's and her physician's decision to terminate her pregnancy. Again, the Court recognized a right of noninterference.

Many people apparently thought that the Court had also recognized a positive right—i.e., a right to have aid and assistance from the state and others in abortions, for they were surprised when the Court in 1977 ruled on legal and constitutional grounds that federal and state governments do not have to provide funds for nontherapeutic abortions; federal and state governments do not have a duty to provide such funds, and pregnant women who are seeking nontherapeutic abortions do not have a right to financial assistance. It appears to us that the Court's decisions are not inconsistent: they affirm a negative right and deny a positive right on legal and constitutional grounds. Although it is possible to argue that the Court *should* have found a positive right as well as a negative right, there is no inconsistency over rights.

Opponents of the most recent decisions may, however, charge that these decisions embody a different order of inconsistency in that they affirm a positive right to financial assistance for bringing a pregnancy to term while they deny a *positive* right to terminate a pregnancy. Some opponents contend that abortion and birth are two legitimate alternative ways to deal with the condition of pregnancy. One of the strongest arguments for the view that the legislature morally ought to provide funds for poor women who seek abortions appeals to a principle of justice (Cf. Chapter 6): It is unfair not to assist poor women in obtaining abortions, when other women can easily obtain them; and it is unfair for the society to try to salve its conscience about abortion by forcing poor women to complete pregnancies that others can terminate or by forcing them to seek inexpensive and risky abortions in unsafe surroundings.

The abortion controversy may also be analyzed by reference to the distinction between the statements (1) "S has a right to do Y" and (2) "S acts rightly in doing Y." The distinction is between "rights" (or "a right") and "right conduct" as well as between "rights" and their "right exercise."[31] Sometimes when we say that a person has a right to do X, we mean that he or she does no wrong in performing X. But often our statement that someone has a right to do X implies nothing about the morality of the act; it only means that we believe that others have no right to interfere with the act. Thus, one can affirm that a woman has a moral or a legal right to have an abortion without affirming that she acts rightly in those circumstances. A society might create a legal right to abortions, because of the bad consequences of criminal prohibition (e.g., women seek illegal abortions under unsafe conditions); and one might argue that there is a moral right to an abortion for the same reasons. Nevertheless, it is not inconsistent to say that a woman who has this legal and moral right to have an abortion is not acting rightly in having an abortion. For example, one might argue that her reasons are not strong enough to warrant an abortion. To say that she has a right is to say that we should not try to stop her forcibly, but it need not imply that she acts rightly.

As the controversy over abortion makes clear, many of the disputes that plague obligations and duties reappear in discussions of rights. For example, is there a right of privacy, and does the fetus have a right to life? How much weight do we assign to these different rights? When they come into conflict, which right takes precedence? Answers to these questions, which may finally be unanswerable to everyone's satisfaction, can only come through the framework of systematic reflection on moral principles and rules, including duties, obligations, and rights. We shall examine the relevant principles and rules in subsequent chapters.

Notes

1. Jeremy Bentham, *An Introduction to the Principles of Morals and Legislation* (New York: Hafner Publishing Co., 1948). Cf. Chapter I.3.
2. John Stuart Mill, *Utilitarianism, On Liberty, and Essay on Bentham*, ed. with an Introduction by Mary Warnock (Cleveland: World Publishing Co., 1962), pp. 256–78.
3. G. E. Moore, *Principia Ethica* (Cambridge: Cambridge University Press, 1962), pp. 90f.
4. J. J. C. Smart, *An Outline of a System of Utilitarian Ethics* (Melbourne: University Press, 1961), and "Extreme and Restricted Utilitarianism," *The Philosophical Quarterly* VI (1956), as reprinted in M. Bayles, ed., *Contemporary Utilitarianism* (Garden City: Doubleday Anchor Books, 1968), especially pp. 104ff in the latter source.
5. David Hume, *A Treatise of Human Nature*, ed. L. A. Selby-Bigge (Oxford: Oxford University Press, 1888). Book III, Parts I and II, especially pp. 494–500. Richard B. Brandt, "Toward a Credible Form of Utilitarianism," in Bayles, ed., *Contemporary Utilitarianism*, pp. 143–86.
6. Moral Code Utilitarianism also may provide a way of circumventing a prominent objection against the act/rule distinction that has been advanced by David Lyons in *Forms and Limits of Utilitarianism* (Oxford: Clarendon Press, 1965). He argues that whatever would count for an act utilitarian as a reason for *breaking* a rule would count equally for a rule utilitarian as a good reason for *emending* a rule—and hence the two come in practice to the same theory. It would be very difficult and perhaps impossible to emend an entire code with the frequency with which a rule could be validly broken by act utilitarians.
7. See W. D. Ross, *The Right and the Good* (Oxford: Clarendon Press, 1930); *The Foundations of Ethics* (Oxford: Clarendon Press, 1939); and John Rawls, *A Theory of Justice* (Cambridge, Mass.: Harvard University Press, 1971).
8. See Alan Donagan, *The Theory of Morality* (Chicago: University of Chicago Press, 1977).
9. Immanuel Kant, *Groundwork of the Metaphysic of Morals*, translated by

H. J. Paton (New York: Harper and Row, Harper Torchbooks, 1964), pp. 90–91.

10. Ross, *The Right and the Good,* pp. 22, 41–42.

11. Rawls, *A Theory of Justice,* Pars. 8, 11, 51, especially pp. 339–40.

12. See Ross, *The Right and the Good* and *The Foundations of Ethics.* Some rule deontologists writing in contemporary biomedical ethics are Paul Ramsey and Robert Veatch. See Ramsey, *The Patient as Person* (New Haven: Yale University Press, 1970) and *Ethics at the Edges of Life: Medical and Legal Intersections* (New Haven: Yale University Press, 1978); and Veatch, *Death, Dying and the Biological Revolution* (New Haven: Yale University Press, 1976). For an analysis of Ramsey and Veatch, see James Childress, "Ethical Issues in Death and Dying," *Religious Studies Review* 4 (1978): 180–88.

13. Antony Flew, "Ends and Means," *The Encyclopedia of Philosophy,* ed. Paul Edwards (New York: Macmillan and the Free Press, 1967), vol. II, p. 510.

14. See William Frankena, *Ethics,* 2nd ed. (Englewood Cliffs, N.J.: Prentice-Hall, 1973).

15. Richard B. Brandt, *Ethical Theory* (Englewood Cliffs, N.J.: Prentice-Hall, 1959), p. 404.

16. See Lyons, *The Forms and Limits of Utilitarianism.*

17. "Toward a Credible Form of Utilitarianism," in Bayles, ed., *Contemporary Utilitarianism,* p. 166.

18. G. J. Warnock, *The Object of Morality* (London: Methuen and Co., 1971), p. 33.

19. Donald Evans, "Paul Ramsey on Exceptionless Moral Rules," *American Journal of Jurisprudence* 16 (1971): 184–214. See also Sissela Bok, *Lying: Moral Choice in Public and Private Life* (New York: Pantheon Books, 1978), pp. 13–16.

20. Richard C. Cabot, "The Use of Truth and Falsehood in Medicine: An Experimental Study," *American Medicine* 5 (1903): 344–49; reprinted in Stanley Joel Reiser, Arthur J. Dyck, and William J. Curran, eds., *Ethics in Medicine: Historical Perspectives and Contemporary Concerns* (Cambridge, Mass.: MIT Press, 1977), p. 213.

21. See Robert Nozick, "Moral Complications and Moral Structures," *Natural Law Forum* 13 (1968): 1–50.

22. See Joel Feinberg, *Social Philosophy* (Englewood Cliffs, N.J.: Prentice-Hall, 1973), p. 67. Feinberg prefers the narrower term "validity" to the broader term "justification," since validity "is justification of a peculiar and narrow kind, namely justification within a system of rules."

23. David Braybrooke, "The Firm but Untidy Correlativity of Rights and Obligations," *Canadian Journal of Philosophy* 1 (March 1972): 351–63.

24. Feinberg, *Social Philosophy,* p. 61.

25. Mill, *Utilitarianism,* p. 305.

26. *Ibid.* It is still largely undecided whether we should ascribe rights to non-persons, such as trees and animals. We have a duty not to be cruel to animals,

for example, but is it appropriate to ascribe rights to them? The answer to this question will obviously depend upon one's theory of rights and their foundation. According to one recent theory, only entities capable of having *interests* can have rights, and therefore trees and vegetables cannot have rights. However, since both animals and future generations can be said to have interests they can be said meaningfully to have rights. See Joel Feinberg, "The Rights of Animals and Unborn Generations," in *Philosophy and Environmental Crisis,* ed. W. T. Blackstone (Athens, Ga.: University of Georgia Press, 1974).

27. Act utilitarians, by contrast, seem committed to the translation of rights into interests and needs in order to facilitate utilitarian calculation; but rule utilitarians need not resort to this maneuver. The utilitarian critique of natural rights offered by Bentham is well-known: "Natural rights is simple nonsense: natural and imprescriptible rights, rhetorical nonsense—nonsense upon stilts." That critique, however, was aimed at the epistemology of *natural* rights, not at any use of the language of rights or at any development of a theory of moral rights. Bentham's invectives were directed against "naturalistic" theories rather than "rights." Bentham, *Anarchical Fallacies,* in *The Collected Papers of Jeremy Bentham,* vol. 2, ed. John Bowring (Edinburgh, 1843), as reprinted in *Human Rights,* ed. A. I. Melden (Belmont, Cal.: Wadsworth Press, 1970), p. 32.

28. Ronald Dworkin, *Taking Rights Seriously* (Cambridge, Mass.: Harvard University Press, 1977), pp. 96–97. See also Richard Flathman's justification of the practice of rights in *The Practice of Rights* (Cambridge: Cambridge University Press, 1976).

29. Feinberg, *Social Philosophy,* p. 59.

30. The relevant decisions are: *Roe v. Wade* 410 U.S. 113 (1973), *Doe v. Bolton* 410 U.S. 179 (1973), *Planned Parenthood of Missouri v. Danforth* 428 U.S. 52 (1976), *Beal v. Doe* 432 U.S. 438 (1977), *Maher v. Roe* 432 U.S. 464 (1977), *Poelker v. Doe* 432 U.S. 519 (1977).

31. See A. I. Melden, *Rights and Right Conduct* (Oxford: Basil Blackwell, 1959).

3

The Principle of Autonomy

Diverse figures in philosophy, including Kant, Nietzsche, Sartre, R. M. Hare, and Robert Paul Wolff, have held that morality in some sense requires autonomous persons. Their views are different, however, because they select different themes from a family of ideas associated with autonomy: freedom of choice, choosing for oneself, creating one's own moral position, accepting ultimate responsibility for one's moral views, etc. Because of these divergent interpretations, we shall examine the concept of autonomy before trying to develop a moral principle of autonomy and sketching its implications for biomedical ethics.

The concept of autonomy

The autonomous person

Autonomy is a form of personal liberty of action where the individual determines his or her own course of action in accordance with a plan chosen by himself or herself. The autonomous person is one who not only deliberates about and chooses such plans but who is capable of acting on the basis of such deliberations, just as a truly independent government has autonomous control of its territories and policies. A person's autonomy is his or her independence, self-reliance, and self-contained ability to decide. A person of diminished autonomy, by contrast, is highly dependent on

56

others and in at least some respect incapable of deliberating or acting on the basis of such deliberations. Institutionalized populations such as prisoners and the mentally retarded may have diminished autonomy. A form of psychological incapacitation afflicts the retarded, while a severely restricted social environment curtails the autonomy of prisoners. The most general idea of autonomy is that of being one's own person, without constraints either by another's action or by a psychological or physical limitation. The term "autonomy" is thus quite broad, for it can refer to both *the will* and *action in society;* and both internal and external constraints on action can limit autonomy.

Two figures in the history of philosophy have shaped our understanding of autonomy as, respectively, freedom of the will and freedom of action. These figures are Immanuel Kant (a rule deontologist) and John Stuart Mill (a utilitarian). In his *Groundwork of the Metaphysics of Morals* and other writings, Kant contrasted heteronomy (rule by other persons or conditions) and autonomy. Autonomy is governing oneself, including making one's own choices, in accord with moral principles which are one's own and which are universalizable, i.e., can be willed to be universally valid for everyone. Under "heteronomy," Kant included both external and internal determinations of the will, but *not* moral principles. While one's own self-imposed rule obliges one to so act, one is only complying with a self-legislated rule. Coerced actions are obviously heteronomous, but Kant also regarded acting from desire, impulse, and habit as heteronomous. Thus, a person who acts out of desire, rather than reason, is not acting autonomously, for heteronomy is subjection of the will to any rule or motive outside itself.

Whereas Kant was largely concerned about the autonomy of the *will,* Mill was more concerned about the autonomy of *action.* As Mill recognized, the latter is more difficult to justify than the former. In *On Liberty,* Mill argues that social and political control over individual actions is legitimate only if necessary to prevent harm to other individuals affected by those actions. He construes the principle of utility to permit all citizens to develop their potential according to their own convictions, as long as they do not interfere with a like expression of freedom by others. The promotion of autonomous expression in his view maximizes the benefits for all concerned. Conformity to established patterns reduces individual productivity and creativity which, if developed, could benefit the society. The society thus benefits in proportion as individuals develop their own natural talents and facilities for judgment. In his discussion of individuality, Mill holds that a person "without character" is one who is controlled by his environment—church, state, parents, family, etc.—whereas a person with true character is one of genuine individuality who takes from the culture only what he finds valuable. The latter person can make new discoveries and develop new practices.

For our purposes, Kant's main contribution to a theory of autonomy is his discussion of self-legislation: the reasons for actions for autonomous persons are their own reasons, and they are principled rather than arbitrary reasons. This notion of self-directed action based on a rational principle accepted by the agent is the central ingredient in "autonomy" in the remainder of this chapter. "Acceptance by the agent" needs emphasis. Kant is often interpreted as holding that each individual person must *make* (author or originate) his own moral principles. Because this extreme interpretation denies much that we know about the moral life, we will here understand Kant to mean that each individual must *will the acceptance* of his principles. Finally, while Mill's views on autonomous choice in many ways parallel Kant's, Mill's concerns about the tyranny of society led to idealistic notions about freeing oneself from society and becoming virtually a sovereign, except where others are involved. In this discussion of autonomy and subsequently in our treatment of paternalism in Chapter 5, we will see both the importance and the limits of this ideal.

Respect for autonomy and the principle of autonomy

It is one thing to be autonomous and to apprehend that others are acting autonomously, but quite another to be *respected* as an autonomous agent and to respect the autonomy of others. To respect autonomous agents is to recognize with due appreciation their own considered value judgments and outlooks even when it is believed that their judgments are mistaken. To respect them in this way is to acknowledge their right to their own views and the permissibility of their actions based on such beliefs. And to grant them this right is to say that they are entitled to such autonomous determination without limitations on their liberty being imposed by others. This conclusion follows from Mill's views on individualism and social liberty, but it also has an important basis in Kant's thought. To respect autonomy for Kant is bound up with conceiving the other person as having unconditional worth, solely because persons are ends in themselves determining their own destiny and are not to be treated merely as means. To treat a person merely as a means always involves a violation of autonomy for Kant, because the person is then being treated in accordance with rules not of his own choosing. To show a lack of respect for an autonomous agent, then, is either to reject that person's considered judgments or to deny him the freedom to act on those considered judgments. For Kant a moral relation between persons is always one where there is mutual respect for autonomy—where both are autonomous, of course. It is hard to find fault with this particular point in his argument.

The moral notion of respecting the autonomy of other persons can, for our purposes, be formulated as a *principle of autonomy* that should guide our judgments about how to treat self-determining moral agents. It follows from the views advanced by Mill that insofar as an autonomous agent's actions do not infringe the autonomous actions of others, that person should be free to perform whatever action he wishes—even if it involves serious risk for the agent and even if others consider it to be foolish. We shall later in this chapter discuss those occasions on which a rational agent expresses an autonomous wish to take his own life and those occasions on which it might be permissible to restrain such autonomous actions. Whether or not there are limits to the valid expression of autonomy, Mill is surely right to insist that in self-regarding actions we ought to be as free as possible to do as we wish. (See Chapter 5 for some possible qualifications.) This is the first aspect of the principle of autonomy.

The second aspect follows from Kant's position: in evaluating the self-regarding actions of others we ought to respect them as persons with the same right to their judgments as we have to our own. This aspect of the principle of autonomy is often referred to as the principle of respect for persons, because it demands respect not for a utilitarian or any other reason except that another is a person and therefore rightfully a rational determiner of his or her own destiny. So far as our actions in regard to others are concerned, it is doubtful that the approaches taken by Mill and Kant lead to significantly different courses of action. Mill's view leads to a moral demand of noninterference with the autonomy of others in society, while Kant's leads to a moral demand that certain attitudes of respect be framed about the personhood and beliefs of others. In the end these two very different philosophers present views of autonomy which are both acceptable and in no major respects incompatible.

It is important, however, that the principle of autonomy not be interpreted either as absolute or as too broad in scope. Some persons are not in a position to act in a sufficiently autonomous manner, perhaps because they are immature, incapacitated, ignorant, coerced, or in a position in which they can be exploited by others. Infants and irrationally suicidal individuals are typical examples. The actions of such nonautonomous persons may be validly obstructed in order to protect them from harms that might result from their own actions. Those who defend autonomy have never denied that this interference is valid, because they regard such actions as substantially nonautonomous. The principle of autonomy thus applies exclusively to persons capable of autonomous choice.

Autonomy and authority

It is sometimes held that autonomy is such a supreme value that it is inconsistent with the authority of the state, social groups, or individuals who function in special contexts as authorities and who make decisions over the lives of autonomous agents. This radical position would reject, for example, the legitimacy of governmental implementation of restrictive public policies intended to protect and promote health. It also entails that medical authorities can never validly intervene in the lives of autonomous patients. One argument for this position is that the autonomous person is one who self-determines his actions through moral deliberation *totally unimpeded by any authority's influence.*[1] In this theory, because autonomous persons must act on their own reasons, they should never submit to another person or authority simply because the other utters an imperative. Obviously a conflict between autonomy and all authority results, for it is a necessary condition of authority that a person be obeyed merely because that person occupies a position of authority; and it is a necessary condition of autonomy that a person must refuse all heteronomous influence by authorities.[2] Because this conclusion might seem to follow from the philosophies of both Mill and Kant, it is worth considering whether autonomy is radically inconsistent with authority in the way this theory suggests.

We think there is no fundamental inconsistency, because the very notions of autonomy and authority employed in this theory are eccentric and indefensible. Common conceptions of nondictatorial political and social practices generally assume that provision of reasons is part of, not distinct from, the process of legitimate authoritative command. That is, reasons which justify commands are not regarded as isolated from command circumstances. Dutiful citizens are not expected to comply with authoritative commands without provision of reasons and merely because authorities have spoken. In democratic theories of the state, for example, authorities are not envisioned as issuing commands without justification. And the legitimacy of any command is regarded as contingent upon the command's not exceeding the limits of autonomously delegated authority. Moreover, we often gratefully appeal to authorities when we know of no other place to turn. If we want to know what should be done about an irregular heartbeat, or how to play tennis better, or whether an automobile's mileage rating is accurate, we consult with an authoritative individual and willingly—autonomously—rely on that person's determinations.

Moral principles are not disembodied rules, cut off from their cultural setting. Most, if not all, of our moral beliefs have arisen from shared experiences and tacit social agreements and arrangements. Morality is by its very nature not an individual-centered phenomenon, as even Kant and Mill usually acknowledge. The notions of virtuous conduct, acceptable forms of loving, kinds of respect owed others, and many other moral views have been adopted largely, and willingly, from cultural arrangements. In some cases a principle could not be a *moral* principle and stand in abstraction from such an arrangement. It would then just be an individual principle. Codes of medical ethics, for example, do not allow individual authorship, and to act against them merely on grounds of individual principle is to act immorally by the standards of that community, unless there is something about the codes incompatible with morality itself.

One can, of course, act autonomously by rejecting all these social understandings of morality. This action would be, as Nietzsche put it, a transvaluation of values. But, as we have seen, it does not follow that because it is an autonomous action it is morally acceptable or even morally principled. It also does not follow that when one acts on a principle widely shared in society that one acts nonautonomously. Autonomy is perfectly compatible with authority, as long as the authority is autonomously accepted—whether it be a social, political, or religious authority. As Kant rightly pointed out, autonomy is compatible even with a rigid understanding of the objectivity and authority of all moral principles (as a system that applies to everyone). To this it may be added that autonomy is compatible with moral traditions, even if these traditions can never be taken as conclusive authorities in and of themselves. Autonomy is thus far more closely linked to the notion of reflective individual choice or acceptance of a view than it is to the notion of rejection of authority and traditional views.

This conclusion about the compatibility of autonomy and both delegated authority and moral tradition holds for medical contexts as well as for political ones. The authority assumed by medical professionals presents many of the difficulties about autonomy and consent that arise in the medical setting. We shall see that a number of interesting paradoxes of autonomy emerge in medical contexts because of the condition of the subject, on the one hand, and the authoritative position of the medical professional, on the other. There will be a number of occasions (both here and in the section on paternalism in Chapter 5) where we may doubt that authority and autonomy are in fact compatible. These contexts will usually be ones, however, where authority either is not delegated or is itself questionable as an authority.

Informed consent

The voluntary consent of the human subject is absolutely essential.

This means that the person involved should have the legal capacity to give consent; should be so situated as to be able to exercise free power of choice, without the intervention of any element of force, fraud, deceit, duress, overreaching, or other ulterior form of constraint or coercion; and should have sufficient knowledge and comprehension of the subject matter involved as to enable him to make an understanding and enlightened decision. This latter element requires that before the acceptance of an affirmative decision by the experimental subject there should be made known to him the nature, duration, and purpose of the experiment; the methods and means by which it is to be conducted; all inconveniences and hazards reasonably to be expected; and the effects upon his health or person which may possibly come from his participation in the experiment. (*Nuremberg Code,* Rule 1; See Appendix II)

The horrible story of experimentation in concentration camps led to serious concern about the use of nonconsenting subjects in questionable and sometimes brutal experiments. Indeed, since the Nuremberg trials the issue of informed consent has received more attention than any ethical issue in biomedical research involving human subjects. The Nuremberg

Code cited above is one result, but controversies about informed consent have also arisen in other quarters. In American law, for example, the doctrine of informed consent has gradually emerged from malpractice cases involving nonconsensual touching of the patient's body—a form of intentional interference qualifying as battery. Touching without consent, where patients are capable of consent, has been found unacceptable, irrespective of considerations of the quality of care. As a rough generalization, it can be said that most recent discussions of informed consent can be traced historically to two sources: (1) Standards for medical *practice* have derived from case law, and (2) standards for *research* have grown from their roots in both the Nuremberg Code and the Declaration of Helsinki.

The functions of informed consent

In recent years virtually all medical and research codes of ethics have held that physicians must obtain the informed consent of patients before undertaking significant therapeutic or research procedures. While these consent measures have largely been designed to protect the autonomy of patients and subjects, they also serve other functions. Alexander Capron has helpfully identified several important functions:[3]

(1) The promotion of individual autonomy
(2) The protection of patients and subjects
(3) The avoidance of fraud and duress
(4) The encouragement of self-scrutiny by medical professionals
(5) The promotion of rational decisions
(6) The involvement of the public (in promoting autonomy as a general social value and in controlling biomedical research)

Capron correctly argues that informed consent serves each of these several functions, but, both historically and contemporarily, the primary function it serves is the protection of individual autonomy. Autonomy is fostered by informed consent procedures in at least two ways. First, at the level of the unique relationship between patients or subjects and medical professionals, autonomy is protected because persons are granted the right to make decisions affecting their lives, even though the health professional may possess far more information and training. A second and rather different way of protecting autonomy was suggested by Mill.

By establishing mechanisms in society that promote individual thought and initiative, Mill believed that the interests of both society and the individual would be enhanced. An extension of his argument is the following: to the extent violations of autonomy are institutionally condoned, we all stand to suffer, because the right to make such choices will in general be impaired or even eliminated by this institutional arrangement. This latter consideration, as advanced by Mill, will become of major significance in Chapter 5, where the subject of paternalism is investigated.

The justification of informed consent

The *functions* of informed consent mentioned by Capron can also be reconstructed as formal *justifications* of the requirement that informed consent be obtained. Thus, one justification of the requirement is that of protecting patients and subjects by preventing harm to them—a justification based on the principle of nonmaleficence. This justification is especially appropriate for legal requirements governing consent. As we shall see, the law of battery protects against unauthorized touching; and the law of negligence holds researchers responsible for certain deviant procedures they might employ.[4] Second-party consent, or consent on behalf of a person given by another, can be similarly justified. Nonetheless, this justification in terms of the principle of nonmaleficence is not fundamental to moral justifications of first-party consent. While a person's own decision may *indirectly* function to prevent harm, he may also autonomously choose a greater risk than others would choose for him. The principle of autonomy justifies allowing a person this option of greater risk.

Another important justification for informed consent is based on the principle of utility: informed consent will maximally protect and benefit *everyone* in society, including health professionals, patients, and the institutions of medical practice and research themselves. Rules of consent serve to protect and benefit patients and professionals, to allay public fears (especially about research), to encourage self-scrutiny by physicians and investigators, and to maintain relations of trust. This justification is closely related to Capron's fourth and sixth functions.

Even though both the justification based on utility and the justification based on nonmaleficence are appropriate for some consent requirements, neither is the primary justification of informed consent. Both the historical roots and the primary justification of informed consent are located in the principle of autonomy—not in the principles of nonmaleficence or utility. There is a moral duty to seek a valid consent *because* the consenting party is an autonomous person, with all the entitlements that status confers. By contrast, neither utility nor nonmaleficence leads to this strong conclusion, for both would justify not seeking consent in some circumstances—utility when it would not maximize the social welfare and nonmaleficence when no apparent harm would result. When informed consent is justified by the principle of autonomy, it is introduced, as Robert Veatch puts it, "not to facilitate social benefits, but as a check against them,"[5] for persons have rights independent of such considerations as immediate social utility and risk to patients or subjects.

This view has long-standing appeal in the law, where it is somewhat more fully developed than in writings on moral philosophy. Justice Cardozo's statement in behalf of autonomy is well known: "Every human being of adult years and sound mind has a right to determine what shall be done with his own body; and a surgeon who performs an operation without his patient's consent commits an assault, for which he is liable in damages. . . . This is true except in cases of emergency where the patient is unconscious and where it is necessary to operate before consent can be obtained."[6] An updated and in some ways even stronger view of this sort is found in the landmark *Natanson v. Kline* opinion, where it is argued that

Anglo-American law starts with the premise of thoroughgoing self-determination. It follows that each man is considered to be master of his own body, and he may, if he be of sound mind, expressly prohibit the performance of lifesaving surgery, or other medical treatment.[7]

In short, the fact that we would often seek to obtain informed consent, even when it does not maximize immediate social utility and even when subjects and patients are not being protected against risk, indicates that autonomy and not some other principle is the basic justifying principle.

As previously mentioned, nonautonomous persons must sometimes be protected by securing the informed consent of a second person who is appropriately related to the patient or subject. Parents, legal guardians, and perhaps a patient-designated friend all might qualify as a second party whose consent or permission is morally valid. The need for this derivative form of consent arises both when persons are incapable of consenting, e.g., when comatose, or in infancy, or emotionally distraught, and also when an informed consent is only doubtfully present. In the case of patients who are mentally ill, for example, we may on occasion reasonably doubt the validity of consent; and for classes of persons such as children and prisoners the ability of individuals to give a free and informed consent to biomedical or behavioral research may at times be doubtful. In these cases, where we might fall into error, it seems best to err on the side of ethical conservatism: we should strive not to deny an important medical benefit when a person is incapable of knowledgeably accepting it, even if—after careful examination—we are uncertain about the validity of a consent or refusal. By contrast to the justification for obtaining first-party consent, which is based on protecting autonomy, the justification for obtaining second-party consent derives largely and perhaps exclusively from the moral demand that subjects and patients be protected from harm—a demand derived from the principles of non-maleficence and beneficence. (See Chapters 4 and 5.)

The elements of informed consent

Whether first parties or second parties are in question, it is generally agreed that informed consent must be solicited whenever a procedure is intrusive, whenever significant risks might be run to persons, and whenever the purposes of the procedure might be questionable. But there is controversy concerning the elements that constitute informed consent.

Medical and research codes, as well as federal regulations, have traditionally emphasized that the act of consent must be genuinely *voluntary* and that there must be adequate *disclosure* of information; but there are actually several distinct elements of informed consent, each containing its own separate issues. The information element of informed consent refers to adequate disclosure of information and adequate comprehension by patients or subjects of what is disclosed, while the consent component refers to a voluntary decision on the part of a competent person. But how much and what types of information must be imparted, and how well must it be understood? Is consent valid if it is given under conditions of social pressure or if the consent is irresponsible? Underneath these questions is the need for a detailed analysis of the concept of informed consent that raises the moral problems unique to each element. Ac-

cordingly, each of the following four elements and the issues each raises
will now be discussed:

I. Information Elements
1. Disclosure of Information
2. Comprehension of Information
II. Consent Elements
3. Voluntary Consent
4. Competence to Consent

Each of these four components should be understood as a necessary
condition of valid informed consent. However, this broad generalization
will have to be qualified and refined as each of the elements is studied. We
begin with the last of the four elements in the above chart.

Competence

Competence to consent could perhaps be more appropriately described as
a *presupposition* of informed consent than as an *element* of informed
consent. Logically, competence is a precondition of acting voluntarily and
apprehending information. It is fundamental in biomedical contexts,
because certain physical and mental defects can result in a situation where
patients and subjects are not—in psychological fact or in law—able to
give informed consent. Obviously many conditions external to an agent
may inhibit voluntary action, but many internal conditions may also limit
voluntary consent. It is usually the latter that give rise to questions about
competence. For example, minors commonly are not capable of responsible actions, while the mentally disabled and the comatose present even
more troublesome cases.

The concept of competence is a multidimensional one. Competence and
incompetence are often assessed by diverse and even inconsistent theories
of comprehension, rationality, freedom, physiological state, etc., and
judgments of incompetence often apply to a limited range of decision
making, not to all decisions made by a person. Some persons who are
legally incompetent may be competent to conduct most of their personal
affairs, and vice versa. The same person's ability to make decisions may
vary over time, and the person may at a single time be competent to make
certain practical decisions but incompetent to make others. For example,
a person judged incompetent to drive an automobile may not be in-

competent to decide to participate in medical research, or may be able to handle simple affairs easily, while faltering before complex ones. Accordingly, the notions of *limited* competence and *intermittent* competence are useful, because they require a statement of the precise decisions a person can make, while avoiding the false dichotomy of "either competent or incompetent." Use of these notions would preserve maximum autonomy, justifying intervention only in those areas where a person clearly is of questionable competence.

Each class of possible subjects who might be classified as incompetent should therefore be considered separately, especially where unfair evaluations might occur. For example, from the fact that persons have been admitted to institutions on grounds of incompetence, it does not follow that they *are* incompetent. Questions of the need for their consent, and of its validity, depend in complex ways on the precise nature of their incompetence to consent, their previous declarations, and on the precise constraints characteristic of their conditions of life. Some patients and research subjects, such as children, have inherent limits on their capacity to understand and consent. Still other subjects may not be capable of understanding information, while successfully assimilating part of the information. It is easy to violate the autonomy of members of such groups, and sometimes extraordinary measures must be taken in order not to invalidate the consent process. For example, those who have a severely limited capacity to understand may want to consult with other persons, who may also have to be informed and ultimately may become the consenting party.

Two cases included in the Appendix (#13 and #8) illustrate the difficulties often encountered in attempting to judge competence. In one case a sixty-eight-year-old man with kidney disease and multiple additional problems also develops intermittent psychotic behavior. The psychiatric diagnosis is that of chronic psychotic organic brain syndrome resulting from cerebral arteriosclerosis. Nonetheless, two psychiatrists declare the patient competent to make fundamental decisions affecting his treatment, based on behavioral and psychiatric indications. Because the patient exhibits what his attending physician regards as erratic and irrational behavior, the psychiatrists' declaration of competence is reluctantly accepted by the physician and by certain members of the family. In this difficult case the patient's behavior is perhaps best understood in terms of limited and intermittent competence. In the second case, a man who generally exhibits normal behavior patterns is involuntarily committed to a mental institution because of certain bizarre actions that follow from his unique and unorthodox religious beliefs. Because the man's religious beliefs lead to serious self-destructive behavior (pulling out an eye and cutting off a hand), he is judged incompetent, despite his generally competent behavior and despite the fact that his peculiar actions follow "reasonably" from his—many would say, equally peculiar— religious beliefs. While this puzzling case probably cannot be understood in terms of intermittent competence, it may be that the notion of limited competence again applies.

Perhaps the major question in recent years about competence centers on *standards* for its determination. Conventional standards isolate various abilities to comprehend information and to reason about the consequences of one's actions. In particular, a person is said to be incompetent unless both capable of processing a certain amount of information and capable of choosing both ends and the means to those ends. The most promising headway toward a useful definition has come through criminal and civil law. Courts have disagreed on which of the following three properties is most crucial to a determination of competency:[8] (1) capacity to reach a decision based on *rational reasons,* (2) the reaching of a *reasonable result* through a decision, or (3) the *capacity to make a decision* at all. Without attempting to distinguish all the arguments and possible reasons for adopting any one of these three standards, it seems reasonable to combine them as follows: a person is competent if and only if that person can make decisions based on rational reasons. In biomedical contexts this standard entails that a person must be able to understand a therapy or research procedure, must be able to weigh its risks and benefits, and must be able to make a decision in the light of such knowledge and through such abilities, even if the person chooses not to utilize the information.

But what about those who are *incompetent?* It is here that the problem of justifying second-party consent arises. The matter is relatively simple for therapeutic treatment: the second party is designated to act in the best interests of the incompetent person. However, in cases of research that does not hold out the prospect of direct benefit to subjects—e.g., infants—how can their involvement be justified? The general justification for such research is utilitarian: the promotion of the interests of all members of society through the research. Those appointed as second parties will be called upon to consider the significance of research procedures in the light of this goal when deciding whether or not to allow incompetents to become involved. In effect they are designated to decide about the involvement of incompetents on the same basis as any of us might consider our own involvement, while protecting any special interests or views held by the incompetent.

A further problem is that the term "competence" often functions to hide a significant value judgment about another person. A person who appears to others to be irrational or unreasonable might be declared incompetent in order that "treatment" may be provided. Such a declaration readily hides a value judgment about what a rational person ought to consent to do, presented in the guise of an empirical determination of incompetence. Jeffrie Murphy has recently argued for a presumably objective theory of competence based on the idea that a person may be incompetent in various ways if the person is so ignorant, compulsive, or devoid of reason that he cannot make important decisions. Still more important is Murphy's recognition that all such theories have troublesome borderline cases:

[T]he vast majority of cases that confront us will be borderline—cases in that greyish area between full competence and obvious incompetence. The real problem that will face us, then, is what to do in the borderline cases. When in doubt, which way should we err—on the side of safety or on the side of liberty? It is vital that we do not adopt analyses of "incompetence" or patterns of argument that obscure the obviously moral nature of this question.[9]

It is thus seldom a simple *empirical* question as to whether a person is or is not competent. If precise criteria were available for making such determinations, the grey area would vanish. But since such criteria are not available, *moral* judgments about what to do with possibly incompetent persons cannot be avoided.

Disclosure of information

Most medical and research codes specify conditions under which a person can be said to have sufficient information on the basis of which he or she could make an informed choice. Commonly mentioned as necessary items of disclosure are contemplated procedures, alternative available procedures, anticipated risks and benefits, and a statement offering the person an opportunity to ask further questions and to withdraw at any time (in the case of research). Several writers on the subject of informed consent have proposed additional or supplementary conditions—for example, statements of the purpose of the procedure, the uncertain risks involved, persons in charge, and, if research is involved, how subjects were selected. Such lists could be indefinitely expanded, but many possible inclusions are not applicable to all areas of medical research and practice. Expansive lists of conditions are sometimes appropriate, while in other contexts they would waste precious time and might even prove to be damaging to patients or subjects. Accordingly, it is more important to determine which primary moral standards should govern the disclosure of information. We shall concentrate on this topic.

Standards of disclosure. One major question is how the distinction is to be drawn between adequately informed consent, on the one hand, and partially informed or even uninformed consent, on the other hand. Three general standards of disclosure have emerged in legal and ethical writings on informed consent: (A) What is operative in the biomedical professions, (B) What the reasonable person would want to know, and (C) What individual patients or subjects of research want to know. In the past there has been a strong reliance on (A). For example, it was only recently reported that

> The view accepted by the majority of American jurisdictions bases the duty to disclose on a community standard; it requires only such disclosures of risks as is consistent with the practice of the local medical community. Expert medical testimony is required to show a breach of local medical standards.[10]

This standard was devised under the conviction that the doctor's proper role is that of acting in the patient's best medical interest. The obligation to disclose information is in effect subservient to a medical judgment of what is in the patient's best interest. Medical care standards, rather than patients' rights, are thus considered the operative guidelines governing proper disclosure. For this reason many have come to think—rightly, in our view—that this standard strips away too much autonomy from patients.

Lately this standard has been declining in significance, even in the courts, for two primary reasons. First, the amount of material information a person needs to make a decision is not a technical medical judgment, and is perhaps better within the comprehension of an average juror than an average physician. Second, medical custom often expresses the values and goals of the medical profession, but information provided to patients and subjects should be as free as possible of the values and goals of medical professionals, especially those doing research. The latter are more likely than most to believe in the scientific merit and social worth of their procedures; and they may well see risks and benefits in a quite different perspective than would others.

The reasonable person standard (B) now seems the prevalent criterion, and certainly it is an improvement over (A). But before the standard of the reasonable person can be accepted as the operational standard of disclosure for both research and practice, we need to know more precisely what it involves, including its relation, if any, to (C). The best present resource for an answer to this question is case law, which has gradually assembled a set of considerations that explicate the concept of a reasonable person, such as the following:

(1) All material information necessary for a decision must be given, as judged by persons who would compose a jury rather than by expert testimony or by a medical body.[11]

(2) Known risks of significant bodily harm and death must be disclosed.[12]

(3) The reasonable person is a composite or ideal of reasonable persons in society, and the individual subject is not in question. The latter standard might be too subjective and would require too much guesswork by physicians.[13]

(4) Standards of disclosure in medicine are not different from those of other professions where there is a similar fiduciary relationship.[14]

Although somewhat amorphous and open-ended, these legal criteria are useful for purposes of generalizing into moral contexts. However, even this claim is paradoxical. As Judge Robinson noted in *Canterbury v. Spence,* medical duties to disclose, as set forth in the law, are themselves ultimately based on moral considerations of autonomy. The judge calls these considerations "the patient's right of self-decision" and the patient's "prerogative to decide."[15] The point is that duties of disclosure are *at their root* moral rather than legal or medical ones, and these moral duties inform both law and medicine as to the appropriate standards. What has been said, then, about general moral standards based on autonomy and present case law might be focussed into the following minimum standard of disclosure: the patient or subject should be provided with information that a reasonable person in the patient's or subject's circumstances would find relevant and could reasonably be expected to assimilate. In this way the moral requirement to respect autonomy is translated into a consent standard.

Nonetheless, there are special problems about the development of more specific standards and about how the reasonable person standard can actually be employed in the disclosure of information in some areas of biomedical research and practice. One such problem has been suggested on the basis of recent empirical research that attempts to discover whether information disclosed to patients is actually used by these patients in reaching their decisions. For example, data collected in a study by Ruth Faden indicate, among other things, that though ninety-three percent of the patients surveyed believe they benefited from the information disclosed, only twelve percent actually used the information disclosed as the basis of their decision to consent.[16] This study, involving family-planning patients, reaches similar conclusions to an earlier study by Fellner and Marshall of persons consenting to be kidney donors.[17] In both studies data indicate that patients make their decisions largely prior to and independent of the actual process of disclosing information. These data do not in any way show that patient decisions were *uninformed* or that disclosed information was *irrelevant*, for the patients may have only believed that the additional information was not such as to shake their prior commitment to a particular course of action. For example, a kidney donor could very reasonably decide that the eventual death of his brother far outweighs any information disclosed by a physician. Nonetheless, the above empirical findings do throw into open question what should count as facts that are material to the decision-making process for actual *individual* patients, as contrasted to *average reasonable* patients.

Based on the above considerations, we suggest that the average reasonable-person standard presently operative in law should be supplemented by a standard which takes account of the independent informational needs of actual reasonable persons in the process of making a difficult decision. Yet an entirely subjective standard—(C) above— seems inappropriate, because patients often do not know what information would be relevant for their deliberations. Perhaps the best solution is a compromise standard, combining (B) and (C): whatever a reasonable person would judge material to the decision-making process should be disclosed, and, in addition, any remaining information material to an individual patient should be offered through a process of asking a patient what else he or she wishes to know and providing truthful answers to any questions asked. Autonomy is not adequately protected unless some more rigorous criterion of this general description is adopted. If subjects fail to have an adequate idea, given their own concerns and needs, of what they are deciding, then there is no *informed* consent, even if they do possess all the information a disembodied "reasonable person" would possess. And since the protection of autonomy is the central justification of informed consent requirements in morals and the law, this modified, more stringent version of the reasonable-person standard seems morally required.

Intentional nondisclosure. This proposal involves practical difficulties, however. For example, in clinical medicine there is the legal doctrine of therapeutic privilege. According to this doctrine, a physician may intentionally and validly fail to disclose information, based on a judgment that to divulge the information would be potentially harmful to the patient or would otherwise be infeasible. When such practices involve deception or incomplete disclosure, ethical problems arise about autonomy and consent. For similar reasons, courts have increasingly curtailed physician latitude of judgment, just as they have increasingly required the use of the reasonable-person standard over standards operative in the medical professions. This trend, of course, holds only for patients capable of informed consent and not for patients who are unconscious or otherwise incapable of communicating. It also does not apply to cases where there is a severe impracticality of communicating with patients. Thus the doctrine of therapeutic privilege, judiciously interpreted to deal with such cases, is not intrinsically objectionable.

Two main types of incomplete disclosure have raised important issues. First, there is the use of randomized clinical trials—random assignment to treatment categories where there are alternative treatments—in which some patients receive placebos or an experimental therapy, e.g., a drug, while other patients receive a standard or alternative therapy. Such procedures are blind, at least in that the patient does not know which treatment or placebo is received. Second, certain research, especially in psychology, appears to require overt deception for its successful completion without biasing its results. The major moral problem is how much information, if any, ought to be disclosed in both types of cases.

Consider first the use of randomized clinical trials. It has been argued, on the one hand, that patients and subjects should not be informed that randomization is involved, because completion of the trial with adequate information would be rendered impossible[18] and, on the other hand, that both the fact of randomization and the progress of the trial itself should be divulged to participants.[19] At a minimum it seems to us that the following should be said about such practices: the procedures involved should be carefully scrutinized—by investigators and review committees—to determine that several possibilities are explored. For example, the probability of generating resentment on the part of subjects and of destroying relations of trust, the possibility of humiliation, and the benefits of the research should be considered. In order that autonomy not be violated, information that a subject would need in order to make a decision about participation—as judged by the revised standard of the reasonable person—would have to be provided. So long as a subject comprehends the sorts of procedures envisioned, as well as what is commonly done in such research, consent can be reasonably said to be informed. However, it is not enough simply to assert that "Where scientific or humane values justify delaying or withholding information, the investigator acquires a special responsibility to assure that there are not damaging consequences for the participant," as the Code of Ethics of the American Psychological Association reads.[20] Still, general information provided to patients—such as the information that the procedure involves a randomized clinical trial and that the results will later be divulged to the subjects—may in many cases be sufficient.

This approach to incomplete disclosures in randomized clinical trials can be more sharply formulated. Such research is justified only if:

(1) There is no satisfactory alternative methodology which avoids the problem of withholding information.

(2) The subjects are informed that they are involved in a randomized clinical trial and might be receiving a placebo or a nonvalidated therapy.

(3) The research is well designed, including provisions for the evaluation of the alternative therapies.

(4) All therapies to be included have no substantial disparity in their prior probabilities of benefit.

(5) Risks to patients are fully detailed prior to their consent and are minimal (e.g., not beyond the risk involved in a standard physical examination) if there is a risk that cannot be divulged.

(6) Consent safeguards, such as a surrogate consent system, have been put in place wherever appropriate.

This list specifies only necessary conditions of justified randomized clinical trial procedure and consent. The conditions are not, however, sufficient to justify all such research, for many subtle problems may require further conditions to be satisfied before the research would be justified. Nonetheless, it seems wrong to maintain that patients and subjects *cannot* be adequately protected in such research. So long as principles of non-maleficence, beneficence, and autonomy are not violated in carrying out the research, the procedures are not inherently objectionable. Nonmaleficence and beneficence can be handled by careful scrutiny of possible harms that might result, and autonomy can be protected by insuring that subjects have an adequate idea of what they are accepting even if they do not have information about all possible details.

On the other hand, the six conditions listed above are not met in most of the biomedical and psychological research that involves intentional deception. Much of this research involves minor risk and only minor deception; but the deception is nonetheless often resented by subjects subsequent to their involvement. If the research is important, it might be argued that minor deception and minimal risks are outweighed by substantial benefits. The justification of such research would thus turn on a risk/benefit analysis. However, when substantial deception and/or substantial risk are present, justification becomes more problematic. Stanley Milgram's well-known experiments in which subjects were falsely informed that they would be supplying electroshock to other subjects provide examples of this sort.[21] Another and perhaps more fascinating case is #4 in the Appendix. In this case a social scientist using substantial deception placed homosexual subjects at risk of public disclosure and embarrassment and invaded their privacy. Also a remarkably revealing sociological study of the practices of Italian priests in hearing confessions of sexual sins—published in English as *Sex and the Confessional*[22]— involved the deception of priests and the taping of their questions and advice. While these cases are more social-scientific than biomedical, they illustrate the point that deception (and resulting risk) can and does occur in the world of research.

Can research of this sort be justified? We do not see how it is possible to do so when significant risk is involved, unless subjects can be informed that they are being placed at risk and consent to this placement. The critical question is thus whether subjects accept the risk of involvement in deceptive practices. If they do not, it seems too fundamental a violation of the principle of autonomy *both* to place them at risk and to deceive them. This conclusion is far from innocuous, since much research of this description has been carried out in the past and is still being considered by and in some cases approved by research review committees. Still, this conclusion does not imply that research involving deception cannot justifiably be undertaken. Relatively risk-free and significant research—especially in behavioral psychology and sociology—could not in some cases be undertaken without deception or incomplete disclosure. Examples would include studies of visual and other perceptual responses. Cases in which disclosure would invalidate the research should be distinguished from cases in which disclosure would be inconvenient, time consuming, or expensive. Generally, deception should be permitted only if essential to obtain important information, when there is insubstantial risk, and when no other moral principles are violated.

Comprehension of information

Just as a sufficient quantity of information is needed for a consent to be informed, so adequate comprehension of the information by subjects or patients is a necessary condition of a valid informed consent. Without sufficient comprehension a person cannot use the information in making decisions—should he or she elect to use the information. Many conditions other than mere lack of sufficient information can limit comprehension. Irrationality and immaturity can do so, for example. But even if there were no problems about competence, problems about adequate comprehension would remain, for information may be presented in a distorted way or in unsuitable circumstances so that communication of the information fails to occur.

It is sometimes argued that a patient or subject cannot comprehend enough information to give informed consent. Franz Ingelfinger argues, for example, that "the chances are remote that the subject really understands what he has consented to,"[23] and Robert Mulford similarly argues that "the subject is ordinarily not qualified to evaluate the true risks and expected benefits."[24] This position is based on an inadequate view of so-called "full" disclosure. So long as one clings to the ideal of complete disclosure of all possibly relevant knowledge, such claims about the limited capacity of subjects will be given credence. But if this ideal standard is replaced by an acceptable reasonable-person standard, there should no longer be any temptation to succumb to the Ingelfinger-Mulford form of pessimism. From the fact that we are never *fully* voluntary, fully informed, or fully autonomous persons, it does not follow that we are never *adequately* informed, free, and autonomous. A different lesson is to be learned: because comprehension is both limited and difficult, we should strive harder in biomedical and educational contexts to foster information and to avoid undue influence. Apprehending one's medical situation is not substantially different from apprehending one's financial situation when consulting with a CPA, or one's legal situation when consulting with a lawyer, or even one's marital situation when consulting with a marriage counselor. The shades of understanding are manifold, but various degrees of apprehension may nonetheless be adequate for an informed judgment.

Another problem is whether we ought to recognize waivers of informed consent. What are we to say about those idiosyncratic individuals who choose to have less information than would a "reasonable" person? Robert Veatch has argued that anyone who refuses to accept as much information as the reasonable person would accept cannot be said to have apprehended the relevant information and, therefore, cannot be said to have given an acceptable consent—at least not to involvement in research.[25] But is this view correct? Some persons do not want to know anything about what will be done. Indeed, some studies claim to show that over sixty percent of patients want to know virtually nothing about procedures or the risks of the procedures,[26] and other studies, as we have seen, indicate that only about twelve percent of patients use the information provided in reaching their decisions.[27]

There seem to be two major alternative ways of treating such persons. First, it might be maintained that when the reasonable-person standard is not being met, the contemplated procedure cannot be undertaken until sufficient information has been imparted, notwithstanding the person's autonomously expressed desire not to be informed. According to this approach, persons should be coerced against their autonomous wishes into receiving undesired information. Second, a contrasting view is that when a patient or subject has been sufficiently informed to know whether or not further information is wished, and when the right to further information has been waived, no further information should be provided. In this second view, the person's informed waiver is itself sufficient to constitute *valid* consent to therapy or research, even if it is not an *informed* consent to that procedure.

Either alternative presents risks. On the one hand, forced information is a prima facie violation of autonomy, and many circumstances can be imagined in which information waivers would be justified. For example, if a deeply committed Jehovah's Witness were to inform a doctor that he wishes to have everything possible done for him, but does not want to *know* if transfusions or similar procedures would be employed, it is hard to imagine a moral argument to the conclusion that he must be told. On the other hand, to consider the second alternative, the fact must be faced that patients commonly have an inordinate trust in physicians, and the general recognition of waivers of consent in research and therapeutic settings could make patients more vulnerable to those who would use far too abbreviated consent procedures merely because they are convenient.

There probably cannot be any general theoretical solution to this problem of waivers. Each case of consent and the possibility of a waiver will have to be considered in its own complexity. There may, however, be a procedural way to resolve the problem. There could be rules against allowing waivers, but these rules could be considered as specifying prima facie duties which can be relaxed after special consideration by deliberative bodies, such as institutional review committees and hospital ethics committees. Such rules would be developed to protect patients and subjects, but if protective bodies themselves were to find that the person's interest in a particular case was best protected by a waiver, they could allow the waiver. This procedural solution is not a mere avoidance of the problem. It would be easy to violate autonomy and to fail to live up to our responsibilities by inflexible rules which either permit or prohibit waivers. This procedural suggestion at least provides a flexible arrangement for meeting such problems.

A similar and related problem arises when patients or subjects reach their decisions on irrelevant grounds, even though they have been adequately informed. Such persons comprehend the relevant information but reach their decision based on emotional, irrational, or false views. For example, a person might falsely and irrationally believe that a doctor will not fill out his insurance forms unless he consents to a procedure the doctor has suggested; and he might persist in this belief even when informed of its falsity. Similarly, a sufficiently informed psychiatric patient capable of consent might consent to involvement in a nonpsychiatric, nontherapeutic research procedure under the false assumption that it is therapeutic. In these cases the adequate information that is both disclosed and apprehended plays no role in the decision to be involved in the research or to accept the therapy. The question then arises whether autonomous subjects should be coerced into giving up their false beliefs and irrational tendencies in order that they may decide on the basis of pertinent information alone.

In a general statement about the coercion of information, H. Tristram Engelhardt has argued that "One cannot try (nor should one) to force subjects who can be rational free agents to use that rationality and freedom to its fullest,"[28] because informed consent only entails that patients and subjects make their own free and rational assessments. Robert Veatch has similarly argued that where subjects specifically object to further information or persuasion, the information should not be imposed.[29] While these statements set forth commendable ideals, they do not imply that we should never coerce patients or subjects to further information. When a patient's or subject's autonomy is clearly limited by his own ignorance, as in the case of false belief, it may be legitimate to promote autonomy by attempting to impose the information. In this respect these cases resemble the waiver cases just discussed. In both, unsatisfactory apprehension leads to the problem, and, as with the waiver cases, the best general solution is probably a procedural one.

It might be argued that these conclusions about apprehension hold for therapeutic settings but do not fit research settings where persons would be involved in nontherapeutic research. In the therapeutic environment the physician acts to the end of a patient's best interests, but in research settings the person is used as a means to the investigator's ends. Nonetheless, we believe this distinction between the two settings largely irrelevant to the points made in this section about deficient apprehension. Factors such as the amount of risk involved and the person's identification with the purposes of research could make a decisive difference as to whether he should be involved, quite independent of whether it is a clinical or a research setting. Moreover, by participating in research, subjects might derive certain benefits which they could appreciate and which would be important to them, even though they consented on what the "reasonable person" would judge to be irrelevant grounds.

Voluntariness

Voluntariness connotes the ability to choose one's own goals, and to be able to choose among several goals if a wide choice is offered, without being unduly influenced or coerced to any of the alternatives by other persons or institutions. The mere *absence* of constraining influences may, however, not indicate that a subject is acting *freely*. On some occasions the person may have to be provided with the means to realize a chosen end, as well as given freedom of choice. For example, it makes no sense to say that a person is free to choose a nonvalidated therapy instead of a validated one, if only the validated one is actually made available. In contexts of informed consent, voluntariness is optimal when there is adequate disclosure, adequate comprehension, and a subject capable of choice who in fact chooses a specific action. However, the primary *meaning* of "voluntariness" is exercising choice about an action free of coercion or undue influence by another person.

How shall we understand the notions of coercion and undue influence? Coercion occurs when one person intentionally uses an actual threat of harm or forceful manipulation to influence another. The harm could be physical, psychological, economic, etc. By contrast, undue influence occurs whenever someone uses an excessive reward or irrationally persuasive technique to induce a person to a decision the person might otherwise not reach. If admission to a hospital of persons needing care were made contingent upon their enrollment in a research protocol that was unrelated to their illness, undue influence would have been exerted. But if the only temptation inviting enrollment in a nontherapeutic research project is time off from one's work at no extra pay for the duration of the experiment, no undue influence would have been exerted. Coercion and undue influence are points on a continuum, and it is probably not possible to locate these points precisely.

Mere influence or pressure to make a decision, however, contrasts sharply with coercion and undue influence. We almost always make decisions in a context of competing wants, needs, familial interests, legal obligations, persuasive arguments, etc. Many inducements will thus be pressures but not unduly influential ones—though no sharp boundary line can perhaps be drawn in some cases between pressure to decide and undue influence. For example, a person may be pressured by an office solicitor to make a blood donation. The solicitation would normally be acceptable, but could become unacceptable if salary or year-ending bonus considerations were brought into the picture as inducements. Consent to therapy and research may therefore be voluntary and valid even when some pressures play a significant role in the decision.

Many examples indicate how these distinctions can be brought to bear on practical contexts of informed consent. In Case #26 hepatitis research was being done on mentally retarded children in New York. One allegation surrounding this case is that the parents were "coerced" into "volunteering" their children. Allegedly they were coerced—or, as some would prefer to say, unduly influenced—because there was a waiting list for admission to the school and parents were told that their children could be immediately admitted if they were "volunteered" for the hepatitis study. If this allegation of manipulative tactics were true, which is still in doubt, it would be a clear case of an unwarranted action. On the other hand, there is nothing about admission to institutions or about institutions themselves which makes unfair influence inevitable. Even in generally coercive environments, such as prisons, it is sometimes possible that informed consent to medical and research procedures can occur. It may be especially important to insure that the right of autonomous determination is defended in such institutions, since there will be a natural presumption that voluntary action is impossible, e.g., in the case of research with prisoners. Yet in environments where many options are foreclosed, not all options need be so. There is no reason why prisoners could not validly consent to medical research—say, in the form of drug testing—if coercive tactics were not specifically involved, and if undue inducements, such as large amounts of money, were not allowed. Thus, a distinction ought to be drawn between generally coercive environments and individual acts of coercion. Informed consent may be valid in the former, but cannot be in the latter.

Refusal of treatment

Occasionally patients who have the capacity to give informed consent to therapies refuse to do so. While these refusals can, of course, occur in non-life-threatening circumstances, the major controversies have emerged from life-threatening contexts. In this section we will concentrate on life-threatening refusals, reserving non-life-threatening decisions for Chapter 5. The major cases to be discussed here involve refusal of some medical therapy presumably necessary to sustain life. Examples include refusal to allow a blood transfusion, or an amputation, or further treatment using kidney dialysis. While patients have refused treatments such as blood transfusions because of their religious convictions, the ethical issues are broader than freedom of religious conscience, for many patients refuse treatments for nonreligious reasons. There are also problems of second-party refusal in the case of children and certain classes of incompetent patients, which we will reserve for the chapter on nonmaleficence. In this section we will concentrate on refusals by competent adult patients, where the critical question is, "What are the implications and limits of the principle of autonomy?"

The "Patient's Bill of Rights" (See Appendix II) holds that "the patient has the right to refuse treatment to the extent permitted by law and to be informed of the medical consequences of his action." Unfortunately, this right of refusal cannot be specified without a discussion of the law, and even then we have to ask whether the law is morally sound, e.g., whether it adequately expresses the principle of autonomy.

While the law is at present tentative and uncertain in this area, courts appear to be moving in the direction of greater latitude of patient choice, unless there is questionable competence. A number of recent legal cases suggest that the patient's informed refusal should be decisive. In *Erickson v. Dilgard*[30] a patient with intestinal bleeding deliberately refused, on religious grounds, a transfusion necessary for continued life. The court upheld the patient's decision on grounds of the protection of individual choice. Similarly, in *In re Estate of Brooks,*[31] it was held that free religious exercise, when there is competent refusal of therapy, is constitutionally sufficient to prevent physicians from compelling the therapy, even when it is known by both patient and physician that death will ensue. In the first case, bodily *self-determination* was regarded as an inviolable right, while in the second, *free exercise of religion* was cited as the basic right. But patient refusal was nonetheless decisive in both.[32]

By examining some cases, we can both illustrate some of the complexities and indicate some conditions under which patient choice may justifiably be restricted. In Case #11, a Jehovah's Witness refused to authorize blood transfusions for herself and her newborn daughter, and her husband also refused to authorize blood transfusions for either his wife or daughter. The judge refused to order transfusions for the woman, but did not accept the parents' proxy (second-party) refusal of therapy for the newborn daughter. In effect, he accepted a first-party refusal, but drew the line at that point and would not accept a second-party refusal for the incompetent child. Legal considerations of jurisdiction over the fate of the infant played a role in this decision, but moral grounds can also be cited for the judge's opinion. As we have seen, the doctrine of informed consent is applied differently to competent and incompetent parties because of considerations of autonomy and nonmaleficence: informed consent functions to protect the right of autonomous choice for competents but functions to protect incompetents from harm. This moral position probably underlies the judge's legal decision in this case.

In some cases a patient's refusal of lifesaving therapy may impose unjustified burdens on or bring excessive harm to others. The *Georgetown College Case* (see Appendix Case #12) is an oft-cited example of a case where the seriousness of the consequences to others might override a patient's autonomous wishes. The court used the following reason, among others, to justify forcing a transfusion on an unwilling patient: "The patient, 25 years old, was the mother of a seven-month-old child. . . . The patient had a responsibility to the community to care for her infant. Thus, the people had an interest in preserving the life of this mother."[33] It has also been argued that the child, even more than the community, is seriously damaged by the mother's decision.[34] While we are uncertain of the actual status of obligations in this dilemmatic case, it provides the *sort* of case where pressing needs might be sufficient to override patient choice. In such circumstances, individual autonomy would seem appropriately overridden only for a moral reason which pertains to the welfare of others and not for paternalistic reasons.[35]

Despite the general endorsement of the patient's right to autonomous choice that we have suggested in this section, the limitations of this view should be appreciated. First, this approach does not consider hard cases of second-party refusals, where someone other than the patient must accept the burden of the decision—e.g., cases where a family member consents to the withholding or cessation of treatment for someone in a vegetative state. (See Chapter 4.) Second, almost all court cases and many common situations in hospitals involve patients of questionable capacity to consent. The conclusions we have reached do not apply to such patients. Only when there is an informed refusal, as judged by our modified reasonable-person standard, should a patient's decision be recognized. In cases of doubtful competence, it is better to err on the side of preserving life. Finally, as just noted, in some cases where persons might be acting irresponsibly and thereby harming another person (usually a dependent), their decisions may be overridden, even when informed and voluntary. Such cases will be rare; but it cannot be determined a priori that sufficient moral grounds for overriding autonomous choices could never be present.

Autonomous suicide

Refusal of therapy in life-threatening circumstances is, of course, not the only way to terminate one's life. It is not even the most common way in some hospital populations, for many patients end their lives by carefully planned suicides. Not all suicides among such populations can correctly be classified as autonomous, but some can be, and in this section we evaluate critically certain views about the morality of autonomous suicide.

There is a rich literature by major figures in the history of philosophy and theology on the morality of suicide. In addition, certain contemporary currents have revived interest in this topic. First, as with refusal of treatment cases, biomedical technology has made it possible for seriously ill and injured persons to prolong their lives beyond the point at which, in former times, they would have died. The suicide rate is remarkably high in some of these populations, and many people have come to think that suicide can be justified in some of these cases. According to the World Health Organization, a reasonable estimate is that in reporting nations approximately 1,000 people commit suicide each day. While health conditions are obviously not always the motivating factor, they figure prominently in many suicides. For example, one study discovered that the incidence of suicide among patients on dialysis is "more than 100 times the normal population." It is not easy, however, to obtain accurate statistics about suicide, in part because many families tend to conceal the fact that a family member's death is a suicide. Even when it occurred under the exigencies of a prolonged illness, and perhaps was rational, families tend to conceal the fact of suicide.

Second, while criminal laws prohibiting suicide have been repealed recently in most jurisdictions in the United States, repeal is currently being debated in others. This debate turns more on moral than on legal considerations. Libertarian arguments have been successfully used to oppose *criminal* sanctions against suicide in most states, but a lively debate continues about the rightness and wrongness of taking one's own life. However, before we can assess this moral controversy, it is necessary to clarify the notion of "suicide" itself.

The definition of suicide

Ordinarily we would think that a death is a suicide if it is an intentionally caused self-destruction and is not forced by the action of another person. However, we have just studied refusal of treatment cases that make it difficult to accept such a simple definition.

When persons suffer from a terminal illness or mortal injury and allow their own death to occur, we find ourselves reluctant to call the act a "suicide." But if a patient with a terminal illness takes his life by an active means, such as a revolver, we generally do refer to the act as one of suicide. The more we have patent cases of agents' actions that involve an intentionally and actively caused death, the more we are likely to classify the act as a suicide; but the more the context is one of merely allowing one's own death where a fatal condition is present, the less inclined we are to call the act a suicide. For example, if a seriously but not mortally wounded burn patient takes a weapon in hand and intentionally brings about his death, it is a suicide. But if a seriously burned patient is suffering terribly from a terminal wound and refuses yet another tubbing or blood transfusion, we are not likely to regard the death as a suicide. The passive nature of the death in the second case makes us reluctant to label it a suicide, whereas the active character of the death in the first case renders the death a suicide.

However, our concept of suicide is not quite as clear as these examples might suggest, for this analysis of suicide in terms of taking active steps seems mistaken in some cases. For example, a patient with a terminal condition might easily avoid dying for a long time but might choose to end his life immediately by not taking cheap and painless medication. We are not sure what to say in such cases, but it can be explained why our concept of suicide leaves us in this state of uncertainty.

Terms in their ordinary meaning often contain evaluative accretions from social attitudes that render them difficult to analyze. The meaning we have located for "suicide" appears to be a premiere instance of this problem. Because self-caused deaths are often revolting and inexplicable, an emotive meaning of disapproval has been incorporated into our use of "suicide." Because of this already attached disapproval, we find it hard to view acts of which we approve, or at least do not disapprove, as suicides. For this reason we have been led to the semantic exclusion of such actions from the realm of suicide. For example, when coercion, refusal of treatment, or sacrifice are present we are inclined not to attach the stigma of the label "suicide," and so generally exclude these actions. Terminal illness and altruistic reasons for suicide play a similar role. Because self-caused deaths under the latter conditions commonly are understandable, acceptable, and perhaps even laudable, semantic exclusion of them from the realm of the suicidal is tempting and is a *fait accompli* in the English language. We thus by the very logic of the term prejudice any pending moral analysis of the action of a suicide as being right or wrong, let alone praiseworthy or blameworthy.

Because this prejudicial feature infects our ordinary understanding of "suicide," it needs to be replaced by a more objective, even though stipulative, meaning for purposes of moral thinking. It will not be easy to employ a standard term in a nonstandard way in the discussions that follow, but our investigations of the morality and rationality of suicide will be enhanced by acceptance of an uncorrupted term. We propose, then, that suicide occurs if and only if one intentionally terminates one's own life—no matter what the conditions or precise nature of the intention or the causal route to death.

The morality of suicide

How are we to determine whether a particular act of suicide is or is not immoral? As with other moral issues, this question should be answered by reference to those moral principles that permit us to take a consistent position on the issues. We want to suggest, without further argument, that three moral principles are directly relevant to discussions of suicide.

(1) The first of these principles is *the principle of autonomy* itself. As we have seen, to show a lack of respect for an autonomous agent is either to show disrespect for that person's deliberate choices or to deny that person the freedom to act on those choices. It would, therefore, be a showing of disrespect to deny autonomous persons the right to commit suicide when, in their considered judgment, they ought to do so.

(2) A second principle often appealed to in discussions of suicide may be called *the principle of human worth* (or the sanctity of human life). According to this view human life has an intrinsic value irrevocably destroyed by suicide, which is therefore an act of killing that is morally wrong. As this principle is usually construed, it is permissible to *allow*

someone to die instead of attempting heroic efforts to save them, but it is not acceptable to *kill,* because one then becomes morally responsible for an active destruction of life. From this view, the act of killing is wrong not because it produces social disutility and not because it violates autonomy. It is wrong merely because it is an intentional, active termination of human life. The principle is thus taken as independent of the principles previously discussed in this chapter, though it may be derivative from the principle of nonmaleficence. (See the discussion of the killing/letting die distinction in Chapter 4.)

One could have a number of different reasons for holding this second principle. It might be believed that life is a gift from God, and therefore is only to be terminated at God's own appointed moment. Or one might think that human life has a dignity that sets it apart from all nonhuman creatures. However, these views coalesce into a single deontological belief: human life has intrinsic value, and it is always a wrong-making characteristic of any action that it is an intentional termination of a human life. Still, there are stronger and weaker ways of interpreting this principle. On the strongest possible view, it is always wrong intentionally to terminate any human life, whatever the circumstances—whether in capital punishment cases, or as an act of self-defense, or by abortion, or by suicide, or by any means whatever. A markedly weak version of the principle would be that the intrinsic value of life itself is always a consideration when one is contemplating the intentional termination of a life—but it is only a consideration and not necessarily the most important or overriding consideration.

Few people would now defend either the strongest or the weakest version of this principle. A middle position—basically the construal that those who now defend this principle would support—is that killing is prima facie wrong and so permissible only if it is necessary to save the life of at least one other innocent person or if it is necessary to preserve a morally worthy society.

(3) The final moral principle relevant to discussing the morality of suicide is *the principle of utility.* As we have seen, utilitarians look to the consequences of actions to see what the impact on the interests and welfare of all concerned would be. The interests of the person contemplating suicide, the interests of dependents, the interests of relatives, etc., must all be considered in the calculation of positive values and disvalues. The fact that people love the person contemplating suicide and

that they value the person's contribution to the community are all to be considered in making a moral assessment of the contemplated action. In an overwhelming number of cases a utilitarian calculation would show that more disvalue in the form of grief, guilt, and deprivation would be produced than value gained were someone to commit suicide. Hence the principle of utility would generally dictate that an act of suicide is not justified. However, there are cases where considerations about consequences would not automatically fall on the side of disvalue. For example, imagine someone suffering from apparently untreatable tic douloureux—an excruciatingly painful condition of the trigeminal nerve—and brain cancer as well. Suppose further that this person has neither dependents nor debts, that the suffering of this person's family has been protracted, and that everyone concerned believes death would be a merciful release. An intentional overdose taken by the person could satisfy the utilitarian demand that the greatest possible amount of value or at least the smallest possible amount of disvalue be brought about by the person's action.

Under the assumption that each of the above three moral principles is acceptable, each should be regarded as prima facie binding. That is, the principles assert prima facie duties, in some cases binding a person contemplating suicide and in other cases affecting those who might intervene to prevent suicides. As we discussed in Chapter 2, prima facie duties are more than rules of thumb, because they are always binding unless in conflict with stronger duties. They thus constitute binding moral reasons, even though they do not always prevail over competing prima facie duties. In the present context, this approach to morality may be applied as follows: to the extent the principle of autonomy or one of the other principles just mentioned is relevant, and does not come into conflict with other principles, it is our duty to observe the principle. Thus, if a suicide were genuinely autonomous and there were no powerful utilitarian reasons or reasons of human worth and dignity standing in the way, then we ought to allow the person to commit suicide, because we would otherwise be violating the person's autonomy. A similar analysis could be given for instances falling under each of the principles. This indicates that whether suicide is right or wrong is never a simple or absolute matter. The morality of suicide cannot be determined in abstraction from the facts of a person's own situation.

A ready example of the use of prima facie reasoning about suicide is

found in a famous essay on the subject by the eighteenth-century philosopher David Hume. In this essay he combined the principle of autonomy
with the principle of utility to provide a powerful case in justification of
certain types of suicide—though by no means did Hume draw the radical
conclusion that all suicides can be justified by these two principles. His
strategy was to show that the more one is removed from obligations to the
community and the more one's life is plagued with suffering, the more
justifiable is one's suicide. In the end he advances the largely utilitarian
thesis that if the value of relieving one's misery by taking one's own life is
greater than the value to the community of one's continued existence,
then suicide is justified. This claim might be applied in biomedical contexts by reference once again to the desperate circumstances that often
surround refusal of treatment cases. If one's life has become utterly
miserable and pain management is impossible, while at the same time
one's dignity and ability to relate to others are slipping away, then suicide
would seem to be justified. This is not to say, of course, that it would be
justified to encourage suicide or to assist a person in committing suicide.
These acts present further moral problems. But this conclusion does entail
that suicide under these circumstances is not morally improper and
should not be an object of moral condemnation.

Problems of suicide intervention

If the principle of autonomy is strongly relied upon for the justification of
suicide, then it would seem that there is a *right* to commit suicide, so long
as a person acts autonomously and does not seriously affect the interests
of others. Yet we certainly do not always act as if the suicide has such a
right, for we often intervene to prevent suicide. In days past, for example,
it was not uncommon for several persons to place themselves at risk of
death in order to prevent a person from lying down on subway tracks in
the path of an oncoming train. It is easy to understand why such interventions occur, as acts of humanity. And we may believe that we are
justified in intervening in the lives of such individuals. But if they have a
right to commit suicide, are we really justified? In the case of almost any
other similarly intrusive action, we would agree with the person if he
argued that his autonomy had been violated by those who intervened. For
example, physicians can be successfully sued for malpractice if they
coercively intervene in certain ways in the life of a patient. Yet in the case

of suicide, we feel strongly inclined to say that we have obligations to suicidal persons, even when they are acting autonomously. But can we morally justify the conviction that intervention in the name of saving a life is better than nonintervention in the name of autonomy?

One account of our obligations, by a strong advocate of the principle of autonomy, is the following by Glanville Williams:

If one suddenly comes upon another person attempting suicide, the natural and humane thing to do is to try to stop him, for the purpose of ascertaining the cause of his distress and attempting to remedy it, or else of attempting moral dissuasion if it seems that the act of suicide shows lack of consideration for others, or else again from the purpose of trying to persuade him to accept psychiatric help if this seems to be called for. Whatever the strict law may be (and authority is totally lacking), no one who intervened for such reasons would thereby be in danger of suffering a punitive judgment. But nothing longer than a temporary restraint could be defended. I would gravely doubt whether a suicide attempt should be a factor leading to a diagnosis of psychosis or to compulsory admission to a hospital. Psychiatrists are too ready to assume that an attempt to commit suicide is the act of a mentally sick person.[36]

Yet many do not agree with Williams's estimate. There are two main reasons for disagreement. First, failure to intervene indicates a lack of concern about others and a diminished sense of moral responsibility in a community. Attempts to save a person from suicide in subways are now comparatively rare, and this seems to indicate how times have changed in large cities—and how disastrous the change has been. Second, many believe that most suicides are mentally ill or at least seriously disturbed, and therefore are not really capable of autonomous action. Notoriously, suicidal persons are often under the strain of temporary crises, under the influence of drugs or alcohol, and beset with considerable ambivalence, or simply wish to reduce or interrupt anxiety, while not wishing to die.

Many psychiatric and legal authorities can be cited in support of the belief that suicides are almost always the result of maladaptive attitudes needing therapeutic attention. Their underlying conviction is that the suicidal person suffers from some form of disease or irrational drive to kill himself, and that it is the business of medicine or behavioral therapy to cure the illness and prevent the patient from self-destruction. Freudians even argue that suicide is created by a breakdown of ego defenses and a release of destructive forces. These forces are said to reflect the ambivalent relationship to love objects with whom a person identifies. While no single theory presently suffices for the understanding of the motivation to suicide, many such accounts characterize suicide as substantially nonvoluntary and therefore as nonautonomous. Also, other suicidal persons who are not ill nonetheless may not be in a position to act autonomously, either because they are immature, ignorant, coerced, or in a vulnerable position in which they might be exploited by others.

In all cases these nonautonomous persons are due all the same protections of moral rules afforded to autonomous persons. One way of respecting them as persons is by direct intervention in their lives intended to protect them against harms resulting from their illness, immaturity, psychological incapacitation, ignorance, or possible exploitation—e.g., by coercively preventing their suicide. These might be medical interventions, coercive institutionalizations, or some other method of prevention. Those who are defenders of autonomy have never denied that this interference is valid, because they regard such suicidal actions as nonautonomous. They regard the principle of autonomy and the derivative right to commit suicide as extending only to those capable of autonomous choice. On the other hand, some suicides are genuinely autonomous suicides; yet we still may feel compelled to intervene in order to prevent the potential suicide from taking his life. Because virtually everyone is agreed that nonautonomous suicidal actions should be prevented by intervention, the only controversial question is whether these *autonomous* suicides should be similarly prevented. This issue properly falls under the problem of paternalism, a problem to be treated in Chapter 5. We shall, therefore, defer further discussion of the morality of suicide intervention until this future discussion of paternalism.

Conclusion

Our analysis of suicide leads to the conclusion that there are good reasons for suicide in some circumstances, but that suicidal action may be cowardly and even morally wrong in other circumstances. In some cases one may have moral obligations not to commit suicide, while in other cases one may have the right or even a moral obligation to commit suicide—though the last situation would be extremely rare. This conclusion can be analyzed in terms of the account of prima facie duties discussed in Chapter 2. For example, merely because one has *some* obligations not to commit suicide, it does not follow that when all interests are taken account of, the actual obligation will be to abstain from suicide. Moreover, weak duties are sometimes overridden not only by stronger moral duties but also by strong prudential interests. Even though a daughter might beg her terminally ill father to stay alive for his last remaining month, his agony may nonetheless be sufficient to override the daughter's interest in his remaining alive. One valid reason for taking one's life in one's last days is to prevent a loss of one's own dignity, while at the same time sparing a family grief and financial loss. In doing so one may be maximizing not only one's own interests but the interests of all concerned.

At the same time, in determining whether to commit suicide, it is easy to exaggerate the direness of one's situation. One's desires, sufferings, and hopes in the present moment tend to overwhelm consideration of what one's desires, sufferings, and joys may be at future times. In the case of terminal illness, which provides one of the strongest justifications of suicide, an optimistic frame of mind is not likely to be cultivated. Indeed, the matter is likely to become worse daily. And in the case of depression— where there is not a terminal illness—from which the majority of suicides are committed, it is easy to miscalculate by substituting present feelings for rational calculations of future possibilities. The reason for this speculation about depression is the following: it is one thing to reach the conclusion, as we have, that autonomous suicide may be justified, but quite another to frame a realistic appraisal of the circumstances and of the actual state of mind of many persons who commit "autonomous" suicide. Ideally, a person contemplating suicide would take account of all relevant variables and future possibilities, but such contemplation often does not occur. Thus, questions about our obligations to prevent suicides will always be difficult because of our uncertainty as to whether they are or are not truly autonomous.

In any final assessment of the wrongness of an act of suicide, it is important to analyze two different judgments that might be reached. First, we might say that a suicide is seriously mistaken, and even morally wrong, but not blameworthy. Second, we might say that the suicide is both morally wrong and blameworthy. These judgments derive from the moral view that some wrong suicides may be excused.[37] We can excuse some suicides if they act on false information, if they are of temporarily unsound mind, or when depression or some other psychological state overwhelms a person of an ordinarily even disposition. Perhaps the most compelling cases are those where a person acts altruistically but on false information in committing suicide. For example, a person might falsely believe that he has a disease that will produce prolonged agony and leave his family in financial ruin. We can sometimes say not only that such a person acted wrongly though excusably, but even that he acted *commendably* (though wrongly). Many who would absolutely forbid suicide fail to distinguish the objective wrongness of an action from the moral excusability and even praiseworthiness of that same action. One virtue of our analysis of suicide is that it permits us to make these important distinctions and to adjust our moral judgments about suicide accordingly.

Notes

1. Cf. Robert Paul Wolff, *In Defense of Anarchism* (New York: Harper and Row, 1970). See also Wolff's even stronger claims in his article, "On Violence," *The Journal of Philosophy* 66 (October 2, 1969).
2. Wolff, *In Defense of Anarchism,* pp. 4–6, 13f. In "On Violence" (p. 608), Wolff maintains that "obedience *is* heteronymy [sic]. The autonomous man is *of necessity* an anarchist" (our italics). We can only understand this necessity as logical necessity.
3. "Informed Consent in Catastrophic Disease and Treatment," *University of Pennsylvania Law Review* 123 (December, 1974): 364–76.
4. Cf. Charles Fried, *Medical Experimentation* (New York: American Elsevier, 1974), pp. 18ff.
5. Robert M. Veatch, "Three Theories of Informed Consent: Philosophical Foundations and Policy Implications." National Commission for the Protection of Human Subjects of Biomedical and Behavioral Research, *Appendix: Volume I. Belmont Report: Ethical Principles and Guidelines for the Protection of Human Subjects of Research* (Washington: DHEW Publication No. (OS) 78-0013, 1978).
6. *Schloendorff v. New York Hospital.* 211 N.Y. 125, 127, 129; 105 N.E. 92, 93 (1914).
7. *Natanson v. Kline.* 186 Kan. 393, 350 P.2d 1093 (1960), rehearing denied, 187 Kan. 186, 354 P.2d 670 (1960).
8. We are indebted to Professor Donald Bersoff of the University of Maryland Law School for suggesting this tripartite approach.
9. Jeffrie Murphy, "Incompetence and Paternalism," *Archiv für Rechts-und-Sozialphilosophie* 50 (1974): 465–86.
10. "Informed Consent and the Dying Patient," *The Yale Law Journal* 83 (1974), p. 1637. Much the same point is made in *Canterbury v. Spence,* 464 Federal Reporter, 2nd Series, 772, where the standards operative in the biomedical professions are analyzed as of two types: (1) good medical practice standards, and (2) what a reasonable practitioner would disclose under the circumstances. See the excerpt from the case reprinted in Tom L. Beauchamp and

LeRoy Walters, eds., *Contemporary Issues in Bioethics* (Encino, Calif.: Dickenson Publishing Co., 1978), p. 143. (Hereafter this anthology is abbreviated B-W.)

11. Cf. *Wilkinson v. Vesey,* 110 R.I. 606, 626; 295 A.2d 676, 688 (1972).

12. Cf. *Cobbs v. Grant,* 8 Cal. 3d 229, 502 P.2d 1.

13. Cf. *Canterbury v. Spence,* 464 Federal Reporter, 2nd Series, 772, as reprinted in B-W, p. 144 (and also fn. 8). *Cobbs v. Grant,* however, seems more subjective in that it appeals to "the patient's need" to know as a critical standard.

14. Cf. *Berkey v. Anderson,* 1 Cal. APP. 3d 790, 805; 82 Cal. Reporter 67, 78 (1969).

15. *Canterbury v. Spence,* in B-W, p. 144.

16. Ruth R. Faden, "Disclosure and Informed Consent: Does It Matter How We Tell It?" *Health Education Monographs* 5 (1977): 198–215; and Ruth R. Faden and Tom L. Beauchamp, "Informed Consent and Decision Making: The Impact of Disclosed Information," *Social Indicators Research* (1979).

17. C. H. Fellner and J. R. Marshall, "Kidney Donors—The Myth of Informed Consent," *American Journal of Psychiatry* 126 (1970): 1245.

18. See some examples of randomized clinical trials in Chapter 7 below and also Thomas C. Chalmers, "The Ethics of Randomization as a Decision-Making Technique and the Problem of Informed Consent," as reprinted in B-W, pp. 426–30.

19. See Fried, *Medical Experimentation,* pp. 25–36.

20. *Ethical Principles in the Conduct of Research with Human Participants* (Washington, D.C.: American Psychological Association, 1973), p. 2. Principle 8.

21. Stanley Milgram, "Behavioral Study of Obedience," *Journal of Abnormal Psychology* 67 (1963): 371–78; "Some Conditions of Obedience and Disobedience to Authority," *Human Relations* 18 (1965): 57–76; *Obedience to Authority* (New York: Harper & Row, 1974).

22. Norberto Valenti and Clara di Meglio, *Sex and the Confessional* (New York: Stein and Day, 1974).

23. Franz J. Ingelfinger, "Informed (but Uneducated) Consent," as reprinted in B-W, pp. 434–35.

24. Robert D. Mulford, "Experimentation on Human Beings," *Stanford Law Review* 20 (November 1967): 106.

25. Veatch, "Three Theories of Informed Consent."

26. Cf. Ralph J. Alfidi, "Controversy, Alternatives, and Decisions in Complying with the Legal Doctrine of Informed Consent," *Radiology* 114 (January 1975), as reprinted in B-W, p. 148.

27. Cf. the articles in footnote 16 above.

28. "Basic Ethical Principles in the Conduct of Biomedical and Behavioral Research Involving Human Subjects." National Commission for the Protection of Human Subjects of Biomedical and Behavioral Research, *Appendix: Vol. I. Belmont Report,* p. 8–22. (see footnote 5 above).

29. Veatch, "Three Theories of Informed Consent."
30. 244 Misc. 2d 27, 252 N.Y.S. 2d 705 (Sup. Ct. 1962).
31. 205 N.E. 2d 435 (1965), 32 Ill 2d 361.
32. These cases, as well as other similar ones, are intelligently discussed in a comprehensive article on the subject by Robert M. Byrn, "Compulsory Life-saving Treatment for the Competent Adult," *Fordham Law Review* 44 (1975): 1–36.
33. *Application of the President and Directors of Georgetown College, Inc.,* 331 F. 2d 1000, p. 1008. Cf. also Byrn, op. cit., p. 33. These same issues are posed in *In re Osborne.* On some interpretations of the decision in *George-town College,* the judge's verdict was reached as much on grounds of questionable competence as on the utilitarian grounds cited above.
34. Norman Cantor, "A Patient's Decision to Decline Life-Saving Medical Treatment: Bodily Integrity Versus the Preservation of Life," *Rutgers Law Review* 26 (1973): 228, 251–54.
35. A case which in our judgment is paternalistic and unjustifiable for this reason is *John F. Kennedy Hospital v. Heston* 58 N.J. 576, 279 A 2d 670 (1971). A reversal of this approach is found in the appellate court decision in *In re Estate of Brooks 32* Ill. 2d 361, 205 N.E. 2d 435 (1965), though the latter preceded the former by six years. In the former case, see especially pp. 584f, and in the latter, especially pp. 440f.
36. "Euthanasia," *Medico-Legal Journal* 41 (1973): 27.
37. In this analysis we have drawn heavily from Brandt's useful discussion of the subject in "The Morality and Rationality of Suicide," in S. Perlin, ed., *A Handbook for the Study of Suicide* (New York: Oxford University Press, 1975), p. 124.

4

The Principle of Nonmaleficence

The Hippocratic Oath expresses the duty of nonmaleficence alongside the duty of beneficence: "I will use treatment to help the sick according to my ability and judgment, but I will never use it to injure or wrong them." Generally, the concept of nonmaleficence is associated with the maxim *primum non nocere*—"above all, do no harm"—which has wide currency in discussions of the responsibilities of health care professionals, particularly physicians. The origins of this maxim, however, are obscure. Scholars have been unable to locate it in the Hippocratic corpus, and the venerable statement "at least, do no harm" may not be the most accurate translation of a passage appearing in the Hippocratic corpus.[1]

A duty of nonmaleficence is recognized in most rule-deontological and rule-utilitarian theories. One of its classic formulations appears in W. D. Ross's *The Right and the Good,* where it is distinguished from the duty of beneficence. However, not all philosophers identify nonmaleficence and beneficence as distinct or separate duties. For example, William Frankena holds that the principle of beneficence includes four elements:

(1) One ought not to inflict evil or harm (what is bad).
(2) One ought to prevent evil or harm.
(3) One ought to remove evil.
(4) One ought to do or promote good.[2]

He acknowledges that the fourth element may not be a duty at all, and that these elements appear in a serial arrangement so that the first takes precedence over the second, the second over the third, and so forth. When these elements come into conflict, he appeals to the principle of utility as a heuristic maxim: maximize good or minimize evil.

It is difficult to separate nonmaleficence and beneficence in this volume because many issues of biomedical ethics involve both, e.g., risk-benefit analysis, which we will discuss in the next chapter. But there are reasons for distinguishing them and considering them as separate though related principles. First, to confuse them is to obscure distinctions that we make in ordinary moral discourse. Second, ordinary moral discourse expresses the defensible conviction that we have certain duties not to injure others that are not only distinct from but also more stringent than our duties to benefit others. For example, our duty not to push someone who cannot swim into deep water seems stronger than our duty to rescue someone who has accidentally strayed into deep water. It is morally incumbent on us to take moderate risks with our own safety in many cases in order to avoid endangering others, but it is less obvious that moderate risks are morally required to benefit others. Even if a philosopher tries to encompass the ideas of benefiting others and not injuring them under the principle of beneficence, he or she will still be forced to distinguish, as Frankena does, between stronger and weaker requirements of this principle that correspond roughly to what we call nonmaleficence and beneficence. Therefore, it seems to be more satisfactory to consider them as distinct principles that may, on occasion, come into conflict, as the notion of risk-benefit analysis suggests.

The concept of nonmaleficence

Exactly what does "nonmaleficence" involve? First, it must be distinguished from nonmalevolence, which describes a moral virtue or motive rather than a moral action. Second, nonmaleficence is frequently explicated by the terms "harm" and "injury." Both terms are somewhat ambiguous. "Injury" may refer to harm, disability, or death, on the one hand, or to injustices and wrongs, on the other. Even Ross views "not injuring others" as a synonym of "nonmaleficence" and includes under the duty of nonmaleficence a number of prohibitions from the Decalogue, including the rules against killing, stealing, committing adultery, and bearing false witness.[3]

Some definitions of "harm" are so broad as to include injuries to reputation, to property, and to liberty. For example, if the object of harm is always an *interest,* it is possible to have various interests that could be violated or damaged, such as health, property, domestic relations, and privacy.[4] Then it would be possible to distinguish trivial and serious harms by the order and magnitude of the interests involved. Some philosophers use a narrow definition of harm, distinguishing physical—and mental—harms from injuries to other interests such as property and liberty. Whether the broad or narrow definition of harm succeeds is not critical for our discussion, for we will concentrate on physical harms, including pain and suffering, disability, and death, without denying the importance of mental harms and other injuries. In particular, we will emphasize intending, causing, permitting, and imposing the risk of death, although we will also refer to other harms along the way.

The duty of nonmaleficence encompasses both intentional harm and the risk of harm. An example of intentional harm is physical assault, while an example of the risk of harm is driving an automobile too fast. The line between risk of harm and intentional harm is not always clear, however. For instance, the line between negligence, defined as "conduct which falls below a standard established by the law for the protection of others against unreasonable harm," and intent to harm becomes harder to draw as the probability of harm to another becomes greater.[5] Substantial certainty of harm is often viewed as indistinguishable from an intent to harm. Even though the distinction becomes blurred in some cases, it is both possible and important to distinguish the intentional infliction of harm from the imposition of risks of harm.

Under the prima facie duty of nonmaleficence, intentional harm is prohibited except under very special conditions, such as self-defense, while risking harm is allowed under many conditions as long as the goals of the conduct are sufficiently important. In cases of risk imposition, law and morality recognize a standard of "due care." This standard, which invokes the idea of a "reasonable person," is met when the goals sought are weighty and important enough to justify the risks—both the magnitude of harm and the probability of harm—imposed on others. Grave risks require commensurately important goals for their justification, and emergencies—e.g., a major fire—may justify risks that calculations of good and evil in nonemergency situations will not justify. We will return to these themes when we discuss risk-benefit analysis in Chapter 5.

The duty of nonmaleficence does not merely prohibit intentional harm—except in special circumstances—and require the justification of risks by probable benefits. It also requires that agents be thoughtful and act carefully. Not all harms or risks of harm are intentionally produced. It is possible to violate the duty of nonmaleficence without acting maliciously and even without being aware of or intending the risk of harm. And the violation may involve omission or commission. As Eric D'Arcy emphasizes, this moral requirement to be thoughtful and careful is not separate from other moral rules and principles, such as the duty of nonmaleficence. There is no moral rule against negligence as such. Rather, negligence, which includes the failure to guard against risks of harm to others, "applies to certain types of failure to meet moral obligations" of many different kinds.[6]

For health care professionals, the legal and moral standards of due care include knowledge, skills, and diligence. In making his services available, the physician creates the expectation that he will observe these standards. If his conduct falls below these standards, he acts negligently. Even when the therapeutic relationship proves to be harmful or unhelpful, the patient cannot successfully charge malpractice unless certain standards of care were not met. In *Adkins v. Ropp,* the Supreme Court of Indiana dealt with the claim of a patient that the physician had been negligent in removing foreign matter from the patient's eye and that, as a result, the eye became infected and blinded. The court held as follows:

When a physician and surgeon assumes to treat and care for a patient, in the absence of a special agreement, he is held in law to have impliedly contracted that he possesses the reasonable and ordinary qualifications of his profession and that he will exercise at least reasonable skill, care and diligence in his treatment of him. This implied contract on the part of the physician does not include a promise to effect a cure and negligence cannot be imputed because a cure is not effected, but he does impliedly promise that he will use due diligence and ordinary skill in his treatment of the patient so that a cure may follow such care and skill, and this degree of care and skill is required of him, not only in performing an operation or administering first treatments, but he is held to the like degree of care and skill in the necessary subsequent treatments unless he is excused from further service by the patient himself, or the physician or surgeon upon due notice refuses to further treat the case. In determining whether the physician or surgeon has exercised the degree of skill and care which the law requires, regard must be had to the advanced state of the profession at the time of treatment and in the locality in which the physician or surgeon practices.[7]

With regard to "due care," legal standards and moral standards should be identical.

What constitutes due care, will, of course, vary from time to time and place to place. The practices and policies of the medical profession also in part define the applicable standards. The AMA Code indicates that "Physicians should strive continually to improve medical knowledge and skill . . ." (Section 2). Furthermore, the physician in some circumstances should consult other physicians and specialists: "A physician should seek consultation upon request; in doubtful or difficult cases; or whenever it appears that the quality of medical service may be enhanced thereby" (Section 8). But whatever the practitioner accomplishes, the fallibility of clinical judgment must be acknowledged. Due care cannot eliminate fallibility; it can only diminish the probability of error in diagnosis and treatment.

Albert Jonsen has constructed a typology of uses of the axiom "do no harm" in biomedical ethics.[8] This axiom is used to refer to (1) medicine as a moral enterprise requiring that practitioners develop motives and intentions to serve the well-being of their patients, (2) due care, (3) risk-benefit assessments, and (4) detriment-benefit assessments. Statement (1) is very general and is implicit in this volume, especially in our discussion of the professional-patient relationship and virtues and character (Chapters 7–8); (2) has already been mentioned in this chapter and pervades a number of issues, while (3) will be emphasized in the next chapter, and (4) will be a major subject of this chapter. The major distinction between risk-benefit analysis and detriment-benefit analysis is that the former is concerned with risks of harm, whereas the latter is concerned with the detriments that occur at the time of the procedure or benefit. For example, an amputation not only is subject to the risk-benefit analysis but also to the detriment-benefit analysis, and for the latter, the assessor must be interested in the loss of the limb itself as a detriment.

The detriment-benefit analysis figures prominently in determining when actions that cause or permit death can be viewed as either non-violations or as justified violations of the principle of nonmaleficence and its derivative rules, including the prohibition of killing. When there is an apparent causal connection between our actions and another's death, we have several ways to defeat a charge of moral—if not legal—culpability. First, we might specify the principle of nonmaleficence to prohibit the infliction of harm on an *innocent* person and then try to show that the person we harm or kill is not innocent, e.g., because he is an unjust aggressor. Second, we might contend that the individual is not yet or no longer a person or a human being; e.g., the individual is a four-week-old fetus or one who has been declared dead, although the respirator still induces vital signs. Third, we might argue that the death was merely a foreseen consequence of our actions; it was not direct and intentional. As an indirect and unintentional side effect of an action aimed at a significant good, it does not fall, one might argue, under the prohibitions that flow from the duty of nonmaleficence. Fourth, we might contend that we did not kill the person but only allowed him to die. Fifth, we might appeal to the person's voluntary and informed expression of a desire to die. Sixth, we might hold that death is in the "harmed" person's best interests, e.g., he is suffering from uncontrollable and unmanageable pain, or even that sustaining life under these conditions would violate the principle *primum non nocere*. We will explore some of these options to see if and when they might be morally acceptable responses. We will, however, generally avoid the term "euthanasia" so often used in discussions of these ethical issues in death and dying, because its connotations tend to obscure rather than illuminate the issues.

The principle of double effect

Through a long history, primarily but not exclusively in the Roman Catholic tradition, the principle of double effect has been used to show that an act that has a harmful effect, e.g., death, does not always fall under moral prohibitions, e.g., murder, suicide, or abortion. The harmful effect is seen as an indirect or merely foreseen effect, not the direct and intended effect of the action.

The Roman Catholic position on abortion is a useful initial example of the use of the principle of double effect. Catholic opposition to abortion follows from acceptance of the prohibition against killing innocent human beings and from the conviction that human life begins at conception. Thus, a moral principle is combined with a claim about the beginning of human life (which is as much metaphysical as it is empirical). Despite the prohibition of abortion, considered as the moral equivalent of murder, Catholic teaching acknowledges at least two situations in which the death of the fetus—as a result of the physician's actions—does not lead to the judgment that the physician performed an abortion and thus committed a moral wrong. Both situations involve conditions that threaten the pregnant woman—a cancerous uterus and an ectopic pregnancy. In both, the death of the fetus is held to be the indirect and un-intended effect of a morally legitimate medical procedure. The Catholic position is not that "abortion" is justified in these cases, but that these deaths do not count as abortions because they are indirect and un-intended.[9]

The principle of double effect involves four conditions of a justified action: (1) The action in itself must be good or at least morally indifferent. (2) The agent must intend only the good effect and not the evil effect. The evil effect is foreseen, not intended; it is allowed, not sought. Some philosophers prefer to use Bentham's language of "obliquely intentional" for these foreseen effects. (3) The evil effect cannot be a *means* to the good effect. That is, the good and evil effects must follow immediately from the action. In many cases, this element is the most decisive in determining whether the agent is morally responsible for the harm or death. (4) There must be a proportionality between the good and evil effects of the action.[10]

Let us see how Catholic moralists have applied these conditions to the problem of the removal of a cancerous uterus that results in the foreseen but not intended death of the fetus. The action is the performance of a legitimate medical procedure which has good results, and the medical practitioner intends only the good effect (saving the mother's life), not the evil effect (the death of the fetus). This claim about the agent's intention can be made in part because the fetus' death is not a means to save the mother's life. If the fetus' death were a means, it would be intended along with the end. But saving the mother's life is only contingent upon the fetus' removal, not its death. Its death is an unintended though foreseen effect, and thus is neither an end nor a means to an end. Finally, saving the mother's life is a sufficient reason for the medical procedure and for the death of the fetus; i.e., the good effect outweighs the evil one. Suppose, by contrast, that a physician determines that it is necessary to perform a fetal craniotomy in order to save a woman in labor; the woman will die if the fetus' head is not crushed. Such a craniotomy could not be justified by the principle of double effect, because killing the fetus would be the means to the good end of saving the mother's life, and thus would be part of the intention. The fetus' death would be directly—even if regrettably—willed.

Sometimes the principle of double effect is invoked to justify the deaths of civilians as the indirect result of an attack on a legitimate military target or to justify an agent's acceptance of the risk of death for a good cause. The former would not be considered "murder" and the latter would not be considered "suicide" if the conditions of the principle of double effect were met.

Appeals to the principle of double effect are especially prominent when there is a conflict between obligations or values and it is not possible to meet or realize all of them simultaneously. While these obligations often are to different parties, e.g., obligations to the pregnant woman and to the fetus, two obligations to the same party may be in conflict. Such a situation can occur in the care of terminally ill patients. For example, there is a duty of nonmaleficence, including the duty not to kill, and there is a duty to make the patient comfortable by inducing sleep and alleviating pain. When these duties come into conflict, it may be possible to make the patient comfortable without direct killing only by using measures that may hasten the patient's death. When the conditions of the principle of double effect are met, hastening the patient's death does not count as homicide and is justified. According to the Ethical and Religious Directives for Catholic Health Facilities, "it is not euthanasia to give a dying person sedatives and analgesics for the alleviation of pain, when such a measure is judged necessary, even though they may deprive the patient of the use of reason, or shorten his life."

The principle of double effect has come under attack from many directions.[11] Often critics hold that the conclusions based on the principle are implausible, especially in the instances of abortion and euthanasia. Usually the conclusion is questioned because either the moral principles and rules or the factual premises of the argument are suspect. For example, at least one factual premise involved in the application of the principle of double effect to the deaths of fetuses is widely rejected: it is not clear to many people that the fetus should be considered a human being or person from conception, even if we have certain obligations to it. And this point of view does have credibility, for there are instances of morally justified fetal deaths in addition to those admitted by the restrictive principle of double effect. Regarding death and dying in general, few would dispute the moral justification for the cases of hastening death by relieving pain and inducing sleep that can be brought under the principle of double effect, but the principle simply fails to resolve most of the difficult cases, as we shall see in the next section of this chapter.

Utilitarians, joined by a number of deontologists, commonly argue that the principle of double effect is not morally relevant. First, they contend that it makes no sense to make different moral judgments about the death of a fetus by craniotomy and the death of a fetus that results from the removal of a cancerous uterus when the consequences are identical: a woman's life is saved and a fetus' life is lost. It is not possible to draw the distinction in terms of the degree of probability of the bad result, for the probability of death in at least some removals of a cancerous uterus may be so high as to approach virtual certainty. Second, critics of the principle of double effect contend that it is not possible to distinguish the above two cases of fetal death in terms of the agent's intention, for the physician may not want, desire, or intend the death of the fetus in either case and may regret the death whether he removes a cancerous uterus or performs a craniotomy.

Two different attempts to retain elements of the principle deserve mention. First, some Roman Catholic moral theologians now emphasize the fourth element of the principle—proportionality between good and evil effects—almost to the exclusion of other elements. As a result, it is difficult to distinguish their position as a mode of reasoning from utilitarianism, although, of course, their conceptions of values and disvalues are often different. These theologians are especially interested in avoiding the "physicalism" that the principle of double effect has sometimes encouraged. (Physicalism is the tendency to focus on the physical structure of the act and to hold that this structure makes it intrinsically wrong.) Second, some theologians and philosophers focus primarily on intention rather than on direct and indirect causation; they thus emphasize primary and secondary intentions rather than direct and indirect effects.[12]

Related to the distinctions between primary and secondary intentions and direct and indirect effects is the distinction between killing and letting die, which is equally controversial and deserves separate examination.

Killing and letting die

In Case #14, a sixty-eight-year-old doctor, who is severely suffering from terminal carcinoma of the stomach, collapsed with a massive pulmonary embolism. He survived because one of his young colleagues performed a pulmonary embolectomy. Upon recovery the doctor-patient requested that no steps be taken to prolong his life if he suffered another cardiovascular collapse. He even wrote a note to this effect for the hospital records. He reasoned that his pain was too much to bear given his dismal prospects. He thus asked to be *allowed to die* under certain conditions, but he did not ask to be *killed*. In Case #18, a defective infant needed an operation to remove a duodenal obstruction. The parents and physicians determined that survival was not in this infant's best interests and decided to allow the infant to die rather than to perform an operation. In both cases, we need to ask whether certain actions, e.g., intentionally not taking steps to overcome a cardiovascular collapse and not performing an operation, can be described as "allowing to die" rather than "killing."

For many people, it is important to distinguish killing and letting die and to prohibit the former while authorizing the latter—in some cases. For example, after prohibiting "mercy killing" or the "intentional termination of the life of one human being by another,"[13] the AMA House of Delegates held that cessation of treatment is morally justified under the following conditions: the patient and/or his immediate family, with the advice and judgment of the physician, may decide to withhold or stop the use of "extraordinary means to prolong life when there is irrefutable evidence that biological death is imminent." Although several terms in this statement need careful examination, e.g., "extraordinary," "irrefutable," and "imminent," it is clear that the statement authorizes some instances of allowing to die by withholding or stopping treatment, while it excludes killing. Whether letting particular patients die—e.g., the sixty-eight-year-old man suffering from terminal carcinoma of the stomach and the defective infant needing an operation—is morally acceptable would depend on several conditions, but if their deaths cannot be described as "allowed deaths," they are not justifiable according to the AMA House of Delegates' statement.

In recent years, the distinction between killing and letting die has come under frequent attack. Some critics focus on developments in biomedical technology that appear to make it difficult to classify some acts as killing or letting die, e.g., unplugging the respirator. Other critics dismiss the distinction itself, holding that it is a "moral quibble" without any "moral bite." As we explore the arguments for and against this distinction, it is important to emphasize that acceptance or rejection of the distinction does not necessarily determine conclusions about particular cases. For instance, it is possible to reject the distinction and to hold that some cases of both killing and letting die are right or that all are wrong, and it is possible to affirm the distinction and yet to hold that most cases of letting die and all cases of killing are wrong. Even if the distinction is morally significant it does not dictate a conclusion about a particular case. It is important to avoid the temptation to affirm the moral significance of the distinction and then to accept all cases of letting die as morally fitting. Even instances of letting die must meet other criteria, e.g., the detriment-benefit calculation.

In a widely discussed argument for rejecting both the distinction between active and passive euthanasia and the AMA's policy statement, James Rachels contends that killing is not, in itself, worse than letting die.[14] That is, the "bare difference" between acts of killing and acts of letting die is not in itself a morally relevant difference. Part of his strategy is to sketch two cases that differ only in that one involves killing, while the other involves allowing to die. He contends that if there is no morally relevant difference between these cases, the "bare difference" between killing and allowing to die is demonstrated to be morally irrelevant. In his two cases, two young men want their six-year-old cousins dead so that they can gain large inheritances. Smith drowns his cousin while the boy is taking a bath. Jones plans to drown his cousin, but as he enters the bathroom he sees the boy slip and hit his head; Jones stands by doing nothing, while the boy drowns. Smith killed his cousin; Jones merely allowed his cousin to die. While we agree with Rachels that both acts are equally reprehensible because of their motives and ends, we do not accept his conclusion that these examples show that the distinction between killing and letting die is morally irrelevant.

Several rejoinders to Rachels are in order. First, Rachels's cases and the cessations of treatment envisioned by the AMA are so markedly disanalogous that it is not clear what Rachels's argument shows. In some cases of unjustified acts, including both of Rachels's examples, we are not interested in moral distinctions per se. As Richard Trammell points out, some examples have a "masking" or "sledgehammer" effect; the fact that "one cannot distinguish the taste of two wines when both are mixed with green persimmon juice, does not imply that there is no distinction between the wines."[15] Since Rachels's examples involve two morally unjustified acts by agents whose motives and intentions are despicable, it is not surprising that some *other* features of their situations, e.g., killing and letting die, do not strike us as morally compelling.

Second, while Rachels's cases involve two *unjustified* actions, one of killing and the other of letting die, the AMA statement distinguishes cases of *unjustified killing* from cases of *justified letting die*. The AMA statement does not, however, claim that the moral difference is identical to the distinction between killing and letting die. It does not even imply that the "bare difference" between (passive) letting die and (active) killing is the only difference or even a morally sufficient difference between the justified and unjustified cases. Its point is rather that the justified actions involve (passive) letting die. While "mercy killing" is held to be unjustified in all circumstances, letting die is not held to be right in all circumstances. For an act that results in an earlier death for the patient to be justified, it is necessary that it be describable as an act of "letting die," but this description is not sufficient to justify the act.

Third, in Rachels's cases Smith and Jones are *morally* responsible and *morally* blameworthy for the deaths of their respective cousins, even if Jones, who allowed his cousin to drown, is not *causally* responsible. The law might only find Smith, who killed his cousin, guilty of homicide, but morality condemns both actions because of the agents' motives and their commissions and omissions. While we would not condemn a nonswimmer for failing to jump in deep water to try to rescue a drowning child, we find Jones's actions reprehensible because he (morally) should have rescued the child. Even if he had no other special duties to the child, the duty of beneficence—which we will examine in the next chapter—would require affirmative action. The point of the cases envisioned by the AMA is that the physician is always to be held responsible for killing, but he is not morally bound to preserve life in *all* cases. Indeed, the physician has a right—and perhaps a duty—to stop treatment when the following conditions are met: (1) the life of the body is being preserved by extraordinary means, (2) there is irrefutable evidence that biological death is imminent, and (3) the patient and/or the family consents.

Fourth, even if the distinction between killing and letting die is sometimes morally irrelevant, it does not follow that it is always morally irrelevant. The fact that the difference does not show up in every sort of case does not mean that it is morally unimportant for all cases. Rachels effectively undermines any attempt to rest judgments about ending life on the "bare difference" between killing and letting die, but his target may be a straw man. Many philosophers and theologians have argued that there are independent moral, religious, and other reasons for defending the distinction and for prohibiting killing while authorizing allowing to die in some cases.

One theologian has argued, for example, that we can discern the moral significance of the distinction between killing and letting die only by "placing it in the religious context out of which it grew."[16] That context is the Biblical story of God's actions toward his creatures. In that context it makes *sense* to talk about "placing patients in God's hands," just as it is important not to usurp God's prerogatives by desperately struggling to prolong life when the patient is irreversibly dying. But even if the distinction between killing and letting die originated within a religious context, and even if it makes more sense in that context than in some others, it can be defended on nontheological grounds without being converted into a claim about a "bare difference." However important the religious context was for the origin of the distinction, religious doctrines are not presupposed by the distinction, and independent moral grounds are sufficient to support it.

Some nontheological arguments in favor of the distinction between killing and allowing to die invoke both moral and practical considerations. They hold that the distinction enables us to express and maintain certain principles such as nonmaleficence and to avoid certain harmful consequences. Probably no single reason by itself is sufficient to support the moral relevance of the distinction, and thus to prohibit killing while permitting some intentionally allowed deaths. But several reasons together indicate that the distinction is worth retaining or, in effect, that our current practices should, with some clarifications, be maintained. We now turn to this set of reasons.

The most important arguments for the distinction between killing and letting die depend on a distinction between *acts* and *practices*.[17] It is one thing to justify an act, i.e., to hold that it is right; it is another to justify a practice with its own rules and procedures. As we saw in our examination of rule utilitarianism and rule deontology, many concerns about consequences and principles are applied to practices or rules rather than directly to acts. For example, we might justify a rule of confidentiality because it encourages people to seek therapy and because it promotes respect for persons and their privacy. Such a rule might, however, lead to undesirable results in *particular* cases. Likewise, a rule that prohibits "active euthanasia" while permitting some "allowed deaths" may be justifiable, even though it excludes some acts of killing that in and of themselves might appear to be justifiable. Such a rule would not permit us to kill a patient who suffers from terrible pain, who rationally asks for "mercy" (i.e., to be killed), and who will probably die within three weeks. According to the rule of double effect, we should, of course, use measures to alleviate his pain even though these would hasten his death; we should allow him to die, but we should not kill him. It may be necessary to prohibit some acts that do not appear to be wrong in order to maintain a viable practice that, for the most part, expresses our principles and avoids certain undesirable consequences. Although particular acts of killing may not violate the duty of nonmaleficence and may even be humane and compassionate, a policy of authorizing killing could violate the duty of nonmaleficence by creating a grave risk of harm in many cases.

According to one such line of argument, the prohibition of killing—even for "mercy"—expresses principles and values that provide a basis of trust between patients and health care professionals. Trust involves the expectation that others will respect moral limits. When we trust medical practitioners, we expect them to seek our welfare and, at least, to do us no harm. The prohibition of killing in medical contexts is one expression of the ethos of care for the patient's life and health and of the duty of nonmaleficence. Some claim that it is instrumentally as well as symbolically important, for its removal could weaken a "climate, both moral and legal, which we are not able to do without."[18] David Louisell, for example, contends that "Euthanasia would threaten the patient-physician relationship: confidence might give way to suspicion. . . . Can the physician, historic battler for life, become an affirmative agent of death without jeopardizing the trust of his dependents?"[19]

While this argument has plausibility, it needs to be stated very carefully. It is a wedge or slippery slope argument which may take at least two different forms. One type of wedge argument focuses on moral reasoning and the logic of distinctions between different acts. It holds that there will be no defensible line between acts that we consider legitimate and others that we consider reprehensible, unless we can draw a clear distinction supported by moral reasons. Justification of one sort of act that strikes us as right may have logical implications for the justification of another sort of act that strikes us as wrong. For example, a justification of abortion under some circumstances may also logically be a justification of infanticide under the same circumstances.

This first version of the wedge argument derives its power from the principle of universalizability discussed in Chapter 1. That principle commits us to treating similar cases in a similar way. If we judge X to be right, and we can point to no relevant dissimilarities between X and Y, then we cannot judge Y to be wrong. Because of this principle of universalizability, Paul Ramsey argues, ethical and legal mistakes tend to replicate themselves:

> It is quite clear that at the point of medical, legal, and ethical intersections at the edges of life. . . , the so-called wedge argument is an excellent one. This is true because legal principles and precedents are systematically designed to apply to other cases as well. This is the way the law 'works,' and . . . also the way moral reasoning 'works' from case to similar case.[20]

This first version of the wedge argument, then, focuses on the logical implications of decisions, i.e., what support of one sort of action logically implies for another sort of action, where it is not possible in principle to identify morally relevant dissimilarities.

While we morally justify killing aggressors in various circumstances such as self-defense and war, these killings presumably do not threaten the following rule, derived from the principle of nonmaleficence: do not directly kill innocent persons. These killings are justified because the persons killed are not innocent. If, however, we justify the killing of innocent persons in medical settings, there is no logical way, according to some arguments, to limit the exceptions to those that we consider legitimate, for the principle of nonmaleficence and the rule against directly killing innocent life have been eroded. Such arguments are not, however, compelling. As Rachels contends, "there obviously are good reasons for objecting to killing patients in order to get away for the weekend—or for even more respectable purposes, such as securing organs for transplantation—which do not apply to killing in order to put the patient out of extreme agony."[21]

Some general reasons for justified killing in the medical context might be too inclusive and might also spill over into nonmedical contexts. For example, Drs. Duff and Campbell reported that of 299 consecutive deaths in a special-care nursery, 43 (14 percent) were related to withholding treatment. Those 43 deaths came after parents and physicians "concluded that prognosis for *meaningful life* was extremely poor or hopeless, and therefore rejected further treatment."[22] "Meaningful life" may be too vague and general for use in rules governing either letting die or killing because it may logically compel us to act in cases in ways that we would not find acceptable. But this example also suggests that this version of the wedge argument may be as effective against some reasons for letting die as against some reasons for killing. We will consider these reasons later in this chapter when we examine the distinction between ordinary and extraordinary means.

This first version of the wedge argument thus does not assist supporters of the distinction between killing and letting die as much as they might suppose. Indeed, it can be used against them by critics of the distinction in the following way: if it is rational and morally defensible to allow patients to die under X, Y, and Z conditions, it is rational and morally defensible to kill them under those same conditions. If it is in their best interests to die, it is irrelevant how death is brought about. Rachels makes a similar point when he argues that reliance on the distinction between killing and letting die will lead to making decisions about life and death on *irrelevant grounds*—e.g., whether the patient will or will not die without certain forms of treatment—rather than in terms of the patient's best interests.[23] For example, in Case #18 a baby suffering from several defects needs an operation to remove an intestinal obstruction; otherwise the baby will die. A baby suffering from those same defects but without an intestinal obstruction may be kept alive, while the baby who needs the operation may be allowed to die. It is possible to argue that we need to determine the conditions under which death would be in the baby's best interests and then choose to kill or to let die by determining which means would be more humane and compassionate in the circumstances. In the famous Johns Hopkins Hospital case, the infant with duodenal atresia took two weeks to die, and the dying process was extremely difficult for all the parties involved, particularly the nurses. If a physician and family determine that a patient would be better off dead, why should they violate the patient's interests merely because the patient will not die when artificial treatment is discontinued? A morally irrelevant factor, so the argument goes, is allowed to dictate the outcome in violation of the principle of universalizability.

If the first version of the wedge argument focuses on the logic of moral reasoning—the hammer back of the wedge—the second version (2) focusses on what the wedge is driven into. It examines the culture and society in order to determine the probable impact of changing rules or making exceptions. It may hold that if certain restraints against killing are removed a moral decline will probably result, because various psychological or social forces make it unlikely that people will draw the distinctions that are, in principle, clear and defensible. For example, in some settings, it would be possible to argue that to authorize killing patients for their own benefit when they are suffering excruciating pain or have a bleak future could easily open the door to a policy of killing patients for the sake of social benefits, e.g., in order to reduce the financial burdens, or that voluntary euthanasia would probably open the door to involuntary euthanasia. Obviously, such arguments do not depend on the first version of the wedge or slippery slope, for there are clear and defensible distinctions, rooted in moral principles, between voluntary and involuntary euthanasia and between killing patients for their own benefit and killing them for social benefits. Nevertheless, where there are certain psychological and social forces, e.g., racism or an increasing number of defective newborns or aging persons with vast medical problems requiring an increasing amount of a society's financial resources, the second version of the wedge argument might be compelling. It depends on predicting what will probably in fact happen regardless of what our principles and rules logically imply. Thus, debates about the second version of the wedge argument concern empirical claims rather than the logical matters at issue in the first version.

If rules permitting active killing were introduced into a society, it is not implausible to suppose that the society over time would move increasingly in the direction of involuntary euthanasia, e.g., in the form of killing defective newborns, for social reasons such as the avoidance of social burdens. There could be a general reduction of respect for human life as a result of the official removal of some barriers to killing. Rules against killing in a moral code are not isolated moral principles; they are threads in a fabric of rules that support respect for human life. The more threads we remove, the weaker the fabric becomes. If we focus on attitudes and not merely rules, the general attitude of respect for life may be eroded by shifts in particular areas. Of course, determination of the probability of such an erosion depends not only on the connectedness of rules and attitudes, but also on various forces in the society.

When the second version of the wedge argument is combined with other considerations of consequences, the argument against the authorization of killing is even stronger. It is not a matter of combining several weak arguments in order to build a strong one. Such an approach would be ludicrous. But when there are several good reasons to be suspicious of a proposed policy that offers only limited benefit, the alteration of current practices may not be justified.[24]

In addition to fears of abuse, including abuse of the mentally retarded, and those who cannot consent, there are other legitimate fears. First, easy resort to killing to relieve pain and suffering may divert attention and resources from other strategies that may be effective, such as the hospice movement. Second, consider the following two types of wrongly diagnosed patients:[25]

(1) Patients wrongly diagnosed as hopeless, and who will survive even if a treatment *is* ceased (in order to allow a natural death).
(2) Patients wrongly diagnosed as hopeless, and who will survive only if the treatment is *not ceased*.

If a social rule of allowing some patients to die were in effect, doctors and families who followed it would lose only patients in the second category. But if killing were permitted, at least some of the patients in the first category would be needlessly lost. Thus, a rule prohibiting killing would save some lives that would be lost if *both* killing and allowing to die were permitted. Of course, such a consequence is not a decisive reason for a policy of (only) allowing to die, for the numbers in categories (1) and (2) are likely to be small and the other reasons for killing, e.g., extreme pain and autonomous choice, might be weighty. But it is certainly *a* morally relevant reason alongside other reasons.

Proponents of the practice of killing certain kinds of patients appeal to a range of exceptional cases to show the utility of the practice. One of the strongest reasons for killing some patients is to relieve unbearable and uncontrollable pain and suffering. No one would deny that pain and suffering can so ravage and dehumanize patients that death appears to be in their best interests. Prolonging life and refusing to kill in such circumstances may appear to be cruel and even to violate the duty of nonmaleficence. Often proponents of "mercy killing" appeal to nonmedical situations to show that killing may be more humane and compassionate than letting die—as, for example, in the case of a truck driver inextricably trapped in a burning wreck who cries out for "mercy" and asks to be killed. In such tragic situations we are reluctant to say that those who kill at the behest of the victim act wrongly. Furthermore, juries often find persons who have killed a suffering relative not guilty by reason of temporary insanity.

There are, nevertheless, serious objections to building into *medical practice* an explicit exception to the effect that physicians may kill their patients in order to relieve uncontrollable pain and suffering. One objection is that it is not clear that many, if any, cases in medical practice are really parallel to the person trapped in a burning wreck. The physician may be able to relieve pain and suffering short of killing—even if death is hastened—by means that are not available to a bystander at the scene of an accident. A second objection holds that we should not construct a social or professional ethic based on borderline situations and emergency cases, even if medical practitioners confront some cases of unmanageable pain and suffering. It is dangerous to generalize from emergencies, for hard cases may make bad social and professional ethics as well as bad law. As Charles Fried writes,

The concept of emergency is only a tolerable moral concept if somehow we can truly think of it as exceptional, if we can truly think of it as a circumstance that, far from defying our usual moral universe, suspends it for a limited time and thus suspends usual moral principles. It is when emergencies become usual that we are threatened with moral disintegration, dehumanization.[26]

Third, there are ways to "accept" acts of killing in exceptional circumstances without altering the rules of practice in order to accommodate them. As mentioned earlier, juries often find those who kill suffering relatives not guilty by reason of temporary insanity, as occurred in the Zygmaniak case in New Jersey.[27] In June 1973, George Zygmaniak was in a motorcycle accident that left him paralyzed from the neck down. The paralysis was considered to be irreversible, and Zygmaniak begged his brother, Lester, to kill him. Three days later, Lester brought a sawed-off shotgun to the hospital and shot his brother in the head, after having told him, "Close your eyes now, I'm going to shoot you." Verdicts like "not guilty by reason of temporary insanity" do not *justify* the act of killing a suffering relative. They thus differ from a verdict of not guilty on grounds of self-defense, for self-defense does justify killing at least in some cases. Verdicts like not guilty by reason of temporary insanity thus function to *excuse* the agent by finding that he lacked the conditions of responsibility.

Others have proposed that we maintain the rule against killing even if physicians and others sometimes have to engage in justified civil disobedience. Agreeing with Robert Veatch, Paul Ramsey holds that "[c]ivil disobedience—the courage to go against the rule when morally warranted—may be better than to allow for exceptions in a rule of general practice."[28] But what conditions might justify conscientious refusals to follow the rule prohibiting killing patients? According to Ramsey, when dying patients are totally inaccessible to our care, when our care is a matter of indifference to them because of intractable pain or a deep coma, "there is no longer any morally significant distinction between omission and commission, between standing aside and directly dispatching them."[29] "Total inaccessibility" is a limit of care itself; for care can become totally useless. It is not clear, however, that Ramsey's distinction between dying and nondying can carry his argument. Nor is it clear whether he considers someone in a deep and prolonged state of unconsciousness as dying and, if so, whether such a view is justifiable. In addition, it is necessary to ask whether Ramsey's exception can be limited to the cases that he endorses; it too may be the thin edge of the wedge. Nevertheless, pain and suffering of a certain magnitude can in principle justify active killing, if other conditions are met. They may only justify acts of conscientious refusal to follow the rule of practice, not basic changes in the rule itself.

Finally, which side in the debate has the burden of proof—the proponents or opponents of a practice of selective killing? Antony Flew has argued that supporters of the current practice of prohibiting killing must bear the burden of proof because the prohibition of *voluntary* euthanasia violates the principle of liberty by refusing to respect individual wishes.[30] A policy of voluntary euthanasia, based on either a negative right to die (a right to noninterference) or a positive right to die (a right to be killed), would involve such a change in society's vision of the medical profession and in medical attitudes as to shift the burden of proof to the proponents of change. The prohibition of killing even when it is requested is not arbitrary. It expresses some important moral principles, values, and attitudes whose loss, or serious alteration, could have major negative consequences. Since the practice of prohibiting killing and accepting some "allowed deaths"—as is the case in the medical profession and the law—has served us well, although not perfectly, it should be altered only with the utmost caution. While lines are not easy to draw and maintain, in general we have been able to follow the line between killing and letting die in medical practice. Before we undertake any major changes, we need strong evidence that these changes are really needed in order to avoid important harms or secure important benefits, and that the good effects will outweigh the bad effects. Otherwise, we run the risk of undermining respect for the principle of nonmaleficence and its subsidiary rules.[31]

The distinction between killing and letting die is not, of course, a sufficient basis for medical practice in issues of life and death, for not all "allowed deaths" are morally acceptable. There is considerable debate about when the description "letting die" can be applied and which instances of letting die are morally right. On the one hand, Ramsey clearly limits the application of "letting die" to the *dying;* that is, only those who are irreversibly in the dying process may be allowed to die. On the other hand, Robert Veatch holds that we can justify an allowed death when the treatments are unreasonable even if the patient is not irreversibly dying.[32] What, then, are the conditions under which allowed deaths are justified? To answer this question we need to examine the distinction between treatments that are obligatory and those that are optional.

Optional and obligatory means of treatment

The language of "ordinary" and "extraordinary" means of treatment has a long history, especially in the Roman Catholic context, but it has also been prominent in medical practice and in judicial decisions. The 1973 statement by the AMA House of Delegates holds that the patient and/or his immediate family can decide about the "cessation of *extraordinary means* to prolong the life of the body when there is irrefutable evidence that biological death is imminent." Even more recently, the New Jersey Supreme Court implicitly invoked this distinction when it held that judgments about therapy should be made in terms of the treatment's degree of invasiveness and its chance of success.

Like the distinctions between direct and indirect effects and killing and letting die, this distinction has been employed to determine whether an act that results in death counts as killing, and especially as culpable killing in violation of the duty of nonmaleficence. Historically, the distinction has been applied to decisions of patients, proxies, and physicians. Developed by Roman Catholics to deal with the problems of surgery prior to the discovery of antisepsis and anesthesia, the distinction was used to determine whether a patient's refusal of treatment should be classified as suicide. Refusal of "ordinary" means of treatment was considered suicide, while refusal of "extraordinary" means was not labelled suicide. Likewise, families and physicians did not commit homicide or violate obligations to patients if they only withheld or stopped extraordinary means of treatment.

Unfortunately, a long history does not guarantee clarity, and the distinction between ordinary and extraordinary means of treatment is vague and ambiguous. As a result, several recent commentators have urged that the distinction be replaced by other categories. It is not always clear whether they intend to change only the vocabulary or also the substance of the distinction. We too think that moral discourse would improve if the terms were replaced by such terms as "optional" and "obligatory." "Ordinary" would then be reconstructed to mean morally obligatory, mandatory, required, imperative, etc., while "extraordinary" would be reconstructed to mean morally optional, elective, expendable, etc.[33]

Such a translation is not alien to some traditional discussions of ordinary and extraordinary means of treatment, and it appears to be required because "ordinary" is often wrongly taken to mean "usual," while "extraordinary" is taken to mean "unusual." The "usual/unusual" distinction builds on what is customary in medical practice. Of course, what is customary in medical practice is merely relevant to moral judgments and cannot be construed as always morally acceptable. For example, it may be usual medical practice to treat some disease in a particular way, but whether this usual practice should be repeated for a particular patient depends on the patient's condition as a whole and not merely on what is usual treatment for a particular disease.[34]

It is possible that what is needed is only a replacement of the language of "ordinary" and "extraordinary," while retaining or only partially modifying the substance of the distinction. According to Gerald Kelly, S.J., the distinction can be understood in the following way:

> Ordinary means are all medicines, treatments, and operations, which offer a reasonable hope of benefit and which can be obtained and used without excessive expense, pain, or other inconvenience. Extraordinary means are all medicines, treatments, and operations, which cannot be obtained or used without excessive expense, pain, or other inconvenience, or which, if used, would not offer a reasonable hope of benefit.[35]

Kelly's discussion of the distinction embodies two criteria: for a therapy to be obligatory or required, it must (a) offer a reasonable prospect of benefit, and (b) not involve excessive expense, pain, or other inconvenience. The substance of the distinction is a balance between benefit and detriment, if we assume that "excessive" is to be determined by the probability and magnitude of the benefit. If there is no reasonable hope of benefit, then any expense, pain or other inconvenience is excessive. But if there is a reasonable hope of benefit, the amount of expense, pain, or other inconvenience may be significant without being excessive. Therefore, the point of the distinction and its application turns on a balance between benefits and costs, including immediate detriment, inconvenience, and risk of harm.

We will reserve a systematic treatment of cost-benefit analysis for the next chapter, but it is important now to ask which substantive standards should determine when treatment is obligatory and when it is optional. These standards may vary for competent patients making choices about their own treatment and for second parties making decisions for incompetent patients. Competent and informed patients should have more latitude than second parties in accepting and refusing treatment, because of the incompetent patient's vulnerability to harm. We concentrated on competent patients in our discussion of autonomy in Chapter 3 and shall return to this class of patients in our discussion of paternalism in Chapter 5. Therefore, we shall here consider the substantive criteria of optional and mandatory treatments mainly for incompetent patients. These substantive criteria determine when it is possible to rebut the presumption, based on the principle of nonmaleficence, that the means to prolong life are obligatory.

First, treatment is not obligatory when it offers no prospect of benefit to the patient, because it is pointless. There are several classes of patients for whom treatment will not be efficacious. (a) First, there are those who are dead. It is unfortunate that the impetus for refining the criteria for determining death came from the need for organs for transplantation. There are sufficient reasons for updating the criteria for determining death without considering the interests of potential recipients of organs. If the patient is dead, he can no longer be harmed by the cessation of treatment, and his interests do not dictate treatment. But refined criteria of death will not help in most cases. For example, few people argued seriously during the Karen Anne Quinlan trial that she was dead. Yet among those holding that she was alive, there were moral and legal disagreements about what ought to be done.

(b) Second, there are those whose death is imminent or who are irreversibly dying. The AMA statement, as we have seen, holds that some treatments are optional and may be discontinued when death is "imminent." It is not clear whether this statement holds that all means can be considered "extraordinary" when death is imminent, except those that are palliative, or that only "extraordinary" means can be discontinued when death is imminent. Whatever the intention of the AMA statement, the first interpretation is more defensible. When it can be determined, largely as a matter of medical judgment, that a patient's death is imminent or that a patient is irreversibly dying, such modes of treatment as resuscitation and respiration become optional. Because "ought" implies "can," there is no medical indication for starting or continuing curative treatment if the patient is irreversibly dying and death is imminent. As Ramsey argues, "care means always hoping to cure and to save life until that becomes, in the case of the dying, useless; and care means always abiding with the dying patient until that becomes useless."[36] Optimal care does not mean maximal treatment, and prolonging life is not the same as prolonging dying. Indeed, the paradigm of care for the dying needs to be dramatically revised so that technological interventions do not overwhelm human responses of care.

Second, treatment is not obligatory when its burdens outweigh its benefits for the patient. If it could be argued that objective medical factors are dominant in cases (a) and (b), considerations of value are important and indispensable in another set of cases (c) which would include patients who are in an irreversible vegetative condition, e.g., Karen Ann Quinlan. In (c) cases, patients are not dead, and it is not clear that their deaths are impending, but there is a justifiable prediction of irreversible loss of mentation and unavailability of new therapies that might be efficacious. It might be argued that cases of type (c) actually fall under the principle that useless or pointless treatment need not be continued, but the matter is more complex, for treatment can preserve biological *life* indefinitely in many cases. Hence, the critical question is, "How long should we preserve biological life when there is no reasonable prospect of recovery of cognitive, sapient life?" Answers to this question depend on balancing probable benefits and burdens for the patient.

In a fourth set of cases (d), the patients do not suffer from an irreversible loss of mentation; they are conscious but are so debilitated that they are predicted to be irreversibly unable to make an informed choice, and probably even to be informed. An example might be nonepisodic, senile brain disease of irreversible etiology, with brain shrinkage and scarred cells, resulting in senile psychosis. Still, continued existence could be meaningful to the person, who might be able to enjoy meals, back rubs, etc. Such a case clearly involves balancing probable benefits and burdens to the patient; in this case, treatment may be morally obligatory.

Few decisions are more important than those to withhold or stop a therapeutic procedure that sustains a life. But in some cases it may be unjustified to begin or to continue therapy knowing that it will produce a greater balance of suffering for someone incapable of choosing for or against such therapy. As the Supreme Judicial Court of Massachusetts held in the Saikewicz case (#15), "the 'best interests' of an incompetent person are not necessarily served by imposing on such persons results not mandated as to competent persons similarly situated."[37] An interesting example occurred in the case of *In re Nemser,* where a judge refused to require the amputation of the foot and ankle (a transmalleolar amputation) of an eighty-year-old woman. Her competency was doubtful, and her children sought to consent to the operation for her although it was medically unclear how much benefit could be expected and clear that substantial suffering would be involved. While the operation might actually have cured her, Judge Markowitz held that the substantial hazards and suffering involved outweighed the possible beneficial outcome, though he referred to his decision as "an example of a grave dilemma."[38]

Some of the most difficult questions about the treatment of incompetents involve seriously defective newborns. Some societies have circumvented the duty of nonmaleficence in such cases by purely definitional ploys. For example, the Nuer tribe viewed defective newborns as nonhuman "hippopotamuses" who were mistakenly born to human parents and who should be put in the river, which was viewed as their natural habitat. Such definitional maneuvers are generally excluded in our society as far as newborns are concerned. But it remains important to consider the interests of these newborn human beings and whether maximal treatment is always in their best interests. Some commentators even argue that intensive care for neonates may be "harmful," i.e., violate the duty of nonmaleficence, under three conditions: "inability to survive infancy, inability to live without severe pain, and inability to participate, at least minimally, in human experience."[39] Another commentator has drawn on the duty of nonmaleficence to develop a concept of the "injury of continued existence." While rejecting active euthanasia on prudential grounds, H. Tristram Engelhardt, Jr., has argued that the duty of nonmaleficence may require that death be allowed under some conditions: "The concept of injury for continuance of existence, the proposed analogue of the concept of tort for wrongful life, presupposes that life can be of a negative value such that the medical maxim *primum non nocere* ('first do no harm') *would require not sustaining life.*"[40] Engelhardt may be correct in suggesting that there is a moral *duty* not to sustain life in some circumstances where the burdens seriously outweigh the benefits. However, our intention here is merely to show that under some conditions allowing seriously defective newborns to die is *permissible* because it does not violate the duty of nonmaleficence (and satisfies other relevant justifying conditions).

Consider some candidate cases. It would be justifiable under the conditions mentioned thus far to withhold or to withdraw treatment for some who suffer Tay-Sachs disease—which involves increasing spasticity and dementia and usually results in death by age three or four—and for some who suffer Lesch-Nyhan disease—which involves uncontrollable spasms, mental retardation, compulsive self-mutilation, and early death. Children born with meningomyelocele, however, are more problematic. As in Case #19, it is difficult to know whether to treat vigorously all cases or to treat vigorously only selected cases. The difficulty stems from the fact that while some children with meningomyelocele can have a meaningful life, the chances are slim. Having argued at one point for vigorous and comprehensive treatment for all spina bifida babies, Dr. John Lorber later concluded that such treatment results in only a marginal gain in survival rate and preserves life with severe disabilities and handicaps. He has proposed specific criteria, e.g., the site of the spinal lesion and the degree of paralysis, for determining the level of treatment on the first day after birth. When the decision is made to omit treatment for the disorder, normal custodial care and feeding are provided. The problem is that when these babies survive, they are in worse condition than they would have been had they been treated.[41]

In these and other cases, we should work with a presumption in favor of the prolongation of life. Decision-makers should then try to determine the patient's actual interests and should act accordingly. For a patient who has previously expressed a certain life plan, it may be possible for decision-makers to balance benefits and burdens in terms of that life plan. It might be possible to say that "John Doe would not want to live under those conditions." However, such judgments about a patient's interests in the case of, for example, defective newborns must be made by considering the prospective benefits and burdens as objectively as possible, in the light of the patient's condition, without benefit of his or her previous declarations. The possibility of error is substantial, but no greater than in other judgments in medicine. Because of the possibility of error in diagnosis, prognosis, and judgments about the patient's interests, the prima facie duty to preserve life dictates erring on the side of sustaining life, at least in cases of doubt about the evidence.

Debates about whether treatment is optional or obligatory often involve standards of the "quality of life." In the Saikewicz case (see #15) a sixty-seven-year-old man, with an I.Q. of 10 and a mental age of approximately two years and eight months, suffered from acute myeloblastic monocytic leukemia. Chemotherapy would have produced considerable suffering and possibly serious side effects. Remission under chemotherapy occurs in only 30 to 50 percent of such cases and typically only for between two and thirteen months. If not given chemotherapy, Saikewicz could expect to live for a matter of weeks or, perhaps, several months. If the disease were allowed to run its course, he would not experience great pain and suffering. In not requiring treatment, the lower court considered "the quality of life available to him [Saikewicz] even if the treatment does bring about remission." The Massachusetts Supreme Court, however, rejected this formulation *if* it equated the value of life with a measure of the quality of life—in particular, with Saikewicz's lower quality of life because of mental retardation. Thus, the Court construed "the vague, and perhaps ill-chosen, term 'quality of life' . . . as a reference to the continuing state of pain and disorientation precipitated by the chemotherapy treatment." It thus balanced the prospective benefit and pain and suffering, finally determining that the patient's actual interests and preferences supported a decision not to provide chemotherapy. From a moral as well as a legal standpoint, we would agree that this decision was justified. However, we object to its procedural requirements in the next section of this chapter.

Because such slogans as "quality of life" and "sanctity of life" mislead more often than they illuminate, they should be replaced by more careful statements of substantive positions, such as those attempted by Paul Ramsey and Richard McCormick. Opposing any judgments about quality of life, Ramsey contends that what is important in the ordinary/extraordinary distinction can be "reduced almost without significant remainder to a medical indications policy."[42] According to Ramsey, to determine which treatment is obligatory and optional for incompetent patients, it is only necessary to determine which treatment is medically indicated. For the *dying,* the relevant choices are between further palliative treatments and no treatments. For unconscious or incompetent *nondying* patients, there is an obligation to use the treatment medically indicated. Ramsey contends that we are moving toward a policy of active, involuntary euthanasia for unconscious or incompetent nondying patients. Against such a policy, he asserts an "undiminished obligation first of all to save life and, in the second instance, to use palliative treatments where possible."[43] Above all, quality of life judgments are to be avoided, he argues, because they violate the principle of *equality* of life.

Ramsey's approach concentrates on medical factors that are objective even though they cannot be infallibly determined, e.g., criteria used in the classification of patients as dying and nondying and in the determination of treatment as medically indicated. It is not clear, however, that these objective medical factors will carry the weight he intends. In particular, it is not clear that these factors can be used apart from values that inspire, control, and limit them. For example, Richard McCormick contends that it is impossible to determine what will benefit a patient without *presupposing* a standard of quality of life. He believes that even the language of "medically indicated" presupposes judgments about the patient's condition, and "among the objective conditions of the patient to be considered, one of the most crucial is the *kind of life* that will be preserved as a result of our interventions."[44] Any attempt to make "life"—as metabolism and vital processes—good in itself is "vitalism" and should be rejected in favor of a view that life is a conditional value. While the person is "an incalculable value," the maintenance of physical life should not automatically be considered a benefit to the person. Although McCormick does not spell out his criteria of the quality of life, he offers a minimal condition: the capacity for experience or social interrelating. If this minimal condition is not met, as in anencephaly, treatment is not required.

Ramsey has objected that such a quality of life approach shifts from the question whether *treatments* are beneficial to patients to the question whether patients' *lives* are beneficial to them. The latter question, he insists, opens the door to active, involuntary euthanasia.[45] He appeals to the wedge argument (in its first version) and contends that quality of life criteria logically commit us to active, involuntary euthanasia. The critical question is whether the criteria of "quality of life" or, as we prefer, the criteria for determining the patient's best interests, can be stated with sufficient precision and cogency to avoid the dangers stressed by both versions of the wedge argument. We think that they can, but the vagueness of terms such as "dignity" and "meaningful life" is a cause for concern, and the increasingly widespread practice of allowing defective newborn infants to die when their "allowed deaths" are not justified (e.g., in Case #18) provides a good reason for caution.

Some factors can be excluded from consideration. Just as the Massachussetts Supreme Court in the Saikewicz case found it inappropriate to include mental retardation in a determination of the quality of life, we too contend that this factor is irrelevant in determining whether treatment would be in the patient's best interests. Jonsen and Garland correctly urge that "a baby with Down's syndrome, although sure to be mentally deficient, should be given life-sustaining therapy as a rule whenever needed; an anencephalic baby (born without a developed brain) should not be resuscitated or sustained."[46] Unfortunately, the "gray area" between these two extremes is less easily handled by such a general pronouncement.

There is some debate about the relevance of burdens to the family and to the society in determining whether treatment is mandatory or optional. Robert Veatch appears to hold that when second parties make decisions for incompetent patients, only the incompetent patients' burdens are relevant, while competent patients may include any burdens they find valid. He says emphatically that treatments are reasonable only if they do not give rise to "patient-centered objections." His position is not as restrictive as it appears, however, for the category of "patient-centered objections" is broad—"patient-centered objections based on physical or mental burden; familial, social or economic concern; or religious belief."[47] He may mean that only some "patient-centered objections" are relevant, but it is not clear, for example, how he would treat the "patient-centered objection" that the treatment would be so expensive as to exhaust all the uninsured patient's funds. Apparently he would permit the competent patient to refuse treatment for this reason. But it is uncertain whether he would allow this same objection to be used *by family members* in order to refuse treatment for a patient whose imminent loss of resources directly affects them. Our contention is that such an objection should not be decisive in determining whether treatment is optional or obligatory. Rather, the patient's interests should be decisive, and these may conflict with the interests of the family. To allow familial and social burdens to be determinative would open the door to a dangerous practice. Still, in situations of scarcity, difficult allocation questions do emerge, and we will consider them in our discussion of justice in Chapter 6.

Two final points need to be made. First, the distinction between *with-*

holding treatment that was never started and *withdrawing* treatment already started is morally irrelevant to determining whether treatment is obligatory or optional. In many cases, it is necessary to begin and vigorously pursue certain kinds of treatment in order to diagnose the patient's condition with precision. Diagnosis and prognosis often require time that can only be gained by such vigorous efforts as resuscitation, respiration, etc. If it is determined that treatment is optional because of the patient's interests, as analyzed through a benefit-detriment calculus, treatment may be discontinued. The moral grounds for withdrawing are the same as for withholding treatment. The critical issue is not that of an act versus an omission, for the description "allowing to die" is consistent with such acts as turning off the respirator. Second, no particular treatment procedures can be classified as "obligatory" or "optional." These terms do not refer to the *nature* of the treatment procedures or to customary medical practice, but rather pertain to the patient's condition and interests. Even critical treatments such as intravenous feeding may be optional in some cases, as perhaps in the Karen Anne Quinlan case. Whether a particular treatment is *obligatory* depends on whether it serves the patient's interests, including interests in his comfort and in seeing that his autonomous wishes are carried out.

Who should decide?

In many areas of biomedicine, especially in cases of terminal care, the question "Who should decide?" remains controversial. In this chapter we have concentrated on the question "What are the criteria of right decisions?" Answers to that question only partially form the basis for determining who should make the decisions.

John Rawls has argued that there are at least three possible relationships between procedures and right results or decisions. (1) Perfect procedural justice: there is an independent standard of a right outcome or decision, and it is possible to devise a procedure to ensure this outcome. An example is ensuring a fair distribution of a birthday cake at a children's party by having the child who cuts the cake take the last piece. (2) Imperfect procedural justice: there is an independent standard of a right outcome, but the procedures are imperfect in that they cannot ensure the desired outcome. For example, in criminal trials, we have an independent standard of a right outcome—the guilty and only the guilty should be convicted—but we lack a procedure that will produce this outcome in all cases. (3) Pure procedural justice: there is no independent standard of right results, and any result of the procedure is correct if the procedure has been followed. Gambling is an example.[48]

If our earlier argument in this chapter is correct, the most we can hope for in life and death decisions in medical practice is imperfect procedural justice. There are, we have argued, some independent standards, but there is no procedure to guarantee that decisions or outcomes will match those standards. Consider two significantly different situations. First, consider situations in which sick or dying patients make their own decisions. If the patient is competent and can make informed and voluntary choices, the principle of autonomy requires that we recognize the patient's right to make the decision even if he or she exercises that right wrongly. Nonetheless, we should not view the patient's decision as correct simply because the patient exercised it under conditions of rationality, understanding, and voluntariness. Nor should we view the patient's right to make the decision as absolute. Thus, this first type of situation cannot be viewed as one of pure procedural justice.

A second type of situation involves incompetent patients who cannot make their own decisions about withholding or withdrawing treatment. In such cases, the principle of nonmaleficence requires that we establish procedures to protect their interests, and yet no procedure will *guarantee* that their interests will always be protected. At best, this state of affairs is an instance of imperfect procedural justice. Some have argued, however, that some procedures are justified by principles and values other than or in addition to nonmaleficence and are preferable for that reason. For example, Dr. Raymond Duff argues that the family, in consultation with the physician, should make the decisions about the treatment or non-treatment of defective newborns, not only because the family can be expected to act in the infant's best interests—which would express the principle of nonmaleficence—but primarily because the family needs to gain a sense of control over its destiny in the face of this misfortune.[49] Nevertheless, judgments about decision-makers and procedures for incompetents should be made first of all in terms of the principle of nonmaleficence: if it can be determined that any particular decision-maker cannot be counted on to seek the patient's interests, that decision-maker should be replaced. Thus, it is important to determine whether classes of decision-makers and particular decision-makers can render rational and impartial judgments about the patient's best interests independent of conflicts of interests.

Four major classes of decision-makers have been proposed and actually used in cases of withholding and ceasing treatment of incompetent patients: families, physicians, committees, and courts. We believe that families of patients should be given first priority as the primary decision-makers. They should receive the advice and counsel of physicians, who should appeal to the hospital committee or to the courts to protect the patient's interests when they have reason to think that the patient would be harmed by a family decision. In effect, we are proposing a structure of serial decision making, with the family as the central agent whenever the patient cannot make the decision. The family's role should be primary because of the presumed identity of interests with the patient, and intimate knowledge of his or her wishes and wants. Nevertheless, that role should not be final or ultimate, because families do not always know or seek the best interests of their members. In this unhappy event, the physician(s) should attempt to persuade the family to reach a different decision. Should their attempts fail, they should invoke institutional procedures established to resolve such conflicts, e.g., an ethics committee in the hospital, and, if appropriate, the courts.

Arguments for giving primacy to some decision-maker other than the family usually appeal to the importance of fair and impartial decisions. Such arguments frequently hold that families cannot be fair and impartial, because prolonged extension of a relative's life may put a serious strain on financial, emotional, and other familial resources. Thus, so these arguments go, fair and impartial judgments about patients' interests, and actions in accord with the principle of nonmaleficence, require independent decision-makers. Such arguments also depend on empirical determinations. Is it true, for example, that patients' interests will likely be violated by allowing family members to make decisions? In the absence of convincing evidence that the principle of nonmaleficence will be more closely approximated by decision-makers other than family members, there are good reasons for allowing family members to make the decisions.

The consultative role assigned to physicians and other health care professionals cannot, however, be reduced to the mere provision of information. In Robert Veatch's analysis, the physician should only present information for the patient's or family's consideration and then should withdraw if he or she cannot comply with their request. Underlying his recommendation is a worry about societal acceptance of the fallacy of the "generalization of expertise"—the view that those who have technical knowledge also have moral insight. While it is true, as Veatch argues, that technical knowledge does not entail moral insight, it does not preclude moral insight.[50] Physicians and other health care professionals should engage in moral discussions of the options with patients and their families, and they should have the right to withdraw from cases when they cannot in good conscience act on a second party's decisions for treatment or nontreatment. We will discuss such cases of conscientious refusal by physicians and other professionals in Chapter 8. It is important, however, to emphasize here that withdrawal is not always morally acceptable if there is a high probability that there would be consequences seriously detrimental to the patient's interests. The duties of nonmaleficence and beneficence require that physicians and other health care professionals actively pursue measures to prevent such violations.

In the Quinlan case, the New Jersey Supreme Court recognized Joseph Quinlan as Karen Ann Quinlan's guardian and thus recognized his right to make decisions about her treatment, after consultation with physicians of his choice.[51] The Court held that when the guardian and attending physicians concur that life-support systems should be discontinued because there is no reasonable possibility that the patient will return to a cognitive, sapient state, they should then consult the hospital "ethics committee." Because its designated function is merely to confirm the patient's medical prognosis, the "ethics committee" is surely misnamed. More importantly, it is not clear why this additional layer of decision making is required unless there is either uncertainty about the prognosis or disagreement between family and physicians.

Expressly departing from the Quinlan decision of the New Jersey Supreme Court, the Supreme Judicial Court of Massachusetts held in the Saikewicz case (see Case #15) that questions of life and death require the "process of detached but passionate investigation and decision that forms the ideal on which the judicial branch of government was created."[52] Achieving this ideal is the courts' responsibility and is "not to be entrusted to any other group." The Massachusetts Court held that probate courts should make these decisions after considering all viewpoints and alternatives, including those of an ethics committee. Saikewicz, as noted above, was sixty-seven and had an I.Q. of 10 and a mental age of approximately two years and eight months. He had lived in state institutions since 1923.

Only two members of his family could be located—two sisters who did not want to become involved.

In such cases, where there is no family, or when the family is not interested, it is necessary to find some other decision-maker—either the physicians, a committee, or the courts—although there may also be other alternatives. There is nothing inherently objectionable about an appeal to probate courts as decision-makers in such cases, although there is no evidence to suppose that physicians and hospital committees, including laypersons, would be inadequate for most cases of this sort. The Massachusetts Court may, however, have mandated a procedure for other sorts of cases even where the families are involved and where there is no evidence of prejudicial decision making. If so, the outcome is unfortunate. The decision may have also had the effect of establishing a procedural presumption in favor of treatment, resuscitation, etc., until the probate judge specifically authorizes cessation. As we have seen, there should be a substantive presumption in favor of treatment until it no longer serves the patient's interests. However, a procedural requirement of treatment unless and until the probate judge acts may not serve the patient's interests. Such a procedural requirement is not needed unless there are conflicts of interests or reason to suspect abuse, as might often occur in the case of wards of the state and other vulnerable parties.[53]

Who, in conclusion, should make final decisions in life and death matters? The principle of autonomy requires that the competent patient be allowed to make his or her own decisions. While there may be some extreme cases that would justify familial or medical intervention against the patient's will, these are likely to be cases where there is reason to think that the patient is in some important respect incompetent, uninformed, or acting involuntarily. The principles of nonmaleficence and beneficence require that incompetent patients be protected against various harms. Decision-makers, procedures, and processes should be designed to protect the patient's interests, although at best they can only be instances of imperfect procedural justice. Apart from evidence to the contrary, families may be presumed to have the patient's best interests at heart and to have a firm grasp of those interests. Thus, they should be the primary decision-makers for incompetent patients. Physicians and other health care professionals, however, remain morally responsible in these settings, not only to provide information, but to engage in moral counseling, to withdraw when they cannot satisfy their consciences, and to take active measures to prevent abuses of patient's interests. Health care professionals, hospital committees, and the courts should function to protect the patient's interests when there are conflicting judgments or evidence of abuse.

Notes

1. W. H. S. Jones, *Hippocrates I* (Cambridge, Mass.: Harvard University Press, 1923), p. 165. See also Ludwig Edelstein, *Ancient Medicine* (Baltimore: The Johns Hopkins University Press, 1967). Extremely useful for our purposes is Albert R. Jonsen, "Do No Harm: Axiom of Medical Ethics," *Philosophical Medical Ethics: Its Nature and Significance,* ed. Stuart F. Spicker and H. Tristram Engelhardt, Jr. (Dordrecht, Holland: D. Reidel Publishing Co., 1977).
2. Frankena, *Ethics,* 2nd ed. (Englewood Cliffs, N.J.: Prentice-Hall, 1973), p. 47.
3. *The Right and the Good* (Oxford: Clarendon Press, 1930), pp. 21–22.
4. See Joel Feinberg, *Social Philosophy* (Englewood Cliffs, N.J.: Prentice-Hall, 1973), pp. 25ff.
5. William L. Prosser, *Handbook of the Law of Torts,* 4th ed. (St. Paul, Minn.: West Publishing Co., 1971), pp. 145–46.
6. Eric D'Arcy, *Human Acts* (Oxford: Clarendon Press, 1963), p. 121.
7. Quoted in Angela Roddy Holder, *Medical Malpractice Law* (New York: John Wiley and Sons, 1975), p. 42.
8. Albert R. Jonsen, "Do No Harm," pp. 27–41.
9. See David Granfield, *The Abortion Decision* (Garden City, N.Y.: Doubleday, 1969).
10. For some of the literature on double effect, see Joseph T. Mangan, S.J., "An Historical Analysis of the Principle of Double Effect," *Theological Studies* 10 (1949): 40–61; Richard A. McCormick, S.J., *Ambiguity in Moral Choice* (Milwaukee: Marquette University, 1973); Paul Ramsey and Richard A. McCormick, S.J., eds., *Doing Evil to Achieve Good: Moral Choice in Conflict Situations* (Chicago: Loyola University Press, 1978). For criticisms see Jonathan Bennett, "Whatever the Consequences," *Analysis* 26 (1966): 83–102; Philippa Foot, "The Problem of Abortion and the Doctrine of Double Effect," *Oxford Review* 5 (1967): 5–15; and Susan Nicholson, *Abortion and the Roman Catholic Church, JRE Studies in Religious Ethics,* II (Knoxville, Tennessee: Religious Ethics, Inc., 1978).
11. See the critical literature mentioned in footnote 10.
12. For the emphasis on proportionality, see McCormick, *Ambiguity in Moral Choice;* for the emphasis on intention, see Charles Fried, *Right and Wrong* (Cambridge, Mass.: Harvard University Press, 1978).
13. It is a mistake to view these expressions as synonymous, though the AMA statement appears to.

14. James Rachels, "Active and Passive Euthanasia," *The New England Journal of Medicine* 292 (January 9, 1975): 78–80.

15. Richard L. Trammell, "Saving Life and Taking Life," *Journal of Philosophy* 72 (1975): 131–37.

16. Gilbert Meilaender, "The Distinction Between Killing and Allowing to Die," *Theological Studies* 37 (1976): 467–70.

17. See John Rawls, "Two Concepts of Rules," *The Philosophical Review* 64 (1955): 3–32.

18. G. J. Hughes, S.J., "Killing and Letting Die," *The Month* 236 (1975): 42–45.

19. David Louisell, "Euthanasia and Biothanasia: On Dying and Killing," *Linacre Quarterly* 40 (1973): 234–58.

20. Paul Ramsey, *Ethics at the Edges of Life* (New Haven: Yale University Press, 1978), pp. 306–7.

21. James Rachels, "Medical Ethics and the Rule Against Killing: Comments on Professor Hare's Paper," *Philosophical Medical Ethics: Its Nature and Significance*, ed. S. F. Spicker and H. T. Engelhardt, Jr., p. 65.

22. Raymond S. Duff and A.G.M. Campbell, "Moral and Ethical Dilemmas in the Special Care Nursery," *The New England Journal of Medicine* 289 (1973): 890. Italics added.

23. Rachels, "Active and Passive Euthanasia," pp. 78–80.

24. For an important debate about these issues, see Yale Kamisar, "Some Nonreligious Views Against Proposed 'Mercy-killing' Legislation," *Minnesota Law Review* 42 (1958) and Glanville Williams, "'Mercy-killing' Legislation—A Rejoinder," *Minnesota Law Review* 43 (1958), reprinted in Tom Beauchamp and LeRoy Walters, eds., *Contemporary Issues in Bioethics* (Encino, Calif.: Dickenson Publishing Co., 1978), pp. 308–23.

25. We owe most of this argument to James Rachels.

26. Charles Fried, "Rights and Health Care—Beyond Equity and Efficiency," *The New England Journal of Medicine* 293 (July 31, 1975): 245.

27. For a discussion of this case, see Paige Mitchell, *Act of Love: The Killing of George Zygmaniak* (New York: Knopf, 1976).

28. See Paul Ramsey, *Ethics at the Edges of Life* (New Haven, Conn.: Yale University Press, 1978), p. 217; Robert Veatch, *Death, Dying, and the Biological Revolution* (New Haven, Conn.: Yale University Press, 1976), p. 97.

29. Ramsey, *Ethics at the Edges of Life,* pp. 195, 214, 216; cf. Ramsey, *The Patient as Person,* pp. 161–64.

30. Antony Flew, "The Principle of Euthanasia," in A. B. Downing, ed., *Euthanasia and the Right to Death: The Case for Voluntary Euthanasia* (London: Peter Owen, 1969), pp. 30–48.

31. For other discussions by the authors of the main ideas in this section on Killing and Letting Die, see Tom L. Beauchamp, "A Reply to Rachels on Active and Passive Euthanasia," *Ethical Issues in Death and Dying,* Tom L. Beauchamp and Seymour Perlin, eds. (Englewood Cliffs, N.J.: Prentice-Hall, 1978), pp. 246–58; James Childress, "To Kill or Let Die," *Bioethics and Human Rights,* Elsie Bandman and Bertram Bandman, eds. (Boston: Little, Brown,

1978), pp. 128–31; Childress, "On Ending Life," *Criterion* (Summer 1978): 4–8.

32. See Ramsey, *Ethics at the Edges of Life* and Veatch, *Death, Dying and the Biological Revolution.*

33. See Ramsey, *Ethics at the Edges of Life,* p. 153, and Veatch, *Death, Dying and the Biological Revolution,* Chapter 3. For an analysis of these books, as well as some other recent literature, see James F. Childress, "Ethical Issues in Death and Dying," *Religious Studies Review* (June 1978): 180–88.

34. See Ramsey, *The Patient as Person,* p. 120.

35. Gerald Kelly, S.J., "The Duty to Preserve Life," *Theological Studies* 12 (December 1951): 550.

36. Ramsey, *Ethics at the Edges of Life,* p. 219. In cases involving those who are dead (a) and those who are dying (b), objective medical factors are primary, and the role of expert judgment is central. Expert judgment about objective medical factors is not, of course, infallible. The possibility of error should lead to preserving life in cases of serious doubt about death or dying as a way to fulfill the duty of nonmaleficence. Another problem is the difficulty of specifying some of the criteria such as "imminence." While this term "imminent" allows physicians latitude of judgment, it suffers from vagueness, for it could mean, for example, "any second now" or "in less than one year." A similar problem plagues attempts to classify patients as either dying or nondying.

37. *Superintendent of Belchertown v. Saikewicz,* Mass. 370 N.E. 2d 417 (1977).

38. 51 Misc. 2d 616, 273 N.Y.S. 2d 624 (Sup. Ct. 1966).

39. Albert R. Jonsen and Michael J. Garland, "A Moral Policy for Life/Death Decisions in the Intensive Care Nursery," in *Ethics of Newborn Intensive Care,* Albert R. Jonsen and Michael J. Garland, eds. (Berkeley: University of California, Institute of Governmental Studies, 1976), p. 148.

40. Engelhardt, "Ethical Issues in Aiding the Death of Young Children," in *Beneficent Euthanasia,* Marvin Kohl, ed. (Buffalo, N.Y.: Prometheus Books, 1975), p. 187. Emphasis added.

41. See R. B. Zachary, "Ethical and Social Aspects of Treatment of Spina Bifida," *Lancet* 2 (1968): 274–76; John M. Freeman, "To Treat or Not to Treat: Ethical Dilemmas of Treating the Infant with a Myelomeningocele," *Clinical Neurosurgery* 20 (1973): 134–46; John Lorber, "Selective Treatment of Myelomeningocele: To Treat or Not to Treat?" *Pediatrics* 53 (1974): 307–8; several articles in Chester Swinyard, ed., *Decision Making and the Defective Newborn* (Springfield, Ill.: Charles C. Thomas, 1978); and articles on "Ethical Perspectives on the Care of Infants" and "Public Policy and Procedural Questions" in the *Encyclopedia of Bioethics.*

42. Ramsey, *Ethics at the Edges of Life,* p. 155.

43. Ibid., p. 165.

44. McCormick, "The Quality of Life, the Sanctity of Life," *The Hastings Center Report* 8 (February 1978): 32. See also "To Save or Let Die: The Dilemma of Modern Medicine," *Journal of the American Medical Association* 229 (1974): 172–76.

45. Ramsey, *Ethics at the Edges of Life,* p. 172.

46. Jonsen and Garland, "A Moral Policy for Life/Death Decisions," p. 148.
47. Veatch, *Death, Dying and the Biological Revolution*, p. 112.
48. John Rawls, *A Theory of Justice* (Cambridge, Mass.: Harvard University Press, 1971), pp. 85–86.
49. See Duff, "On Deciding the Use of the Family Commons," *Developmental Disabilities: Psychologic and Social Implications,* ed. Daniel Bergsma and Ann E. Pulver (New York: Alan R. Liss, 1976), pp. 73–84.
50. Veatch, "Generalization of Expertise," *Hastings Center Studies* 1 (May 1973): 29–40.
51. *In re Quinlan,* 70 N.J. 10 (1976).
52. *Superintendent of Belchertown State School v. Saikewicz,* Mass. 370 N.E. 2d 417 (1977).
53. See Richard A. McCormick and Andre E. Hellegers, "The Specter of Joseph Saikewicz: Mental Incompetence and the Law," *America* (1978): 257–60. Contrast George J. Annas, "The Incompetent's Right to Die: The Case of Joseph Saikewicz," *The Hastings Center Report* 8 (February 1978): 21–23. Annas holds that the adversary proceeding the court recommends is the most likely way to get a correct resolution of the difficult questions about a patient's interests and will.

5

The Principle of Beneficence

The concept of beneficence

Morality requires not only that we treat persons autonomously and not harm them but also that we contribute to their health and welfare. Such actions to benefit others are commonly placed under the heading of beneficence. While there probably are no sharp breaks or transition points on the continuum from the noninfliction of harm to the production of benefit, the principle of beneficence is generally thought to be more altruistic and farther-reaching than that of nonmaleficence because it requires positive steps to help others. Nonmaleficence, as we saw in the previous chapter, refers to the *noninfliction* of harm on others. Sometimes in moral philosophy nonmaleficence is used to refer more broadly to the *prevention* of harm and also to the *removal* of harmful conditions. However, since prevention and removal generally require positive acts that assist others, we shall use the term "beneficence" to refer to acts involving prevention of harm, removal of harmful conditions, and positive benefiting, while "nonmaleficence" will be restricted to the noninfliction of harm.

The term "beneficence" actually has an even broader usage in English, including among its meanings the doing of good, active promotion of good, kindness, and charity. But in this chapter beneficence will be understood as a *duty,* and thus as distinct from mere kindness or charity.

In its most general meaning, it is the duty to help others further their important and legitimate interests when we can do so with minimal risk to ourselves. The duty to *confer* benefits and actively to prevent and remove harms is important in biomedical and behavioral contexts, and of equal importance is the duty to *balance* the good it is possible to produce against the harms that might result from doing or not doing the good. It is thus appropriate to distinguish two principles under the general heading of beneficence: the first principle requires the *provision* of benefits, and the second requires a *balancing* of benefits and harms. The first may be called the principle of positive beneficence, while the second is already familiar to us as the principle of utility.

The principle of positive beneficence

Firmly established in the history of medicine is the belief that the failure of practitioners to increase the good of others when they are in a position to do so—and not simply failure to avoid harm—is morally and professionally wrong. The Hippocratic Oath requires that physicians benefit patients, as well as avoid harm to them, and one major justification of biomedical research is the production of positive benefits for society. Preventive medicine and active public health interventions provide other obvious examples. For instance, once methods of treating yellow fever and cowpox were discovered in early modern medicine, it was universally agreed that it would be immoral not to take positive steps to establish preventive programs. At present, to take a more current example, research in the area of gene therapy is said to be justified on the basis of its promise to provide a therapy more beneficial than its alternatives (a cure that is genotypic as well as phenotypic).

Perhaps the clearest cases in the clinical practice of medicine of acting on the duty of beneficence involve extremely dependent patients needing social assistance. Case #21 in the Appendix provides an example. Here a bill has been introduced in a state legislature that would establish community-based homes for the care and education of the mentally retarded. The bill is intended to provide medical facilities for thousands of persons who live in unpleasant, impoverished, and medically unsatisfactory facilities. There are, of course, always questions about precisely how much should be allocated by society to provide care to such persons; but that we are morally obliged to be as beneficent as possible, within our means, has seldom been at issue in moral and political philosophy, though some have argued that the *state* is not the appropriate means of beneficence.[1] Controversies usually arise only concerning how beneficent society can afford to be. Here allocation rules and decisions quite properly function to restrain or at least to place limits on beneficence. The problem of beneficence in this form converts to the problem of how, in a situation of scarcity, goods and services should be distributed in society, if they should be distributed at all. This problem should be situated under the larger umbrella of distributive justice—a topic to be considered in Chapter 6.

Because beneficence potentially demands extreme generosity in the moral life, some moral philosophers have argued that it is *virtuous,* but not a *duty,* to act beneficently. They have treated beneficent actions as akin to acts of charity or acts of conscience. From this perspective the positive benefiting of others is based on personal ideals beyond the call of duty, and thus is supererogatory rather than obligatory. There is considerable merit in this view, since we are not *always* morally required to benefit persons, even if we are in a position to do so. For example, we are not morally required to perform all possible acts of charity. In what respects and within what limits, then, is beneficence a duty?

That we normally tend to think of some beneficent actions as demanded by social duties can be seen by reference to public support of biomedical research. The obligation to benefit members of society other than those who are involved as research subjects, including future generations, is often cited as the primary justification of scientific research. For example, we do not believe that children who serve as research subjects will each individually benefit from the research in all cases. And yet we believe that at least some research involving children that presents minimal or only slightly more than minimal risk is justified. Children are often the only subjects that can be used if we are to help other children through the study of childhood disorders and child development. Research on infants, for example, has proved highly beneficial in learning about correct levels of fluids, nutriments, and oxygen in the treatment of newborns. This knowledge is generally of benefit only to succeeding generations.

In the Willowbrook case (see Appendix, Case #26), we find precisely this justification advanced by those who conducted hepatitis research that involved institutionalized and mentally retarded children. Administrators at Willowbrook used the argument that successful research would eventuate in generalizable knowledge about hepatitis that could benefit all potential victims of the disease. While it is controversial in this case whether such children should have been involved in the research at all, it is generally agreed that both individual and concerted social actions intended to benefit others are sometimes morally justified, even though they involve certain risks.

Still, it is one thing to maintain that actions or programs are morally *justified* and quite another to maintain that they are morally *required*. Thus, we have not yet demonstrated that beneficent actions are *duties*. Several proposals have been offered in moral philosophy to resolve this problem.

A first proposal involves only weak support for beneficence as a duty. William Frankena has argued that, "Even if one holds that beneficence is not a *requirement* of morality but something supererogatory and morally *good,* one is still regarding beneficence as an important part of morality— as desirable if not required."[2] This contention is of little assistance for our purposes. No one really denies that beneficent acts are morally praiseworthy when they *exceed* what is morally required. If one repaid a debt by returning even more money than one agreed to return, one would obviously have performed a morally praiseworthy and generous action. It adds little to say that it is an important "part of morality" when the whole issue is whether a different "part of morality" makes beneficence a duty. Frankena's point is that to say we "ought to do" something may mean that we ought to do it because it is a *moral* duty, or it may mean that we ought to do it because of a *self-imposed* requirement. As Feinberg[3] has put it, we should distinguish between two senses of "required": (1) required by a moral duty and (2) required by some self-imposed stricture, such as a rule of conscience or a commitment to charity. By using such distinctions, both Frankena and Feinberg leave it an open question whether beneficence is a strict moral requirement or is rather more akin to an optional act of charity.[4]

A second and more substantive proposal is that the idea of obligatory beneficent actions can be grounded in a requirement to "prevent what is bad." This approach has been suggested by Peter Singer, who relies heavily on a distinction between preventing evil and promoting good:

> I begin with the assumption that suffering and death from lack of food, shelter, and medical care are bad. . . . I shall not argue for this view. People can hold all

sorts of eccentric positions, and perhaps from some of them it would not follow that death by starvation is in itself bad. . . .

My next point is this: if it is in our power to prevent something bad from happening, without thereby sacrificing anything of comparable moral importance, we ought, morally, to do it. By "without sacrificing anything of comparable moral importance" I mean without causing anything else comparably bad to happen, or something that is wrong in itself, or failing to promote some moral good. . . . This principle seems almost as uncontroversial as the last one. It requires us only to prevent what is bad, and not to promote what is good. . . .[5]

This argument may appear to be an instance of the widely held view that society cannot legitimately impose affirmative duties to promote the good but may impose negative injunctions not to cause harm. For example, we would generally agree both that a corporation creating health hazards because of poor pollution-control devices has an obligation to cease such harm-causing activities and that this obligation is much stronger than any corporate obligation to promote social welfare—*if* the corporation has the latter obligation at all. But this distinction does *not* quite capture Singer's strategy. He in effect argues that broad commitments of *positive* actions can be grounded in the "prevention of what is bad," without committing us to a still more broadly based promotion of what is good, e.g., in the form of government-sponsored exercise programs to improve health.

While Singer is correct in maintaining that at least some moral duties rest on his principles, his argument leaves us unclear both as to the *scope* of the obligation to be beneficent and as to the moral *grounding* of the obligation to be beneficent. Singer's conception of the scope of the obligation to be beneficent is captured in the above quotation by his contention that we must always act beneficently unless something of "comparable moral importance" must be given up by performing the action. In effect, Singer argues that we must always act positively to benefit others by acting to prevent harm, unless there is a stronger prima facie duty conflicting with and overriding an opportunity to provide such a benefit. But this demand is unrealistic and overly demanding, as Michael Slote has pointed out:

It also seems probable that there are limits to our obligations to help others by preventing harms and evils. To me at least it sometimes seems mistaken to suppose that one has an obligation to go and spend one's life helping sick and starving people in India or elsewhere. Part of the reason for this may be that it can at times seem perfectly understandable, from a moral standpoint, that one should want to lead one's own life and develop one's own plans and potentialities independently of what may be going on, for better or worse, with others outside one's own family. In other words, it can sometimes seem somewhat unfair or morally arbitrary that one's moral freedom to choose one's own special kind of fulfillment in life should be abrogated by the existence of states of affairs for which one was in no way responsible and which would tend not to enter into one's life plans. . . .

It is only when something like a basic life plan has to be sacrificed in order to prevent some evil that we feel any genuine hesitation to make such prevention obligatory. . . .

And so I am saying that the following principle may be true:

It is not morally wrong to omit doing an act if (it is reasonably believed that) doing it would seriously interfere with one's basic life style or with the fulfillment of one's basic life plans—as long as the life style or plans themselves involve no wrongs of commission. . . .

[And we could] add a *principle of positive obligation* to the effect that: One has an obligation to prevent serious evil or harm when one can do so without seriously interfering with one's life plans or style and without doing any wrongs of commission.[6]

There may be unclarities and even serious moral problems in Slote's argument, but it is hard to imagine that pervasive moral rules and practices in contemporary society are more demanding than his principles suggest. Of course one might accept a moral *ideal* of the sort proposed by Singer. Society might even be more advantaged by attempting to make Singer's proposals an obligatory part of morality, but this outcome is far from obvious, given what we know about our actual abilities to live up to such high ideals.

In general we would not say that the duty of beneficence requires the passerby who is a poor and weak swimmer to try to swim a hundred yards to rescue someone who is drowning. If he does nothing, e.g., fails even to run several yards to alert a lifeguard, his omissions are morally culpable. From this and many similar examples we would argue that X has a duty of beneficence toward Y only if each of the following conditions is satisfied: (1) Y is at risk of significant loss or damage, (2) X's action is directly relevant to the prevention of this loss or damage, (3) X's action would probably prevent it, and (4) the benefit that Y will gain outweighs any harms that X is likely to suffer and does not present more than minimal risk to X.[7] To act more generously is morally praiseworthy but also is beyond the call of duty (a supererogatory action). In Rachels's cases discussed in the previous chapter, Jones violated the duty of beneficence when he stood by, doing nothing, while his six-year-old cousin drowned. Singer's cases, by contrast, may exhibit a failure of resolve and an uncertain situation in the balancing of harms and benefits, but he hardly extracts a duty from his analysis.

Despite the insufficiency of the arguments by Frankena and Singer, other important reasons can be offered for construing beneficence as a duty. Suppose hypothetically that a person could be completely abstracted from society as an island unto himself. That person's "right" to autonomous expression would be absolute, for society would have no claim on the person's actions or allegiance. Social claims on an individual—as well as social obligations to respect values such as individual autonomy—only arise in a social context. The duty to benefit others thus arises from complex social interactions. As David Hume pointed out in the eighteenth century:

All our obligations to do good to society seem to imply something reciprocal. I receive the benefits of society, and therefore ought to promote its interests. . . .[8]

This view, which might be called the reciprocity theory of moral obligations, implies that we incur obligations to help others because we have willingly received, or at least willingly will receive, beneficial assistance from them. If a person had not incurred such a reciprocal relation of benefit, then presumably that person would have no duty to act beneficently, as in the case of our hypothetical, isolated individual. The notion that we can actually be free of indebtedness to our parents, to past research in medicine and public health, to educators, to technology, etc., is as hopelessly removed from the reality of the moral life as the idea that we can always act autonomously without affecting others by our actions. One justification, then, for the claim that beneficence is a duty resides in an implicit contract underlying the necessary give and take of social life. Rawls has argued[9] that this duty is one of "fair play," and it would probably be correct to say that Hume's argument *reduces* the duty of beneficence to a duty of fair play. As we shall see, this reduction thesis is too narrow, even though the contractual-fair play grounding is *one* appropriate way of rooting beneficence in basic ethical theory.

Some previously mentioned examples can be further illuminated by this reciprocity account. Consider again the claim that it is ethically acceptable to involve infants and other young children in research. This claim is explained in terms of the conviction that these individuals have received the benefits of past research and therefore have a reciprocal social obligation to contribute to the welfare of future newborns and children. This thesis can easily, of course, be generalized beyond children to all adult members of the community.

However, some of our duties to provide benefits to others derive not from general reciprocity relations but instead from special moral relationships with others. In particular, these duties stem from our previous wrongful acts, and from explicit or implicit commitments, for instance, making promises and accepting positions involving requirements to benefit others, as well as from accepting benefits from others. To focus on the most relevant categories, we often ought to act to benefit someone either because of our "station and its duties" or because our promises require such acts. Thus, the lifeguard who has voluntarily accepted his position has a strong duty to try to rescue a drowning swimmer, even at considerable risk to himself. The claims that we make upon each other as parents, spouses, and friends similarly stem not only from interpersonal encounter but also from fixed rules, roles, and relations that constitute the matrix of obligations and duties.

The aim of the relationship between patients and health care professionals, for example, is to benefit the former. In the Hippocratic Oath, the physician makes a commitment to "come for the benefit of the sick" and to "apply dietetic measures for the benefit of the sick according to my ability and judgment." According to the AMA Code, "the principal objective of the medical profession is to render service to humanity with full respect for the dignity of man." Human needs, actual or perceived, usually form the basis of this beneficial relationship. However, these actual or felt needs are not enough in most circumstances to impose either a legal or a moral duty of service on the health care professional. The AMA Code affirms that "A physician may choose whom he will serve" (Section 5). From a legal standpoint, both the patient (or the patient's representative) and the health care professional must assent to the relationship; the former's need is not sufficient to establish a contract for service.

Of course, one must distinguish different roles a physician or other health care professional may occupy. If one is in private practice, one has no legal duty to see patients even in emergencies where no other physician is available. Thus, a physician has no legal duty even to stop at the scene of an automobile accident or to answer affirmatively when the manager of a restaurant or theater asks "is there a doctor in the house?" But if one is on duty in a hospital emergency room, one may not refuse to care for a patient.

From a moral standpoint, however, the duty of beneficence sometimes creates an obligation or duty even where the law is silent. A request for help or a need for help, as in the case of an automobile accident, imposes a moral responsibility on a health care professional to respond with his or her special knowledge and skills, as long as there is only negligible or minimal risk and no major inconvenience.[10] For example, such a person would not be expected to climb a dangerous mountain to provide aid for a stricken climber or to go several hundred miles to care for someone in need, although he might merit our praise if he did. A physician need not be a "Good Samaritan" but only what Judith Thomson calls "a minimally decent Samaritan."[11]

The principle of utility

Those engaged in medical practice and research know that risks of harm must constantly be weighed against possible benefits. The requirement that there should be a weighing assumes that risks of harm and possible benefits can be measured and balanced. The principle that we ought to bring about the greatest possible balance of value (benefit) over disvalue (harm) is of course one way of formulating the principle of utility. This principle assumes that we not only have an obligation to be positively beneficent and nonmaleficent, but that we also have a moral duty to weigh and balance possible benefits against possible harms in order to maximize benefits and minimize risks of harm. As we saw in Chapter 2, both utilitarians and deontologists need a principle of utility as a principle for balancing benefits and harms, benefits against alternative benefits, and harms against alternative harms. The moral life does not permit us simply to produce benefits and avoid harms, and for this reason a balancing principle is essential. This principle should not be construed as one that *overrides* all other principles, as many utilitarians claim. Rather, it is one principle among others; all equally specify prima facie obligations, and any principle can compete with any other for priority in a particular case.

Accordingly, it should be explicitly noted that the principle of utility should not be construed so that it allows the sacrifice of the rights of individuals to the interests of society as a whole. This inappropriate interpretation of the principle would give it a moral priority over autonomy, justice, etc. In the context of medical research it would thus seem to imply that dangerous research on human subjects could be undertaken, and even *ought* to be undertaken, when the prospect of substantial benefit to society or other individuals outweighs the danger of the research to the individual. This unqualified view of balancing utilities could lead to the sacrifice of patients' and subjects' autonomy and rights. Because in our system utility merely competes with considerations of autonomy, nonmaleficence, and justice, this problem of single-principle priority does not arise. On our construal, the principle of utility is most appropriately used as a principle that balances beneficence and nonmaleficence in conflict situations. That is, possible beneficial actions are balanced against possible harmful actions. This construal of utility is elaborated below in the section on costs and benefits.

The principle of utility is thus one factor to be considered together with positive beneficence, autonomy, justice, and nonmaleficence. For example, the interests of society *are* to be balanced against those of particular individuals in any allocation decision where tax monies are involved, as in the funding of technology, research, and public medical facilities. There can be no certain abstract formulation as to appropriate risks and benefits of, for example, human subjects in research and of society; and so the application and implementation of the principle of utility calls for a sensitive and discriminating analysis of the issues raised in particular cases.

It should also be observed that disputes as abstract as this one about the priority of rights tend to function in a vacuum that is too removed from the actual dilemmas of the moral life. On most occasions when we might question whether individual rights are being sacrificed to some larger public interest, we will be uncertain about the correct answer. This problem is nicely illustrated in Case #20. In this case an army mathematician was kept in a state of suspended animation, intentionally paralyzed by physicians in order to slow his body down to the point where it could fight off pancreatitis and related infections. This patient's hospital costs were approximately $250,000—an expense which would have been borne by the prepaid health maintenance program to which the patient belonged except for a reinsurance arrangement with Blue Cross. Even some physicians questioned the extraordinary treatment provided to this patient—both on grounds of the low probability of success and the virtual certainty of extremely high hospital costs.

It might be argued that the patient's *rights* would have been violated if the treatment had not been provided; for he did, after all, pay into the HMO, and therefore had a right to receive the available benefits. On the other hand, it is clear that no HMO or society can sustain an indefinite number of bills in this range, and if there were *many* such patients society simply could not provide such treatment, because it would be unaffordable. Most controversial disputes about individual rights conflicting with the public good have this character: individuals' needs must at some point be balanced against society's abilities to provide. It is easy in the extremes either to provide a treatment or to deny it, but the intermediate cases carry the stamp of irresolvable dilemmas. Many cases in the Appendix are dilemmatic in this respect, even if there are other ethical dilemmas in these cases that create the major ethical issue. For example, consider cases of defective newborns with diseases such as myelomeningocele (see Appendix Case #19). These cases involve issues about whether society's beneficence should extend to paying for such children and whether surgeons have an obligation to operate (rooted in beneficence) when there is a chance of a favorable outcome but a greater likelihood either of nonsurvival or of survival with multiple defects, including severe mental retardation.

The problem presented in the preceding paragraphs may seem to presuppose that the interests of society can, on balance, come into conflict with and sometimes override substantial individual interests. It is quite plausible, however, to suppose that the interests of society in general are best served by rigid observation of principles protective of individual rights. Whether or not this view is correct, it is arguably the case—to take one example—that the long-term interests of society cannot ever be served by weakening fundamental human rights to be protected against medically risky or scientifically questionable invasions.

Costs and benefits

The principles of positive beneficence and utility are often applied to moral problems when questions arise about the comparison and relative weights of costs—including risks—and benefits. Questions about the most suitable medical treatment are commonly decided by reference to likely benefits, risks, and other costs, while questions about the justification of research involving human subjects are likewise resolved by a showing that the risks are justified by the probable benefits. Such cost/benefit assessments can also play an important role in institutional settings. Members of institutional review committees, and certainly the investigators conducting the research, are expected to describe the risks and benefits for potential subjects prior to the subjects' consent to participation in the research. Investigators are customarily required not only to *array* the risks and benefits but also to determine whether the benefits *justify* the risks imposed on subjects.[12] All such applications of the principle of beneficence to research can, with only slight reformulation, be applied to the treatment of patients and to the delivery of health services.

The nature of costs, risks, and benefits

"Costs" are popularly conceived in financial terms, but in cost/benefit analysis a cost can be anything of negative value that detracts from human health and welfare. In biomedical contexts the specific costs most often mentioned are not quantifiable and already ascertained financial costs but, rather, are risks. Accordingly, we shall often employ the term "risks" rather than "costs" when making a comparison to benefits. For such purposes, the term "risk" refers to a possible future harm, and statements of risk are estimates of the probability of such harms. However, the probability of a harm's occurrence is only one way of expressing a risk and should be distinguished from the magnitude of the potential harm. When expressions such as "minimal risk" or "high risk" are used, they usually refer to the chance of experiencing a harm—its probability—and to the severity of the harm—its magnitude—in the event of occurrence. Of course uncertainty may be present in assessments of either the probability or the magnitude of harm, or both.

The contrasting term "benefit" is sometimes used merely to refer to cost avoidance, but more commonly in biomedicine it refers to something of positive value that promotes health or welfare. Unlike "risk," "benefit" is not a probabilistic term, and hence probability of benefit is the proper contrast to risk, just as benefits are comparable to harms rather than to risks of harm. Accordingly, cost/benefit relations are more precisely expressed through the language of the probability and magnitude of an anticipated benefit and the probability and magnitude of an anticipated harm.

There are many different kinds of risks and benefits. As we have seen, there are risks of physical and psychological harm, but also of damage to other interests such as reputation and property. Case #16 illustrates this range of risk. In this case a baby girl suffers from Seckel or "bird-headed" dwarfism, a recessive genetic disease, as well as multiple other medical complications. The child is at risk of starvation if an operation is not performed, but also is at risk of severe physical and mental suffering, as well as further serious medical complications, if the operation is performed. The family is at risk of psychological harm and perhaps of economic harm (because of the extremely low state per capita funding for institutions that house the retarded). Eventually, the parents decide against the surgery—a decision that in some states might place them at risk of legal harm.

Despite the many envisionable categories of risk of harm, the most likely types of harms to patients and subjects are those of pain and diminished psychological or physical ability. For patients, benefits usually accrue directly from the treatment of illness or behavioral disorders, and risks often must be taken in the hope of receiving these benefits. By contrast, participants in research that does not hold out the prospect of direct therapeutic benefit to them usually become involved in order to benefit society.

Cost/benefit analysis

Cost/benefit analysis is a much discussed but as yet underdeveloped economic and evaluative tool for decision making.[13] It is applied with some frequency to problems of health and safety. It is especially promising as a method for making explicit the overt and covert trade-offs that must be made either as a matter of individual, institutional, or public policy. There are trade-offs, for example, between the benefits of heart surgery with its attendant risks and a life of severely restricted activity without the surgery. Other trade-offs are between lives lost and money expended to save them, between the costs of research and the costs of treatment programs, and between the quality of a product and the quality of the health of those who produce it.

The simple idea behind the cost/benefit approach is that costs and benefits should be measured by some acceptable device, while uncertainties and trade-offs are similarly outlined, in order to present decision-makers with specific, relevant information that can serve as a rational basis for a decision. Although such analysis usually proceeds by measuring different quantitative units—e.g., number of accidents, statistical deaths, dollars expended, and number of persons treated—it attempts in the end to convert and express these seemingly incommensurable units of measurement into a common one, such as money, or at least to bring as many units as possible to commensurate status. This goal of an ultimate reduction gives the method its appeal, because judgments about trade-offs can be made on the basis of perfectly comparable quantities. As it is often metaphorically put, risks and benefits can then be "weighed" and "balanced" and shown to be "in a favorable ratio." Some examples will make this point clearer.

First, consider a well-known study by Klarman of the benefits of eradicating syphilis in the United States.[14] Benefits in this case are the reductions in the costs of, for example, medical care expenditures, economic deprivation from loss of employment, and pain and disablement during and after the disease. In this study the costs incurred in 1962 were measured at $117.5 million. The value of the disease's total eradication would be equivalent to this annual sum projected in perpetuity. By employing discount rates, Klarman argued that the present capital value of this eradication would be several billion dollars. Having arrived at these benefits (based on cost eradication), costs of treatment programs could then be figured for purposes of comparison. Different but parallel studies could also be provided—e.g., cost/benefit calculations based on a control program that achieved a reduction in the *incidence* of the disease but did not eradicate it. Because of the rapid emergence of highly resistant strains, the latter kind of cost/benefit analysis would be the most useful, though Klarman unfortunately did not provide it.

Consider as a second example the issue of proposed standards for occupational exposure to the carcinogen benzene—a case recently under study by OSHA (Occupational Safety and Health Administration), because of reports of excessive leukemia deaths related to benzene in industrial manufacturing plants. In his testimony in this case, Richard Wilson argues both that "an average level of benzene in the work place of 10 parts per million (ppm) is much more acceptable than many other actions" and that the social benefits of the manufacture of benzene at these levels outweighs the risks associated with such production.[15] Wilson recognizes that benzene is a carcinogen and that we must be cautious about the level allowed. His point is that we have no choice except to settle for a conservative estimate of the risks, as determined largely by dose levels generalized from animal studies. If he is correct, we have no rational policy option but to accept a dose level in the vicinity of that point at which we cannot scientifically demonstrate that benzene in such doses produces cancer in humans, even though it demonstrably is a carcinogen. This argument turns on a showing that the entire hazard cannot be banned because too many significant benefits (not directly related to health) would be lost. All manufacture of gasoline, for example, would have to be prohibited. Yet compliance costs at levels less than 10 ppm would be in the hundreds of millions of dollars and would render manufacture nonprofitable—without any evidence that workers would be more, rather than less, protected when all possible harms are taken into consideration.

Although in the benzene case risks beyond the testable level are not known, Wilson's reasoning is not remote from decision analysis that is required elsewhere in biomedicine—for example, in deciding whether to produce the implantable artificial heart, as reported in Case #23 in the Appendix. In both cases we must ask how much society should pay to reduce health-related risks. These risks are continually reducible to lower levels, but at geometrically increasing financial costs. And in both cases the risk of death itself can never be eliminated. The ideal presumably is a level of risk that is socially acceptable, where acceptability is determined by what must elsewhere be given up in the way of benefits in order to achieve the appropriate level. It is this level of acceptability that cost/benefit analyses promise to provide, or at least to help us determine. This claim should not be construed to mean either that all costs and benefits can be fully quantified or that all uncertainties of risk can be eliminated. Rather, it means that there are principles and standards operative in cost/benefit decisions that can often be stated in considerable detail so that *unclarity in the judgmental process is reduced.* It is this reduction of intuitive weighing in the formulation of policy that is of greatest significance in the cost/benefit approach.[16]

The need for this reduction of unclarity has been aptly illustrated in many recent decisions by federal regulatory and administrative agencies (such as the Environmental Protection Agency, the Occupational Safety and Health Administration, and the Food and Drug Administration), whose decisions directly affect the nation's health. An example is found in Case #22 in the Appendix, which recounts the difficulties in, but also the necessity of, making a cost/benefit decision at the National Institutes of Health over how much to budget for cancer research and how much to budget for arthritis research. The frustration of the Director of the National Institute of Arthritis, Metabolism, and Digestive Diseases is directly due to the unavailability of an objective means of assessing the relative worth of funding arthritis research by comparison with cancer research.

Despite the promise held out by the examples mentioned above—and by cost/benefit methodology in general—it will only rarely be possible to use precise quantitative techniques in the ultimate assessment of whether a medical treatment or research protocol is justified, and we must candidly face up to the difficulties that are presented by a purely quantitative model of weighing risks and benefits. This problem is illustrated in Case #24, involving the use of CAT scanning for diagnostic purposes: larger dollar costs of using CAT scans must be weighed against the benefits of the procedure as well as the lower risk presented to patients. In this case both CAT scanning and a less expensive (but more risky, etc.) method will presumably yield the identical diagnostic finding.

Instead of a purely quantitative ideal, then, the proper model for biomedical evaluations is the systematic, nonarbitrary, and nonintuitive comparison of benefits and risks. Such a model demands that justifications of a mode of treatment or a research protocol be thorough in the assimilation and evaluation of information about all aspects of the procedures under consideration, and that those assimilating the data be explicit in stating operative standards and principles as well as quantitative measurements for considering and weighing alternative procedures. When carefully spelled out, cost/benefit analysis can render the entire process of evaluating clinical procedures, research protocols, and preventive measures more rigorous and precise, while at the same time enhancing the quality of information transmitted when informed consent is solicited.

Unfortunately, in some cases the risks and benefits may be fairly well known, and yet one may be incapable of determining whether the benefits *outweigh* the risks. For example, take the case of a premature infant born by Caesarean section after a 34-week gestation period. At birth the baby was "blue, limp, had no reflexes, and a very slow heart rate"—and also had excessive fluid and an enlarged liver and spleen. The parents wanted the child very much, and intense resuscitation measures were initiated. At 14 minutes of age the child was doing poorly and had no spontaneous activity. The doctors feared that "there is an extremely high risk" that a retarded baby (at best) would result from further medical efforts. Physicians and nurses expressed strong differences of opinion as to whether resuscitation efforts should continue, at least if the baby once stopped breathing. Such a dispute can be anchored in considerations other than an assessment of risks and benefits, of course. But how one actually weighs the high risk of mental retardation and the probable disappointment of the parents against the slender possibility of a healthy baby and the parents' known desire to have the child is a matter clearly subject to differences of opinion, even if the probability of harm and the probability of benefit were well established and agreed upon by all. Risk/benefit assessments thus will not function as a panacea for decision-makers.

Nonetheless, risk/benefit analysis can be a useful practical tool. Its immediate utility may be made more concrete by a consideration of how it might be applied in the creation of guidelines for the assessment of research involving human subjects. Those responsible for constructing and evaluating research protocols should, we suggest, employ the risk/benefit approach as follows: There should first be a determination of questionable presuppositions of the research and of the risks that might result from the conduct of the research. Probability, magnitude, and uncertainty should be distinguished with as much clarity as possible in estimations of risk. The method of aggregating risks should similarly be revealed, especially where there is no alternative to the use of such vague categories as small or slight risk. For example, one way of measuring total risk is to multiply the probability of harm, e.g., a statistic based on frequency of past injuries, by the magnitude of harm, e.g., a statistic derived from a scale of ascending numbers corresponding to harms (from minor injuries, such as muscle pains, to deaths). Such measurements in the form of risk indices are useful for comparative purposes, which in turn assist in establishing priorities.

For those persons charged with the review and approval of proposed patient therapies and research protocols, some features of this process will have special importance. Estimates of the proclaimed probability of harm may be too low or estimates of the probability of benefit inflated, as judged by known facts or other available studies in the domain of the research under review. Definitional standards used in the assessment of risk, e.g., a standard of minimal risk, can also be unwarrantably low, even though the estimate reached by the use of such standards is correct.

Finally, even if it were possible to measure all risks and benefits with precision, it would not follow that a favorable or positive net sum of benefits would justify a particular therapeutic intervention or research procedure or that an unfavorable comparison of risks and benefits would render the treatment or research unjustified. Some criteria of the *acceptability* of risk are independent of the analysis and comparison of risks and benefits themselves. In some cases the same level of risk may be acceptable if borne by those who will receive the benefits, but unacceptable if borne by those who will not receive the benefits. Obviously, one major consideration in determining the acceptability of risk is the presence or absence of an informed and consenting individual. In order to show respect for their autonomy, consenting patients and subjects must often, and perhaps always, be allowed to assume risks impermissible for non-consenting persons.

This general problem is present in Case #9, where burn victims, suffering from wounds so severe that their survival is unprecedented, are called upon to make decisions about their treatment. Whereas persons other than the actual victims might elect maximal therapeutic efforts, some patients might reasonably choose only ordinary care, even though the risk of death is thereby increased. The level of risk willingly assumed by a consenting individual may also in some cases permissibly exceed the sum of benefits that persons other than the individual at risk believe likely to occur. A primary consideration in the determination that risk is acceptable is the worth of the therapeutic procedure or the research to the person who stands to benefit from it, especially if that person alone must bear the risk.

Of course, cost/benefit analysis, and the principle of beneficence generally, can be applied not only to individuals but to society as a whole. Determinations of justified medical practice traditionally involve a comparison of risks and benefits only for individual subjects, but determinations of justified research are more complicated. Patients and subjects should always be protected by the scrutiny of risks, but it would not satisfy the principles discussed in this chapter (especially utility) if the need to protect individuals against harm were not balanced against possible benefits of an intervention—in many cases for an entire population. For example, beneficent acts should protect not only against risk of harm to subjects of research but also against the risk of losing the substantial benefits that might be gained from the research. When skillfully done, risk/benefit analysis shows that such complex balancing judgments are generally present in the hard cases.

Cost/benefit analysis has been accused of serious deficiencies for a wide variety of reasons. There are methodological problems in the measurement of values, and especially in rendering commensurable all the units of value that must be compared. This problem can itself lead to arbitrary decision making, and cost/benefit methods as developed in economics have proved difficult to implement concretely. There are also problems concerning how to compute discount rates, psychological effects, and indirect effects of certain personal and social interventions. We have attempted to circumvent these problems in our general presentation of cost/benefit analysis by treating such analysis as encompassing nonquantitative considerations. However, one important ethical problem deserves special attention. Utilitarianism and cost/benefit procedures are commonly said to fail to take account of problems of distributive justice. That is, as a matter of ethics, distribution merely according to the dictates of favorable cost/benefit analyses may produce injustices—as when a study of the costs and benefits of treating mental retardation might show that costs outweigh benefits, and yet justice might demand that special benefits should nonetheless be extended to mentally retarded persons. This important problem will be treated in Chapter 6.

Paternalism

The nature of paternalism

The health care professional or bureaucrat sometimes has a conception of benefits, harms, and their balance that differs from that of the patient. Whose conception of the requirements of beneficence should prevail, that of the health care professional or that of the patient? This issue is complicated by the fact that depressed patients, those on dialysis, and those addicted to potentially harmful drugs may not be likely to reach adequately reasoned decisions. Even patients who are competent and deliberative can make poor choices about courses of action recommended by physicians. Some health care professionals are inclined to respect autonomy by not interfering beyond attempts at persuasion when patients choose harmful courses of action, while others are inclined to protect patients against the consequences of their own choices. The problem of whether or not to intervene in the decisions and affairs of such persons is the problem of paternalism.[17]

Although the *Oxford English Dictionary* dates the term "paternalism" from the 1880's, the idea is much older and, indeed, appears very early in human thought. Its meaning, according to the OED, is "the principle and practice of paternal administration; government as by a father; the claim or attempt to supply the needs or to regulate the life of a nation or community in the same way a father does those of his children." When the analogy with the father is used to illuminate the role of professionals or the state in health care, it presupposes two features of the paternal role: that the father is benevolent and beneficent, i.e., that he has the interests of his children at heart, and that he makes all or at least some of the decisions relating to his children's welfare rather than letting them make these decisions. Paternalism poses moral questions precisely because it involves the claim that beneficence should take precedence over autonomy, at least in some cases.[18]

The problem of paternalism is discernible in outline form in our previous analysis of autonomy, particularly in the discussion of informed consent in Chapter 3. There we studied two alternative models of informed consent, both of which can influence one's perspective on paternalism. According to the first model, which may be called the autonomy model, consent is required because it respects autonomy by granting individuals the right to choose what shall be done to them. According to the second model, which may be called the protection model, consent in medical contexts functions to maximize benefits and minimize harms for individuals. The protection model, based on the duty of beneficence, would support paternalistic intervention, while the autonomy model would generally oppose it. For the autonomy model, the individual's own conception of good should determine what is done to him; for the protection model, not to maximize benefits and minimize harms for individuals, even against their wishes, is to violate the principle of beneficence.

Case #6 illustrates these problems of informed consent and paternalism. A woman had a fatal reaction during urography (visualization of the urinary tract made after injection of an opaque medium). The radiologist had not informed her of a possible fatal reaction to urography on grounds that his duty was to do "what is best for our patients medically." He apparently thought it was best in this case not to inform the patient of risks of death because the information might actually have been "dangerous" instead of protective. In other words, he conceived the doctor's role in informed consent situations as that of making a judgment whether the presentation of information is more or less harmful to the patient. In this particular case he determined that it was not "in the best interest of the patient" to be informed because the risks of death were remote, while the possibility of causing undue alarm was immediate. This attitude is clearly paternalistic and grounded in beneficence, but is it justified to act on such an attitude?

The case just considered is only one of many different types of truth-telling cases involving paternalism. Other cases lie in areas where the news might adversely affect someone's health or lead to suicide, as when a cancer victim is told the truth about his condition. If a patient asks in a sincere manner to be told the truth, it is paternalistic, under most understandings of paternalism, to withhold the truth. There are similar examples outside the scope of serious patient illness—e.g., certain forms of genetic screening programs. If it is known that a woman is opposed to abortion and it is discovered that she has a seriously defective fetus, it might be judged in her best interest to withhold the truth about the fetus on grounds that it would spare her months of grief (and of course the fetus might later be stillborn). Problems of paternalism are not restricted to truth-telling cases. As we shall see, paternalistic intervention extends to many domains of biomedical practice and research, including suicide intervention and the prohibition of dangerous research involving human subjects.

Cases of paternalism involve overriding a person's wishes, wants, or actions in order to benefit or to prevent harm to that person. There are nonpaternalistic reasons for overriding a person's wishes, wants, and actions. Most importantly, we generally believe that it is morally justified to prevent harm to persons when the harm is caused or would be caused by those whose liberty is restricted. This principle, sometimes called the harm principle, was articulated by John Stuart Mill in *On Liberty,* a classic text of antipaternalism:

The object of this Essay is to assert one very simple principle. . . . That principle is, that the sole end for which mankind are warranted, individually or collectively, in interfering with the liberty of action of any of their number, is self-protection. That the only purpose for which power can be rightfully exercised over any member of a civilized community, against his will, is to prevent harm to others. His own good, either physical or moral, is not a sufficient warrant. He cannot rightfully be compelled to do or forbear because it will be better for him to do so, because it will make him happier, because in the opinion of others, to do so would be wise, or even right. These are good reasons for remonstrating with him, or reasoning with him or persuading him, or entreating him, but not for compelling him, or visiting him with any evil in case he do otherwise. To justify that, the conduct from which it is desired to deter him must be calculated to produce evil to someone else. The only part of the conduct of anyone, for which he is amenable to society, is that which concerns others. In the part which merely concerns himself, his independence is of right, absolute.[19]

A second reason, which is rarely if ever satisfactory, is the principle of moralism. This principle proclaims it justifiable to restrict a person's liberty even when no one is harmed, including the individual himself, and when there is no drain on common resources, simply because the action is morally wrong or sinful—as some sexual acts between consenting adults are alleged to be.

Both paternalism and Mill's harm principle arguably rest on the principle of beneficence, because beneficence includes producing good, preventing harm, and removing harm. But in a system such as Mill's, which allows only the harm principle, an individual must be allowed to pursue his own decisions when others are not affected, i.e., when he alone is affected. By contrast, the principle of paternalism authorizes interventions to protect the individual from the consequences of his choices, wishes, and actions. In many cases (e.g., in debates about legislation requiring motorcycle helmets) paternalism and the harm principle are both invoked, but the fact that these and various other principles are relevant to debates about the same case should obscure neither their distinctiveness nor the importance of being clear when a single principle would be sufficient to justify overriding a person's choices, wishes, and actions.

Are paternalistic interventions justified?

In the literature on paternalism, two main positions have been adopted: (1) "Justified Paternalism" and (2) "Antipaternalism." The first of these views has been held by such recent moral philosophers as H.L.A. Hart and Gerald Dworkin, while Mill represents the latter view.

(1) *The justification of paternalism.* Any supporter of the paternalistic principle will specify with care precisely which goods, needs, and interests warrant paternalistic protection. In recent formulations, it has been said that the state is justified in interfering with a person's liberty if that interference protects the person against his or her own choices of actions that are extremely and unreasonably risky, e.g., dangerous self-administered medical experiments, or are potentially dangerous and irreversible in effect, as some drugs are. Supporters of justified paternalism argue nonetheless that it takes a heavy burden of justification to limit free choices and actions by competent persons, especially since there is never direct consent (even if there is second-party consent or direct consent to submit to a paternalistic power). According to this position, paternalism could be justified only if the evils prevented from occurring to the person are greater than the evils caused by interference with his liberty and only if it is universally justified under relevantly similar circumstances to treat persons in this way. Roughly this position is defended by Gerald Dworkin, who argues in an influential article that paternalism should be regarded as a form of "social insurance policy" that fully rational persons would take out in order to protect themselves.[20] Such persons would know, for example, that they might be tempted at times to make decisions that are far-reaching, potentially dangerous, and irreversible, while at other times they might suffer extreme psychological or social pressures to do something they truly believe too risky to be worth performing, e.g., where one's honor is placed in question by a challenge to fight. In still other cases Dworkin believes that persons might not sufficiently understand or appreciate dangers that are relevant to their conduct, e.g., one might not know the facts about research on smoking. Dworkin concludes that we all ought to agree to a limited grant of power to others to control our actions.

A case of the sort that inclines some toward paternalism is found in the Appendix as Case #8. In this case an involuntarily committed mental patient wishes to leave the hospital, though his family is opposed to his release. The patient argues that his mental condition does not justify confinement, yet his history is as follows: He has been confined several times previously. After one confinement he plucked out his right eye. After another confinement he severed his right hand. The patient functions fairly normally in the state hospital, where he sells news materials to fellow patients and handles limited financial affairs. The source of his "problems" apparently is found in his religious beliefs. He regards himself as a true prophet of God and believes that "it is far better for one man to believe and accept an appropriate message from God to sacrifice an eye or a hand according to the sacred scriptures rather than for the present course of the world to cause even greater loss of human life." He acts on this belief, engaging in self-mutilation. According to the paternalist, this person generally functions normally, by usual behavioral or observational criteria, yet needs help. His capacities are too diminished and the substantial threat he presents to himself is too severe to leave him without confinement and custodial care.

(2) *Antipaternalistic individualism.* Some believe that paternalism is never justified, whatever the conditions. This position is basically the one supported by Mill—viz., that the principle of paternalism is not a valid principle for restricting liberty, because it allows too much restriction. The serious adverse consequences of giving such power to the state, or to any class of individuals, such as physicians, motivates antipaternalists to reject the view that the fully rational person would accept paternalism. In addition, they are concerned about the loss of individual liberty, and they generally believe that the autonomous individual more than likely is in a position to ascertain his own best interest more competently than someone who would substitute a judgment about that person's best interest.

Why, from this perspective, ought paternalism to be judged an unacceptable moral principle? The dominant reason offered by antipaternalists is that paternalistic principles are too broad and hence justify too much. For example, Robert Harris has argued that paternalism would in principle "justify the imposition of a Spartan-like regimen requiring rigorous physical exercise and abstention from smoking, drinking, and hazardous pastimes."[21] The more thoughtful restrictions on paternalism proposed by Dworkin would disallow this sort of extreme but, according to antipaternalists, would still leave both unacceptable latitude of judgment in contexts where authoritative controls are likely to be abused and unresolved problems concerning the scope of the principle. On the latter point, suppose that a man risks his life for the advance of medicine by submitting to an unreasonably risky experiment, an act most would think not in his own best interest. Are we to commend him or coercively restrain him? Paternalism suggests that it would be permissible to restrain such a person. Yet if that is so, antipaternalists argue, then the state is permitted in principle to restrain coercively its morally heroic citizens, not to mention its martyrs, if they act—as such people frequently do—in a manner "harmful" to themselves.

The medical example that has the most extensive antipaternalistic literature is the involuntary hospitalization of persons who have neither actually been harmed by others nor actually harmed themselves but are thought to stand in danger of being harmed by others or of harming themselves. These cases involve what might be called double paternalism: a paternalistic justification for commitment and another paternalistic justification for therapy after commitment, e.g., psychotherapy or chemotherapy. A widely discussed case of this sort is that of Mrs. Catherine Lake, included in the Appendix as Case #7. Mrs. Lake suffered from arteriosclerosis causing temporary confusion and mild loss of memory, interspersed with times of mental alertness and rationality. All parties agreed that Mrs. Lake never harmed anyone or presented any threat of danger, yet she was committed to a mental institution because she often seemed confused and defenseless. At her trial, while apparently fully rational, she testified that she knew the risk of living outside the hospital and preferred to take that risk rather than be in the hospital environment. The Court of Appeals denied her petition, arguing that she is "mentally ill," "is a danger to herself . . . and is not competent to care for herself." The legal justification cited by the Court was a statute that "provides for involuntary hospitalization of a person who is 'mentally ill and, because of that illness, is likely to injure himself'. . . ."[22] Antipaternalists resist the reasoning of this Court on grounds that such actions involve an unjustifiable restriction and violation of human liberty. This objection is commonly based on Mill's view that the harm principle alone provides valid grounds for the restriction of liberty. Since Mrs. Lake is not causing harm to others and understands the dangers under which she is placing herself, she should be free to proceed as she wishes, according to antipaternalists.

Strong and weak paternalism

One dividing point between the supporters of a limited paternalism (such as Dworkin) and the opponents of paternalism (such as Mill) is the emphasis placed on the actual capabilities for autonomous action by those making choices. (Cf. the discussion of competence in Chapter 3.)

Supporters of paternalism tend to cite examples of persons of at least slightly diminished capacity—for example, persons on kidney dialysis and those in depression. By contrast, opponents cite examples of persons who are capable of autonomous choice, at least in some contexts—for example, those involuntarily committed merely for eccentric behavior, prisoners not permitted to volunteer for research on drugs, and those who rationally elect to refuse treatment in life-threatening circumstances.

Joel Feinberg's[23] distinction between *strong* and *weak* paternalism illuminates this disagreement. Weak paternalism is explained as follows:

[One] has the right to prevent self-regarding conduct only when it is *substantially nonvoluntary* or when temporary intervention is necessary to establish whether it is voluntary or not.

The class of nonvoluntary actions includes cases of consents that are not adequately informed. Strong paternalism, by contrast, holds that it is sometimes proper to protect or to benefit a person by limiting his liberty even when his choices are informed and voluntary.

Virtually everyone acknowledges that some acts of weak paternalism are justified acts of beneficence, e.g., preventing a person under the influence of LSD from killing himself. But weak paternalism may not be paternalism in an interesting sense because—as Feinberg himself notes—it may not be a liberty-limiting principle that is independent of the harm and autonomy principles. That is, if the justification of so-called "paternalistic" interventions *always* rests on the harm principle or perhaps the autonomy principle, then paternalism is dependent upon and reducible to these other principles. For this reason some writers have rendered "paternalism" synonymous with "strong paternalism."

To the present writers it is difficult and perhaps impossible to justify strong paternalism,[24] though many forms of weak paternalism may be justified. For example, some cases (cf. Case #12) of coercive transfusions of blood are instances of strong paternalism that involve a serious violation of autonomy that cannot be justified by appeals to beneficence and nonmaleficence. Perhaps the most plausible kind of case favoring strong paternalistic interventions under some circumstances would be the following: A psychiatrist is treating a patient like the patient in Case #8 who plucks out his eyes and cuts off his hands for religious reasons. Let us suppose that this patient is not insane and acts conscientiously on his quite unique religious views. Suppose further that this patient asks the psychiatrist a question about his condition, a question that has a definite answer, but which, if answered, would lead the patient to engage in self-maiming behavior in order to satisfy the demands of his religious convictions. Many would be inclined to say that the doctor acts paternalistically but justifiably by concealing information from the patient. Those who believe the physician acts justifiably probably think so because they believe the patient is acting on false religious beliefs and so is uninformed. But suppose the patient were genuinely rational and relevantly informed. Would this case then be an instance of strong paternalism with a plausible claim to justifiability? Paternalism may seem justified in this case for another reason. We may be uncertain about the extent to which the person's actions are voluntary. This uncertainty pervades the cases of strong paternalism that appear to be justified. Moreover, this uncertainty provides one reason why some writers believe that all justified paternalistic interventions are instances of weak paternalism and not of strong paternalism.

There are many examples of justified weak paternalism. Everyone familiar with the practice of medicine knows that some patients who are mentally alert nonetheless can suffer from conditions that affect their behavior, such as depression, drug addiction, and abnormal EEG patterns. Such persons are capable of making judgments that affect their lives, but their limitations can have an important and immediate effect on their decisions. For example, while most everyone would favor allowing children to be consulted about important decisions affecting their lives in medical contexts, almost everyone believes that even the wishes of fairly mature children are sometimes validly overridden in order to provide important therapeutic benefits. If a child bitten by a rabid dog was terrified at the thought of undergoing treatment and refused to submit to it, we would regard the youth's parents and physician as irresponsible if they did not override the child's wishes and force the treatment. Similar cases involving adult patients on dialysis who are suffering from uremia (retention in the blood of toxic urinary constituents) or suicidal patients suffering from serious depression likewise invite paternalistic treatment. To allow persons to die through their own decisions would be callous and uncaring where certain conditions reduce the informed or voluntary character of their actions.

In some of his writings in medical ethics, Robert Veatch has argued that a "priestly model" of medical practice should be set aside in favor of what he calls a "collegial model." For him, informed consent should entirely replace paternalism. He bemoans what he calls a "paternalism in the realm of values" that leads physicians to rely on the principle "benefit and do no harm to the patient" without considering the autonomous expressions of patients.[25] While Veatch's ideal is admirable, it is unrealistic for much of medical practice. The physician is thrust into a paternalistic role on numerous occasions by the questionable condition of his patients, by their enormous regard for his knowledge of their conditions, and perhaps by their unwillingness or inability to make hard decisions. It can be argued that on some occasions the physician actually protects autonomy by overriding the immediate wishes of a patient. For example, in Case #10 a doctor knows that a terminally ill person, who has been his patient for many years, suffers severe and prolonged depression when given distressing news about his health. So deep is the depression when it occurs that the person is effectively incapacitated from making autonomous judgments. While he has shown tendencies in the past to suicide, he is opposed on religious grounds to the taking of his own life and always suffers both a failure of nerve and powerful guilt when he starts to devise a way of ending his life. Though utterly unaware of his terminal condition, he asks his doctor point blank for a complete explanation of a recent physical examination during which the doctor discovered his fatal illness. The doctor tells him that he has never been in better health. Few would say that the doctor made a wrong choice, yet this decision is both paternalistic and a clear-cut case of lying. Moreover, it is particularly interesting since it straddles the boundary between strong paternalism and weak paternalism. Although the patient does act autonomously in making the request for the information, he would not be able to act autonomously if he were given the information.

Such cases illustrate how complex the interactions sometimes become in the attempt to balance considerations of autonomy, beneficence, nonmaleficence, and justice in the treatment of patients. A necessary condition of justified paternalistic actions has already been set forth in rough outline: the paternalistic intervention would have to avoid an extremely risky circumstance where there are potentially serious and irreversible consequences for the patient, as well as no available alternatives that are likely to be more beneficial. Whether it would also be necessary that a state of partial ignorance or partial involuntariness be present—or at least that we cannot ascertain whether such a condition is present—is an unresolved matter of vigorous contemporary debate. This issue is whether strong paternalism is ever justified by balancing an act of beneficence against an invasion of autonomy.

Mill's example of a person about to cross a dangerous bridge provides a promising approach to these problems. If we are unsure whether a person's actions are voluntary or whether the person's judgment is informed, it would be justifiable to intervene temporarily in order to ascertain whether his actions are voluntary and whether he has adequate information. Once adequately informed under conditions of voluntary choice, the agent should be permitted to make the decision. Still, what should be done in those cases of partially voluntary and partially involuntary actions, where it is impossible to satisfy the demands of Mill's proviso? These might be cases involving mental retardation, ongoing psychotic compulsion, or repeated tendencies to suicide. In such cases persons ought to be protected against harms that might result directly from their limiting conditions. To the extent one protects a person from harms produced by causes beyond his knowledge and control, the intervention has plausible claim to being morally justified, for his choices are substantially nonvoluntary. No doubt degrees of control and voluntariness rest on a multilevel continuum, but we can make informed discriminations in most important cases as to the substantial voluntariness or involuntariness of the action.

In conclusion, it should be noted that there are cases where justifications for an action may deceptively appear to be paternalistic, but in fact are based on nonpaternalistic grounds. An example is found in research involving prisoners. In 1976 the National Commission for the Protection of Human Subjects of Biomedical and Behavioral Research issued a report on *Research Involving Prisoners*.[26] It argued that the closed nature of prison environments creates a strong potential for abuse of authority and therefore invites the exploitation and coercion of prisoners. However, a Commission study indicated that most prisoners do not regard their consent to research as obtained under coercion or undue influence. The Commission argued that the inherent coercive possibilities in prisons nonetheless justify regulations prohibiting many types of prisoners from engaging in research, even if they wish to do so.

This justification may appear overtly paternalistic, but closer analysis of the Commission report shows that it is not. The Commission explicitly maintained that if an environment were *not* exploitative or coercive (and if a few other standards were met), then prisoners should be free to choose to participate in research. The Commission's justifying ground was the factual claim that most prisons could not be made sufficiently free of coercion and exploitation by drug companies and prison officials, not the moral claim that prisoners should be protected from their own *freely* chosen actions. Hence the justification is only apparently based on the paternalistic principle. The harm principle provides the real basis: because it is unpredictable whether prisoners will be exploited in settings that render them vulnerable, research to which they might appear to consent validly should nonetheless be prohibited because we cannot adequately monitor the actual validity of the consent. Many decisions about the justification of actions in medical practice and research turn on whether it is the harm principle or some paternalistic principle that actually applies in the circumstances.

We conclude that weak paternalism is a coherent and defensible moral position, though it applies only to a narrow range of cases where patients and subjects are clearly endangered. Strong paternalism, by contrast, is more difficult and perhaps impossible to justify. While some cases of strong paternalism do not seem inherently immoral, the probable abuse of a policy of strong paternalism could outweigh the probable benefits unless the lines could be more carefully drawn then they have been in the past.

Notes

1. Robert Nozick's *Anarchy, State, and Utopia* (New York: Basic Books, 1974) stands in notable exception to the general claim that society is morally obliged to be beneficent to individuals.

2. *Ethics,* 2nd ed. (Englewood Cliffs, N.J.: Prentice-Hall, Inc., 1973), p. 47. Frankena includes moral ideals under the umbrella of "the ingredients of morality" (p. 67f).

3. "The Nature and Value of Rights," *Journal of Value Inquiry* 4 (1970): 243–57, especially 244ff.

4. Frankena later does say (*Ethics,* p. 47) that principles of beneficence specify "prima facie duties," but it remains unclear whether this means that they are moral *requirements* (as Ross's theory of prima facie duties entails that they are), for Frankena allows for an extremely lengthy list of possible prima facie duties (pp. 48, 56). See also Frankena's subsequent essay, "Moral Philosophy and World Hunger," in W. Aiken and H. LaFollette, eds., *World Hunger and*

Moral Obligation (Englewood Cliffs, N.J.: Prentice-Hall, 1977), pp. 66–84, especially pp. 70, 73.

5. "Famine, Affluence, and Morality," *Philosophy and Public Affairs* 1 (1972), as reprinted in T. Mappes and J. Zembaty, eds., *Social Ethics* (New York: McGraw-Hill, 1977), p. 317. This article is updated in "Reconsidering the Famine Relief Argument," in Peter Brown and Henry Shue, eds., *Food Policy: The Responsibility of the United States in the Life and Death Choices* (New York: The Free Press, 1977).

6. Michael A. Slote, "The Morality of Wealth," in *World Hunger and Moral Obligation,* pp. 125–27.

7. Our formulation of these conditions is indebted to Eric D'Arcy, *Human Acts: An Essay in their Moral Evaluation* (Oxford: Clarendon Press, 1963), pp. 56–57.

8. "On Suicide," as reprinted in S. Gorovitz et al., eds., *Moral Problems in Medicine* (Englewood Cliffs, N.J.: Prentice-Hall, 1976), p. 386.

9. John Rawls, "Legal Obligation and the Duty of Fair Play," in Sidney Hook, ed., *Law and Philosophy* (New York: New York University Press, 1964).

10. While the AMA Code grants discretion to the physician in determining whom he will serve, it adds that "in an emergency, however, he should render service to the best of his ability" (Section 5). This principle is annotated: "He should . . . respond to any request for his assistance in an emergency or whenever temperate public opinion expects the service" (1971 edition).

11. Judith Jarvis Thomson, "A Defense of Abortion," *Philosophy and Public Affairs* I (1971), as reprinted in Tom L. Beauchamp, ed., *Ethics and Public Policy* (Englewood Cliffs, N.J.: Prentice-Hall, 1975), pp. 319–21. (Slote acknowledges an indebtedness to this essay for part of his analysis of the duty of beneficence.)

12. The functions and moral obligations of such committees are analyzed in a report on the subject by the National Commission for the Protection of Human Subjects: *Report and Recommendations: Institutional Review Boards,* including a separate *Appendix* (Washington: DHEW Publication Nos. (OS) 78-0008 and (OS) 78-0009, 1978). This study includes considerations of cost/benefit analysis.

13. A comprehensive source for economists' accounts of cost/benefit analysis is E. J. Mishan, *Cost-Benefit Analysis,* Expanded ed. (New York: Praeger Publishers, 1976). On the nature of risk, cf. William W. Lowrance, *Of Acceptable Risk: Science and the Determination of Safety* (Los Altos, Calif.: William Kaufmann, 1976). For applied studies in the area of health and medicine, see John P. Bunker et al., *Costs, Risks, and Benefits of Surgery* (New York: Oxford University Press, 1977) and a special issue of the *George Washington Law Review* 45 (August 1977) devoted to "Risk-Benefit Assessment in Governmental Decisionmaking." For a philosophical critique of cost/benefit reasoning, cf. Alasdair MacIntyre, "Utilitarianism and Cost/Benefit Analysis: An Essay on the Relevance of Moral Philosophy to Bureaucratic Theory," in

K. Sayre, ed., *Values in the Electric Power Industry* (Notre Dame, Ind.: University of Notre Dame Press, 1977). MacIntyre's essay is reprinted with a reply by Tom L. Beauchamp in Tom Beauchamp and Norman Bowie, eds., *Ethical Theory and Business* (Englewood Cliffs, N.J.: Prentice-Hall, 1979), Chapter 4.

14. H. E. Klarman, "Syphilis Control Problems," in R. Dorfman, ed., *Measuring Benefits of Government Investments* (Washington: Brookings Institution, 1965).

15. Richard Wilson. Direct Testimony. *In re Proposed Standards for Occupational Exposure to Benzene* (Washington: OSHA Docket No. H-059, 1977), pp. 10ff.

16. This point has been repeatedly stressed in cases of environmental law that deal with problems of risks to health as balanced against other economic and social benefits. Cf., e.g., Judge David Bazelon's decision in *Environmental Defense Fund v. William D. Ruckelshaus and the Environmental Protection Agency*. 439 F.2d 584 (D.C. Circuit 1971).

17. The term "paternalism" is not wholly felicitous, especially because it is sex-linked. While it might be desirable to use another term, such as "parentalism," the term "paternalism" is established by usage and philosophical discussion.

18. It is important to note, as Frankena has suggested, that "beneficence requires us to respect the liberty of others." *Ethics*, p. 53. Thus we have a conflict of obligations generated by beneficence itself when we attempt both to protect persons *and* to respect their liberty.

19. *On Liberty*, as reprinted in *Essential Works of John Stuart Mill* (New York: Bantam Books, 1961), p. 263.

20. "Paternalism," *The Monist* (January 1972): 64–84. Cf. also Bernard Gert and Charles Culver, "Paternalistic Behavior," *Philosophy & Public Affairs* 6 (Fall 1976): 45–57. The above formulation is indebted to both articles.

21. "Private Consensual Adult Behavior: The Requirement of Harm to Others in the Enforcement of Morality," *UCLA Law Review* 14 (1967): 585n.

22. Cf. Jay Katz, Joseph Goldstein, and Alan M. Dershowitz, eds., *Psychoanalysis, Psychiatry, and the Law* (New York: The Free Press, 1967), pp. 552–54, 710–13.

23. Joel Feinberg, "Legal Paternalism," *The Canadian Journal of Philosophy* 1 (1971): 105–24. See pp. 113, 116. Also, *Social Philosophy* (Englewood Cliffs, N.J.: Prentice-Hall, 1973), p. 33. (Italics added.)

24. This thesis is argued in detail in Tom L. Beauchamp, "Paternalism and Biobehavioral Control," *The Monist* 60 (January 1977): 62–80. Contrast James Childress, "Liberty, Paternalism and Health Care," *Social Responsibility: Journalism, Law, Medicine*, vol. 4, ed. Louis W. Hodges (Lexington, Va.: Washington and Lee University, 1978).

25. Robert Veatch, "Models for Ethical Medicine in a Revolutionary Age," *Hastings Center Report* 2 (June 1972): 5–7, especially p. 6. Cf. also his "Medical Ethics in a Revolutionary Age," *Journal of Current Social Issues* 12

(Fall 1975): especially pp. 14–19. See also, James Childress, "A Masterful Tour: A Response to Robert Veatch," ibid., pp. 20–25.

26. *Report and Recommendations: Research Involving Prisoners* (Washington: DHEW Publication No. (OS) 76–131, 1976).

6

The Principle of Justice

In a short story entitled "The Lottery in Babylon,"[1] Jorge Borges depicts a society in which all social benefits and burdens are distributed solely on the basis of a periodic lottery. Any given person could, at the end of any lottery event, find himself a slave, a factory owner, a priest, an executioner, a prisoner, etc. The lottery takes no account of one's past achievements, one's training, or one's promise. It is a purely random selection system, without regard to contribution, need, or effort. The story is compelling because of the ethical and political oddity of such a "system." We regard it as capricious and unfair, for we think there are *valid principles* of justice which determine how social burdens and benefits ought to be allocated.

When it comes time to state those valid principles with precision, however, we find ourselves in such constant disagreement that our own system of distributing burdens and benefits seems as perplexing as the capriciousness of the lottery method described by Borges. This problem is generally thought to be resolvable only by a theory of justice. Yet the moral requirement that persons be treated justly has proven difficult to analyze. Intuitively we believe that it would be unjust to ask another person to accept an unfair share of the burdens society might impose, but this judgment is not informative unless accompanied by an account of the notion of an unfair share. We may begin work on this problem indirectly, by outlining how the terms "justice" and "distributive justice" are used in contemporary moral philosophy. We can then pass on to more substantive problems about social justice.

The concept of justice

The meaning and types of justice

Some moral philosophers have argued that our basic notion of justice is best explicated in terms of fairness. While there are close conceptual connections between these terms, perhaps the single word most closely linked to the general meaning of "justice" is "desert." One has acted justly towards a person when that person has been given what he is due or owed, and therefore has been given what he deserves or can legitimately claim. If a person deserves to be awarded an M.D. degree, for example, justice has been done when that person receives the degree. What persons deserve or can legitimately claim is based on certain morally relevant properties which they possess, such as being productive or being in need. Similarly, it is wrong, as a matter of justice, to burden or to reward someone if the person does *not* possess the relevant property. It is wrong or unjust of a person to punish his child for knocking another child down, when in fact the person's own negligence led to the incident; and it is unjust to reward a superior for the work of his subordinates when he contributed nothing to the rewardable productivity.

The more restricted expression "distributive justice" refers to the proper distribution of social benefits and burdens. Paying taxes and serving as a subject of nontherapeutic biomedical research are distributed burdens, while welfare checks and research grants are distributed benefits. Recent literature on distributive justice has tended to focus on considerations of fair *economic* distribution, especially unjust distributions in the form of inequalities of income between different classes of persons and unfair tax burdens on certain classes. But there are many problems of distributive justice, including a large number of health-related ones.

Comparative and noncomparative justice

Justice is said to be *comparative* when what one person deserves is determined by balancing the competing claims of other persons against his claims. Here the condition of others in society affects how much an individual is due, e.g., whether a person qualifies to receive a cadaveric kidney transplant. Justice is *noncomparative,* in contrast, when desert is judged by a standard which is independent of the claims of others, e.g., the rule that an innocent person never deserves punishment. This chapter deals exclusively with comparative justice.

Scarcity and distributive justice

Distributive justice applies only to distribution under conditions of scarcity, e.g., where there is competition for benefits. If there were plenty of fresh water for industries to use in dumping their waste materials, and no subsequent problems of disease, then patterns of restricted use need not be established. It is only when we are worried that the supply of drinking water will be exhausted or that public health problems will be affected by the pollutants that limits are set on the amounts, if any, of permissible discharge. Of course, various schemes or patterns could be devised for setting such limits; but this fact is secondary for our present discussion. The point is that there are no problems of distributive justice and no need of principles of distributive justice until some measure of scarcity exists. Even when burdens rather than benefits are being allocated, there is competition for the least disadvantageous distribution.

David Hume pointed out that the concept of comparative justice has been developed in order to handle problems of conflicting claims or interests.[2] As he put it, rules of justice would have no point unless society were composed of persons with limited sympathy for others in the competition for scarce resources. The rules of justice serve to strike a balance between those conflicting interests and also between claims that repeatedly occur in society. Since law and morality are our explicit tools for balancing conflicting claims, there is a close link between the lawful society and the just society. Nonetheless, the law may be unjust; and not all rules of justice are connected to the law or to legal enforcement. Accordingly, parties with conflicting claims often must justify their claims by appeal to basic moral rules.

A compelling example of distributive justice appears as Case #23 in the Appendix. In this case an interdisciplinary panel of distinguished figures in medicine, ethics, and law was assembled in 1972 to consider the merits

and demerits of using modern technology to produce an artificial heart—
the so-called totally implantable artificial heart (TIAH). The alternatives
quickly narrowed to three possibilities in the deliberations of the panel:
(1) produce no heart because it is too expensive, (2) produce a heart
powered by nuclear energy, or (3) produce a heart with an electric motor
and rechargeable batteries. The panel eventually concluded that, on
balance, the battery-powered heart would pose fewer risks to the recipient, his family, and other members of society than would the nuclear-
powered heart. In assessing the implications of each alternative, the panel
considered implications for the quality of life of recipients, the high cost
to society, and even whether it would be too expensive by comparison
with other medical needs that might be fulfilled instead. In the end the
panel concluded (i) that despite the substantial costs, it would be an
injustice not to allocate money for the provision of the artificial heart to
those in need of it (on grounds that comparative justice requires it), and
(ii) that the nuclear-powered heart would distribute too much risk to
society.[3] The kind of weighing of alternatives found in this case, especially
the weighing of risks and benefits, is typical of problems of distributive
justice. In this case decisions would eventually have to be made regarding
two separate problems: whether to allocate money for the production of
the heart and how to allocate the hearts to individuals once technology
makes the hearts available. These two problems of distributive justice are
distinguished later in the chapter as the problem of macroallocation and
the problem of microallocation.

Formal and material principles of justice

Justice in the sense of comparative desert has been analyzed in different
ways in rival theories. But common to all theories of justice is a rather
minimal principle traditionally attributed to Aristotle: equals ought to be
treated equally and unequals unequally. This elementary principle is
referred to as the principle of formal justice, or sometimes as the principle
of formal equality. It is *formal* because it states no particular respects in
which equals ought to be treated the same. It only says that no matter
what respects are under consideration, if persons are equal in those
respects, then they must be treated equally. More fully stated in negative
form, the principle says that no person should be treated unequally,

despite all differences with other persons, unless it has been shown that there is a difference between them relevant to the treatment at stake. In expanded positive form, the principle says that individuals who are equal in the relevant respects should be treated equally, while individuals who are unequal in the relevant respects should be treated differently in proportion to the differences.

The problem with the formal principle is notoriously in its lack of substance. That equals ought to be treated equally, by law and elsewhere, is not likely to stir disagreement. But who is equal and who unequal? Presumably all citizens should have equal political rights, equal access to public services, and should receive equal treatment under the law. But almost all would allow that distinctions based on experience, deprivation, merit, and position sometimes justify differential treatment.

Any plausible theory of justice, then, must specify relevant differences between individuals. And it seems clear enough that not just any proposed criteria are morally fair. For example, if it is judged a good reason for not producing artificial hearts for those in need of them that heart failure victims are often unflatteringly obese, then this introduces a *proposed* relevant difference to distinguish persons who should receive technological advances in medicine from persons who should not. Yet this difference is unacceptable. It allows an injustice based on the morally irrelevant property of unflattering obesity. Some of the most difficult questions about justice arise over how to specify the relevant respects in terms of which people are to be treated equally. Principles that specify these relevant respects are said to be *material* principles of justice, because they put material content into a theory of justice. Examination of some major material principles of distributive justice is therefore in order.

Material principles of justice

Each material principle of justice identifies a relevant property on the basis of which burdens and benefits should be distributed. What makes each principle a plausible candidate is the plausible relevance of the property it isolates. The following is a fairly standard list of the major candidates for the position of valid principles of distributive justice (though longer lists have been proposed[4]):

(1) To each person an equal share
(2) To each person according to individual need
(3) To each person according to individual effort
(4) To each person according to societal contribution
(5) To each person according to merit

There is no obvious barrier to acceptance of more than one of these principles, and some theories of justice accept all five as valid. Most societies use several of them, applying different principles of distribution in different contexts. In the United States, for example, unemployment and welfare payments are distributed on the basis of need (and to some extent on the basis of previous length of employment); jobs and promotions are in many sectors awarded (distributed) on the basis of demonstrated achievement and merit; the higher incomes of wealthy professionals are allowed (distributed) on the grounds of superior effort or merit or social contribution (or perhaps all three); and, at least theoretically, the opportunity for elementary and secondary education is distributed equally to all citizens. While it seems attractive to use all these principles, when they come into conflict a serious weighting or priority problem is created.

Theories of distributive justice are commonly developed by systematically elaborating one or more of the material principles of distributive justice, perhaps in conjunction with other moral principles. *Egalitarian* theories emphasize equal access to the goods in life that every rational person desires; *Marxist* theories emphasize need; *Libertarian* theories emphasize contribution and merit; and *Utilitarian* theories emphasize a mixed use of such criteria so that public and private utility are maximized. The acceptability of any such theory of justice is determined by the quality of its moral argument that some one or more selected material principles ought to be given priority (or perhaps even exclusive consideration) over the others.

Neither principles nor theories of distributive justice can be considered here in detail. Nonetheless, it is important to see how from such meager and abstract beginnings as "the principle of need" both relevant properties and public policies based on justice can be developed. The principle of need declares that distribution is just when it is based on need. But how are we to understand the notion of a need? The term is subject to different interpretations, and a meaning must be fixed before meaningful distribution would be possible. In general, to say that a person needs something is to say that *without it he will be harmed* (or at least detrimentally affected). We can expand this basic idea about need by calling on the formal principle of justice. Conjointly they would require that people of equal need should be treated equally in regard to the satisfaction of these needs, while those who have unequal needs should be treated unequally. There are instructive common sense examples of actions based on this principle which show its relevance to contexts of distribution. In hospital wards patients are given equal amounts of blood and medication when they need equal amounts, and unequal amounts when the amount needed is unequal, while the quality and size of rooms is distributed largely in accordance with the ability to pay. However, this analysis of needs does not take us far, since we are not required to distribute equally for all needs for goods and services, such as needs for pets, athletic equipment, and nightgowns (unless one is prepared to defend a radical form of egalitarianism). Presumably we are interested only in *fundamental* needs, a notion thus far untreated.

To say that someone has a "fundamental need" for something is to say that the person will be harmed or detrimentally affected in a fundamental way if that thing is not obtained. Examples of fundamental harms would be malnutrition, serious bodily injury, and the withholding of critical information. Without nutrition, health care, and education, these harms will befall anyone; hence we say we have a fundamental need for nutrition, health care facilities, and education.

The more the notion of needs is refined, the closer one moves toward the relevant properties necessary for the formulation of a policy position. For example, if people need health care facilities, then it would have to be decided which needs are fundamental and which are not in order to develop a national health insurance policy. Anyone who had such needs would have the relevant properties. While this theoretical refinement cannot be carried out here, it is of vital importance to notice the role of the first step in the argument—the acceptance of the principle of need as a valid material principle of justice. If the principle of need is rejected while accepting, say, only contribution and merit, then one would be opposed in principle to these refinements and their applications to public policy. All public policies based on distributive justice derive ultimately from the acceptance of one or more material principles of distributive justice and from some procedure for refining them.

One of the more intense debates about distributive justice in recent years has focused on the issue of national health insurance. The United States has largely, though not exclusively, operated on the principle that distributions of health care services and goods are best left to the marketplace, where the implicit distributive principle is ability to pay. Some theories of justice challenge this approach. John Rawls's account, which was briefly mentioned in Chapter 2, has sometimes been said to have immediate implications for a national health policy. The following is one interpretation of his views on this subject:[5] Rawls argues that rational and impartial agents would choose principles of justice that maximize the minimum level of primary goods in order to protect vital interests in uncertain but perhaps disastrous contexts. Social allocations to protect everyone's future health and health needs would thus be elected by such agents (if health is a primary good). Such an approach would at least partially supplement the conventional marketplace system of distribution. It would probably also rule out not only *utilitarian* systems (in the form of attempts to produce the highest possible level of health care) but also systems based on distributions to everyone of *equal* sums to be invested in any health commodity the individual wishes.

The implications of this approach to Rawls's theory for national health care would seem to be egalitarian: each member of society, irrespective of wealth or position, would be provided with equal access to an adequate (though not maximal) level of health care for all available types of services. The distribution would proceed on the basis of need, and needs would be met by equal access. Better services, such as luxury hospital rooms and expensive but optional dental work, would be made available for purchase at personal expense by those who wished to do so. But *everyone's* health needs would be met at the level Charles Fried has described as a "decent minimum."[6] This system, however, presents only one of many approaches that might be taken to the vexed problem of national health insurance.

Relevant properties

We have seen that material principles of justice specify relevant properties that one must possess in order to qualify under a particular distributive principle, thereby excluding other respects as irrelevant to the treatment under consideration. These relevant respects are correctly fixed when supported by moral principles and incorrectly fixed when unsupported by moral principles (or when supported by incorrect "moral" principles), as we shall now see.

Established relevance and justified relevance

There are theoretical difficulties in explicating the notion of relevant respects, as well as practical problems in the development of public policies. In some contexts relevant respects are firmly established, perhaps by tradition and perhaps by moral principle. Here it would be generally—though not always—inappropriate to challenge the established relevant respects by attempting to substitute others. For example, trophies are awarded (distributed) at the end of tennis tournaments on the basis of achievement; and how achievement is to be determined is firmly set by the tradition-bound rules of tournament tennis. Similarly, as a moral matter, prison terms are not distributed to those who are not found guilty of crimes, since, as a firm matter of law and morality, guilt is relevant to conviction.

However, in controversial contexts it is morally appropriate either to institute a policy which establishes relevant respects where none has previously been firmly established or to develop a new policy which revises standard "relevant" respects. If a person is chosen to be an ambassador to a foreign nation merely on the basis of wealth, party affiliation, and loyalty to the chief executive, it is arguably the case that these operative (and perhaps even traditionally entrenched) "relevant" properties are from the point of view of justice arbitrary and irrelevant. Here it might be argued that: "You ought to shift your *operative* set of 'relevant' properties to the *right* set of relevant properties, which would include linguistic facility, knowledge of the country, administrative experience, past contribution, etc." The argument is that certain properties accepted as "relevant" are actually irrelevant and that certain properties presumed "irrelevant" are in fact relevant.

A contemporary issue that illustrates this problem, one that is presently unresolved in medical practice, occurs in Case #25, the case of an incompetent donor. In this case a forty-year-old woman in need of a kidney transplant in order to survive has a kidney offered by her fourteen-year-old daughter. The kidney is a fairly good match. However, the woman has a thirty-five-year-old mentally retarded brother who is a somewhat better match. (Some would say the brother is a much better match.) A recent survey of nurses, social workers, and physicians who work with such patients indicates that a majority would seek a court order to take the kidney from the thirty-five-year-old, institutionalized, mentally retarded brother.[7] Here we have a straightforward question about which criteria shall be used to select between these two potential donors—or whether to wait for a cadaveric donor (which is unlikely). The closeness of the match does seem to be a relevant property favoring the use of the brother. On the other hand, the lack of consent from the brother and the apparently knowledgeable consent of the child (a minor) introduces a reason favoring use of the child. There are also reasons against using either potential donor. The child is probably powerfully influenced by the fact that the recipient of her gift is her own mother. The very closeness of the relation and the emotion-laden situation undoubtedly exert pressure on the child—so much pressure that we might call into question the quality of the consent. (Cf. the section on informed consent in Chapter 3.) On the other hand, the class of mentally retarded citizens is particularly vulnerable to misuse and has on occasion been abused for purposes of medical research and practice. This case shows that when rather concrete policies must be formulated, abstract principles of justice provide only rough general guidelines, and further moral argument is needed to fix the specific relevant properties on the basis of which an actual choice can be made.

The role of argument and decision

It is sometimes assumed that relevant properties are fixed independently of moral arguments and human decisions that *establish* them as either relevant or irrelevant. Just as the applicable rules determining the eventual winner of a tennis tournament are valid whether we *know* the rules or not, so it is tempting to think when some moral controversy arises that relevant properties are fixed independently of human cognizance of them. There is something almost certainly right, but something just as certainly misleading, about this thesis. It is true that basic principles of morality control the relevance and irrelevance of properties. If the basic moral principles outlined in previous chapters of this book are not arbitrarily selected and not changeable merely by individual fiat, then the properties which such principles determine to be relevant are also neither arbitrary nor mere matters of individual preference. This important point deserves further explanation.

Consider an issue of research involving adult human subjects. How shall we decide who should become involved in research? If such participation is burdensome, how should this burden be distributed? The formal principle of justice declares that we must treat everyone equally who is alike in the relevant respects. But which respects are here relevant? Suppose the members of one class of adult persons have *consented* to participation, are *informed* regarding the experiments and their risks, and have *voluntarily* given their consent. Suppose, however, that the members of another class of persons either have not consented, or are not informed, or have been coerced. Consent, understanding, and noncoercion are clear cases of nonarbitrary relevant differences (whether or not these properties are sufficient conditions of *justified* research involving human subjects). But *why* are these respects relevant, while properties such as tallness, religious belief, and I.Q. are not relevant? The answer is that their relevance is nonarbitrarily fixed by moral principles. As we have seen, informed consent is relevant because basic moral principles such as autonomy determine its relevance. Or, stated negatively, if consent, understanding, and voluntariness were not present, then human research could easily violate moral rules protecting human welfare and autonomy. No parallel moral constraints require consideration of tallness, handsomeness, and I.Q. This also explains why the language of *morally* relevant properties and *morally* irrelevant properties is often used. We insist that the choice of such properties is neither morally arbitrary nor merely a matter of subjective preference, precisely because their selection is backed by moral principles.

It is a matter of theoretical importance that material principles of distributive justice may be justified by appeal to moral principles other than justice itself. In this book four basic moral principles have been proposed (as the titles in Chapters 3–6 reflect). A tempting account of ethical theory is that nonmaleficence generates its own rules, autonomy its own rules, beneficence its own rules, and justice its own rules. There are, of course, rather direct connections between rules and these basic principles. Rules of privacy and confidentiality, for example, are largely devised to protect autonomy. Material principles of distributive justice, however, do not seem solely connected to any one basic principle, for such principles may be justified on the basis of any one or more of these principles. Thus, there might be utilitarian reasons for a certain distributive principle—e.g., for allocation patterns for certain medical supplies in difficult war zones; and there might be reasons of autonomy for disallowing a particular distributive principle—such as a requirement of mandatory genetic screening.

An illustration of an argument that uses basic moral principles to derive a specific distributive principle of justice, thus showing the relation between principles of justice and other moral principles, is found in a report on research involving children by the National Commission for the Protection of Human Subjects of Biomedical and Behavioral Research. This report recommends that animal and adult studies be completed prior to the use of children, wherever data from animal or adult subjects would be pertinent, and that older children be used prior to the use of younger children. This complex principle of distributive justice is derived in the Commission's report from two further principles: autonomy and nonmaleficence. *Autonomy*—called respect for persons in this report—is said to require obtaining informed consent to involvement as a research subject wherever possible. Since adults and older children can give a more meaningful consent, and since it is easier to inform older children than younger ones, the principle of autonomy (respect for persons) dictates the use of adults and older children first and second in the order of selection. Younger children are to be selected last, and only when results cannot be obtained without their involvement. *Nonmaleficence* (one feature of beneficence in this report) is also invoked because it is easier to avoid doing harm to adult subjects than to children. Young children often do not have a clear grasp of their condition or feelings and hence make inaccurate reports. Investigators are thus less likely to be aware of unusual or untoward occurrences—a fact of childhood that places children at greater risk than adults. These two arguments, based as they are on two moral principles, support the general conclusion that a principle of distributive justice ought to be adopted—as national policy—which allocates research risks first to adults, wherever possible.

On the other hand, there are occasions on which moral principles do *not* unambiguously determine relevant properties. Usually this indefiniteness occurs not because moral considerations are unimportant, but rather because there are conflicting moral demands where no single moral principle is overriding. In such cases a moral *decision* concerning the weight of competing moral claims is required, and this decision in turn fixes the acceptable relevant properties. The words "decision" and "fix" should not, however, be taken to mean that such fixing decisions are arbitrary and without any principled basis. The point is that there is sometimes more than one set of good reasons, but no conclusive or determinative reasons by comparison with others. This problem was discussed in Chapter 1 as the problem of moral dilemmas. Whether members of minority groups formerly discriminated against should be given preferential consideration in hiring is one such issue with important policy implications. Whether 18-year-olds should be allowed to vote is another.

A particularly striking example is found in a current controversy over self-created health problems. Poor diets, high alcoholic intake, and habitual smoking can contribute to high health insurance premiums. Perhaps persons with "clean life-styles" should not have to pay the same health insurance premiums as do those who engage in hazardous activities. Presumably, the only relevant property governing qualification for most group insurance programs is that of being an employee eligible for enrollment in a group plan. However, possession of the property of heavy drug intake seems to throw into open question what the appropriate criteria should be for being enrolled without penalty in such a plan. Perhaps we should consider whether alcohol intake, cigarette smoking, diet, and exercise programs are each relevant or irrelevant to the determination of premium payments. This issue may appear to be either an empirical or a conceptual dispute concerning necessary and sufficient conditions of being "healthy." More plausibly, it is a straightforward moral problem of justice. On the one hand, is it fair to persons who carefully exercise and eat proper foods to allow those with undisciplined habits to cause increases in insurance premiums (without attached penalties)? On the other hand, is it fair to those who know and care little about health maintenance that they be excluded? Such an issue will be decided by considering the weight of moral arguments on each side, and in the end the relevance or irrelevance of drug habits, diet, and exercise programs will be decided by reference to moral standards of fairness.

Numerous moral problems and public policy decisions take this dilemmatic form. There are powerful moral reasons for accepting two or more sets of different and competing properties as equally relevant, even though only one can be adopted. It would be convenient if relevant properties were always fixed in the way tennis rules are established, but often they are not settled in these ways and must be fixed by moral deliberation and decision. Sometimes it is neither unreasonable nor unfair if the final decision favors *either* of two or more competing positions.

Classes of persons

Classes of persons who are the objects of moral concern should be grouped for ethical purposes only by the relevant properties they share in common, though there is often a temptation to group them in terms of convenient but irrelevant properties. Suppose a statute governing jury duty excuses all men but excuses no women, on grounds that there are many more men in the working population than women. Here justice requires us to say that an undue burden is placed on women and an undeserved privilege is granted to men. Being male or female is irrelevant, and so is the sexual grouping. If the relevant property excusing jury duty is employment, then employed men and employed women should be excused without regard to sex. In general, rules and laws are unjust when they make distinctions between classes that are actually similar in what is actually a relevant respect, and/or fail to make distinctions between classes that are actually different in what is actually a relevant respect. This is a simple but important policy application of the formal principle of justice.

One recent issue about justice and classes of persons has emerged from reflection on the selection of human subjects of biomedical research. Three levels of questions are involved. First, should a particular class of subjects be used at all? For example, should prisoners, fetuses, children, and those institutionalized for reasons of mental disability be involved as subjects of research, and, if so, under what conditions? Second, if it is permissible to involve such subjects, should there be some order of selection of subjects within that class, based on different properties possessed by the members of the class? For example, we have seen how, within the class of children, it is morally relevant to distinguish between older and younger children (or, better, between those who comprehend and report their feelings well and those who have diminished capacity to comprehend and report). Typically, these distinctions have policy implications. For example, we might want to establish a national policy that animals, adults, older children, and younger children be used *in that order* when doing biomedical research. Third, on some occasions we may decide that particular individuals within a class may not participate in research at all—not because of some class characteristic they have, but rather because of some morally relevant property not identified with the class under consideration. For example, a child with an amputated leg might be excluded from research on children that involves tests of coordinative skills that are too difficult for this individual child. Having an amputated leg is a morally relevant consideration but has nothing to do with the class of children per se.

These considerations of justice are illustrated by the data included in Case #26 in the Appendix—a case popularly known as Willowbrook. It involves a state institution for mentally retarded children, a portion of whom were used as research subjects in order to develop an effective prophylactic agent against strains of hepatitis which were persistent and continuing in the institution. Some of the experimental research involved exposing children to the resident strain of hepatitis infection. Studies on them were carried out in a special unit which isolated the children and protected them from other infectious diseases. These studies precipitated a series of sometimes emotional debates in various journals on the moral permissibility of using mentally retarded children for this kind of research. At the heart of these discussions are problems about justice to classes of persons. It must first be decided whether it is morally permissible to use children or the retarded or the institutionalized for research. Assuming that it is permissible to use some members of all three of these classes, is it permissible to use the class of children who are institutionalized and retarded? If it is, under what conditions may they be used, and should there be an ordering, such as older members first, or those most severely retarded last?

These questions have been widely debated. The American Bar Association has taken the position that no research can be done on the mentally disabled unless it relates immediately to the etiology, pathogenesis, prevention, diagnosis, or treatment of mental disability itself. This position would not permit studies such as Willowbrook, probably because it is believed that the children involved are already overburdened by their condition and by the somewhat oppressive institutional environments in which they live. Other parties, including an editor of a distinguished medical journal *(The New England Journal of Medicine),* have taken the position that such research is highly valuable for understanding hepatitis, was of potential value to the children in the institution, did not overburden children (because they probably would have contracted hepatitis anyway), and was carried out by very competent investigators. These debates again illustrate how the acceptability of rather concrete and specific principles of distributive justice turns on moral issues such as those of equal and unequal treatment, the minimal obligations owed by all persons to society, and the role of consent. Without a view on these matters, it would be difficult to know which distributive principle should be allowed or disallowed when dealing with classes of persons such as institutionalized, mentally retarded children.

Fair opportunity

Material principles of distributive justice have occupied most of our attention. Consider now those properties which might and often do serve as bases of distribution but which in virtually all contexts are not relevant to distribution, or at least *should not as a matter of justice* be considered relevant. Sex, race, religion, I.Q., and social status are examples. We do in some limited contexts appeal to these properties—e.g., if a script calls for an actor in a male role, then females are excluded. Still, we do not allow distribution of goods and services solely or even primarily on the basis of such properties. But why do we not accept such principles as "to each according to sex" or "to each according to I.Q." as valid principles of distributive justice? The most widely accepted reason why we exclude such properties, and indeed regard them as discriminatory, is because to use such principles would be "to treat people differently in ways that profoundly affect their lives *because of differences for which they have no responsibility*."[8] This reason for excluding the use of various possible distributive principles has important implications, because it implies that differences between persons can fairly be made *relevant differences only if those persons can be held responsible for the differences.*

To see the importance of this point, consider again the distribution of benefits in a state. The fair opportunity principle, as it may be called, says that none should be granted benefits on the basis of their "advantageous" properties, since they are not responsible for such properties; and it also says that none should be *denied* benefits on the basis of their "disadvantageous" properties, since they too are not responsible for such properties. Such properties are never grounds for morally acceptable discrimination between persons *because they are not the sorts of properties that one has a fair chance to acquire or overcome.* Of course in many societies properties such as religion and social status may be acquired and can also be overcome. But race, sex, and I.Q.—those properties that seem to bedevil fair treatment more than any others known to the human species—are not easily alterable.

Consider how the fair opportunity principle could be applied to problems of the institutionalized mentally retarded. If I.Q. is something for which a person is indeed not responsible, and if none should be denied the benefits of the state (or other distributional system) on the basis of any such property, then it would be unjust not to distribute to retarded persons the benefits generally conferred upon all who share in the system of benefits. But this pronouncement is still vague. Consider the more familiar example of a basic education. We confer this benefit on all citizens equally, and we would consider a person deprived or harmed if it were not received. Imagine a community in which an efficient school system gives a uniform opportunity for a high-quality education to all students with basic skills, regardless of sex, race, or religion. Such a system, let us imagine, will not offer an education to students with reading difficulties or mental deficiencies. These students require special training in order to overcome their problems and to receive what for them is a minimally adequate education. If such persons were responsible for their slowness, we might say that they deserve no special training and simply have to expend more effort. But when we discover that they are not responsible, we say they deserve special consideration; and hence we introduce different levels of education for different kinds of students, regardless of the differential in cost (within limits of resources).

At stake is not the *equal* distribution of economic resources. We do not say that the mentally retarded or slow learners with special reading problems should get the same amount of money or training or resources as other pupils because they are not responsible for their condition. Rather, we say they should get what for them is a quality education, even if it costs more, because the principle of fair opportunity *requires* that they receive it. Any other system of distribution would lead to an undue burden on this class of persons. The burden would be undue because it is placed in violation of a principle of justice.

The argument just presented is a sketch of a justification of unequal distribution to certain classes of handicapped individuals. The argument has been that criteria such as effort and merit should not be introduced in cases where a person is handicapped through no fault of his own. Determining a person's due or desert exclusively on the basis of such principles would in fact be morally wrong; for, as applied to the handicapped, such principles do not satisfy the requirements of the principle of fair opportunity. Yet, this finding is paradoxical, because ordinarily we believe that obligations in society are reciprocal, as we discussed in Chapter 5. When a person receives benefits conferred by society, he incurs reciprocal obligations to the society. He ought therefore to promote its interests. And when we promote the interests of others, they similarly are obliged to promote our interests. Where persons cannot reciprocate, through no fault of their own, we apparently make an exception to this reciprocity thesis. The exception is formulated as the principle of fair opportunity.

Still, there are problems with this position. It was earlier said that the term closest to the meaning of justice is "desert"—what a person is due or owed (because deserved). If this term does reflect the meaning of justice, then how can it be said that the retarded and other handicapped persons *deserve* preferential treatment? What, after all, have they done to deserve it? To look at the matter in this way is to miss the point of the fair opportunity principle. Such a question presupposes as appropriate a set of principles of distributive justice (such as merit, effort, and contribution) which in fact are declared inappropriate by the fair opportunity principle. That is, the question understands "deserves" in meritocratic terms, whereas the whole point of the analysis we have suggested is to get away from such an understanding. The claim under consideration is that criteria such as effort and merit cannot be introduced in cases where a person is handicapped through no fault of his own, for fair opportunity must be met before other considerations become relevant.

This conclusion is counterintuitive because we are inclined to think that what a person deserves is a function of performance. If blind chance brings a benefit, then we think the person does not deserve it even if he owns it. And, so described, this judgment is certainly correct. The scoundrel who has a wealthy and dying father does not deserve the wealth he is about to acquire. But in the case of those handicapped through no fault of their own, comparative justice dictates that what they deserve is a function of the available resources in a state. This use of "deserves" is not so counterintuitive. We speak, for example, of giving our children "the high-quality education they deserve" even before they have had the opportunity to display their scholastic abilities. We mean that they deserve the opportunity; we do not mean that they have demonstrated their ability.

Despite our moral conviction that the principle of fair opportunity must be upheld, there are limits to the goods and services that can be provided for the handicapped. Comparative justice demands a fair share, but not an unreasonable share. One of the major continuing controversies in biomedical ethics centers on what a "fair share" is. An illustration of this problem is found in Case #19 in the Appendix. Here a child treated for myelomeningocele, a severe central nervous system anomaly, was examined. Until the late 1950's nothing could be done for such children, who either quickly died or suffered for the remainder of their brief lives. The particular child in this case received partial treatment rather than total care in the expectation that he would die. But he did not die, and over a period of years he was given a series of expensive medical treatments for a variety of problems. At eight years of age he is in a school for the blind. Tests indicate he has an I.Q. of 80, but with serious medical problems in need of constant attention. For such persons it is perplexingly difficult to say what the principle of fair opportunity demands. There can be little doubt that society does not now provide the exceptional medical care and training that such a child would need to receive a "fair opportunity" by comparison with other eight-year-olds. But the moral question remains: How much ought to be provided?

Finally, it should be observed that if one accepts the view of distributive justice suggested by the fair opportunity principle, it will lead to a revisionary perspective on common practices of distribution. For the sake of moral consistency we must say that whenever a person is not responsible for certain "disadvantageous" properties, he should not be denied important benefits simply because he possesses those properties. But suppose, momentarily, that most all of our "abilities" and "disabilities" are a function of what Rawls has referred to as "the natural lottery."[9] That is, suppose that most all of our talents result from heredity and environment and that consequently we are not responsible for them. Suppose that even the ability to work long hours is environmentally produced. Advantageous properties, from this perspective, are not something one deserves any more than are disadvantageous, handicapping properties (though one may deserve certain consequences which result from having such properties[10]). It follows that both the advantageous and the disadvantageous properties are irrelevant for purposes of distributive justice. If this theory of the causal origins of advantageous and disadvantageous properties were accepted, along with the justification based on fair opportunity previously outlined, then one would be led to radically different views about distributive justice than the ones we now generally acknowledge.

It is uncertain what the full implications of this approach would be, though it does seem that something like these assumptions and conclusions are adumbrated in Rawls's *A Theory of Justice,* where he argues as follows:

[The liberal interpretation of] Free Market arrangements must be set within a framework of political and legal institutions which regulates the overall trends of economic events and preserves the social conditions necessary for fair equality of opportunity. . . .

While the liberal conception seems clearly preferable to the system of natural liberty, intuitively it still appears defective. For one thing, . . . it still permits the distribution of wealth and income to be determined by the natural distribution of abilities and talents. Within the limits allowed by the background arrangements, distributive shares are decided by the outcome of the natural lottery; and this outcome is arbitrary from a moral perspective. There is no more reason to permit the distribution of income and wealth to be settled by the distribution of natural assets than by historical and social fortune. Furthermore, the principle of fair opportunity can be only imperfectly carried out, at least as long as the institution of the family exists. The extent to which natural capacities develop and reach fruition is affected by all kinds of social conditions and class attitudes. Even the willingness to make an effort, to try, and so to be deserving in the ordinary sense is itself dependent upon happy family and social circumstances.[11]

At a minimum we would look at the matter of rewards and punishments in a revisionary manner if this approach were accepted. Rather than allowing broad inequalities based on effort, contribution, and merit, as practices in Western nations presently permit, we would tend to regard justice as done when radical inequalities are diminished, so long as "disadvantaged" persons in the state can be advantaged by such a system of conferring benefits. On the other hand, as Bernard Williams has correctly pointed out,[12] this process of reducing inequalities will have to stop somewhere, especially if it is assumed that everything about a person is environmentally controlled. The ideal of absolute equality is untenable. Williams's point forms one of the reasons why it remains uncertain what the *full* implications of the approach Rawls has suggested would be. It may also provide a reason why some would argue that the principle of fair opportunity is in the end not a valid moral principle at all.

It would be inappropriate to pursue these theoretical problems of justice here. The point of considering them to this extent is to show that *if* one accepts a justification of unequal treatment based on the fair opportunity principle, then other areas of social policy will inevitably be affected in significant ways.

Macroallocation

We have thus far encountered a number of problems about justice and biomedicine that are created by a situation of scarce or at least limited resources. We have seen, for example, that debates over a national health insurance policy, debates over unequal distributions of educational advantages to the handicapped, and debates over whether to provide extensive therapies for those afflicted with myelomeningocele all turn on the issue of who shall receive what share of the available goods and services. The same problem recurs for the distribution or allocation of expensive medical equipment, artificial organs, and blood for the treatment of hemophilia. One basic problem underlying these issues of distribution is *economic:* how are these scarce resources to be most efficiently provided? How can more people be helped and how can costs be reduced? But the more basic problems are *ethical:* by what principles, policies, and procedures can justice in the distribution of resources best be ensured? Because these two problems cannot be neatly separated, we should perhaps say that there is both an economic dimension and an ethical dimension to problems of allocation.

Problems of justice in the allocation of resources arise on two different levels: macroallocation and microallocation. At the macroallocation level, decisions must be made as to how much of society's resources should be exchanged for social goods, including health-related expenditures, as well as how priorities are to be established for the distribution of these resources. Such decisions are taken by Congress, state legislatures, private foundations, etc. There usually are two dimensions to such planning: what quantity of our total available financial resources should be allotted to health-related enterprises (medical research, routine services, clinical practice, health education, etc.), and of the total amount so allocated, what quantity should go to which specific projects, e.g., how much to cancer research and how much to dialysis programs? At the microallocation level, health care professionals, hospitals, and other institutions determine which particular individuals shall obtain available resources. We shall discuss macroallocation problems in this section and then conclude the chapter with a discussion of microallocation in the next section.

Macroallocation decisions have become increasingly important because of the heavy federal and foundation involvement in research and treatment programs. There also appears to be a growing recognition that this large expenditure of funds cannot be based solely on economic considerations untempered by principles of justice. Yet it has proved extremely difficult to implement principles of justice in public policy. Not only is it difficult to bring abstract principles to bear on practical realities, but those principles frequently come into conflict, as we have seen.[13]

The problem of whether or not to produce the totally implantable artificial heart again provides a useful example. This problem is analyzable into several discrete issues, some of which are omnipresent in decisions at the health policy level. First, should the government be in the health allocation business at all, instead of leaving the allocation of such goods to the marketplace? Society sometimes allows the principle of ability to pay to determine the distribution of health services and goods, and it constantly considers precisely which goods and services should be distributed in this manner and which should be distributed by different principles.

Second, if the government is in the health allocation business, how much of its budget should be targeted for the protection and promotion of health and how much for other social goods? Health is not our only value. It is not clear that a citizen can complain of injustice if the society puts more money into space programs or defense than into health care. "Wrong" priorities may not be unjust unless there are certain basic needs or rights that must be satisfied for justice to be realized. If there is a right to a minimum of health care, then society would be acting unjustly (at least prima facie) if it did not put enough of its budget into health care to be able to meet that minimum.

Third, what are the most effective and efficient ways to protect and promote life and health (or to prevent death and disability)? Many social goods, such as improved sanitation programs, have direct and indirect impacts on health. Indeed, many of the improvements in health can be traced to improvements in the standard of living rather than to improvements in medical care or technological advancement. Some even argue that to concentrate resources on *medical* care is to misallocate them. For example, Paul Starr contends, "If one wishes to equalize health, equalizing medical care is probably not the most effective strategy."[14] Nevertheless, as long as medical care is important to health or at least increases our sense of security, perhaps we ought to promote equal access to it. Despite the apparent oddity of arguing for equal access to what is partially ineffective, principles of equality may indicate that such a policy is morally defensible and even mandatory.

Fourth, a closely related point is sometimes stated in terms of a conflict between preventive and rescue strategies. Should society concentrate on rescue strategies such as dialysis, kidney transplantation, and the totally implantable artificial heart, or should society concentrate on the prevention of disease and disability? While preventive strategies may hold out the most promise for marked improvements in the nation's health, the appropriate mix of preventive and rescue strategies is difficult to determine because of our limited knowledge. Indeed, it is possible to argue that one of our most pressing needs is for basic research that would help us determine the appropriate policy.

Fifth, which categories of illness or disease should receive priority in the allocation of public resources if it is not possible to fund research and therapy in all areas? When we discuss equal access to medical care, we most often consider need, in contrast to geography, finances, etc., as the relevant property justifying similar treatment. But, from the standpoint of public policy, it may be necessary to give certain diseases priority in research and therapy, and perhaps even to exclude whole classes of cases from a priority list. According to Gene Outka, it is more "just to discriminate by virtue of categories of illness, for example, rather than rich ill and poor ill."[15] Society would not necessarily be unjust if it decided not to allocate much of its budget for certain diseases that are rare and noncommunicable, involve excessive costs, and have little prospect for rehabilitation. For purposes of justice, according to this line of argument, the relevant similarity between persons under conditions of scarcity would be the type of illness rather than medical need as such. While certain forms of treatment would not be developed and distributed for some categories of illness, care would still be provided to all persons and no patient would be abandoned. In trying to determine priorities among diseases, policymakers should take into account the pain and suffering involved, the health costs of various diseases, the ages in life when different diseases occur, etc. It might be appropriate, for instance, to concentrate less on killer diseases, such as some forms of cancer, and more on disabling diseases such as arthritis (cf. Case #22 in the Appendix).

Sixth, different strategies may compromise various values or principles, and this compromise should be acknowledged in formulating public policies. For example, preventive strategies include protecting individuals (e.g., through vaccines), changing the environment, and altering behavioral patterns and life-styles. However, if society emphasizes altering behavioral patterns and life-styles in order to promote health (e.g., through campaigns against cigarette smoking), it must consider limits set by the principle of autonomy. When should the society limit an individual's freedom in order to reduce that individual's risk-taking? One relevant consideration might be the protection of the financial resources of the community. Under a national health insurance scheme, we would expect increased pressure to limit individual liberty to engage in risky behaviors, because citizens will argue that it is unfair to increase their premiums or taxes to pay for the avoidable, self-caused afflictions of others.

A helpful example of the magnitude and complexity of these issues comes from public health policies aimed at preventing disease. Some writers have claimed that our health policies are unjust because we do not allocate more of our resources for preventive measures aimed at protecting those who cannot defend themselves against the onslaughts of disease. They admit that preventive measures will place new burdens and restrictions on the controlling social classes, who have thus far resisted such measures. This resistance is said to be rooted in a free-market conception of justice that emphasizes individual responsibility and personal merit—especially responsibility for one's own health. As one writer has recently developed this thesis,

> The preponderance of our public policy for health continues to define health care as a consumption good to be allocated primarily by private decisions and markets, and only interferes . . . to subsidize, supplement or extend the market system when private decisions result in sufficient imperfections or inequities to be of public concern. Medicare and Medicaid are examples. . . .

> Market justice is a pervasive ideology protecting the most powerful. . . . [But] public health should advocate a "counter-ethic" for protecting the public's health, one articulated in a different tradition of justice. . . .[16]

This "public health ethic" is considered to be a radical counter-ethic by this writer not because it entails a radical political theory but rather because it demands a radically new allocation for preventive health measures.

Programmatic positions of this sort—which are driven by a controlling theory of justice—are subject to attack by the use of arguments that give a different weight to alternative principles of justice. For example, the above theory heavily emphasizes the principle of need. But, as we have seen, the notion of a need is subject to different interpretations and requires considerable refinement to become workable for purposes of public policy. Any such refinement must also explain why need is a more fundamental distributional principle than is, for example, ability to pay. If the principle of need is believed irrelevant for a given context, while contribution and merit, for example, are argued to be the relevant principles, then one would be opposed in principle to the public policies outlined by the above author. Many policy disputes are reducible to a debate of this sort over which principle of justice has primacy in a given context.

Although we have not tried in this section to identify all the important issues that emerge on the level of macroallocation, we have tried to indicate some of the most important conflicts that emerge among various values, principles, and rules, such as the promotion of health and other social goods, effectiveness and efficiency, and principles of justice and liberty. Such conflicts pervade contemporary debates about public policies governing health. As a result, those writers who suppose that it is possible to take an abstract theory of justice or a single principle of justice into the arena of public policy commit the same error as those who would totally exclude considerations of justice. Public policy is invariably multidimensional. Considerations of justice alone rarely determine appropriate policies of macroallocation, in part because principles of justice can conflict. Nonetheless, principles of justice are always relevant, and in some cases they set powerful constraints on what the government may permissibly do in the protection and promotion of health—just as the principle of autonomy and other moral principles also act as constraints.

Microallocation

Not infrequently health care providers, hospitals, and other institutions have to decide which person(s) will receive some scarce preventive or therapeutic procedure. Such microallocation decisions often must be made after a service or good has gained acceptance through an experimental process. Insulin, penicillin, and dialysis are examples. Dialysis, for example, remained a limited resource because of its cost until the Federal Government decided to provide almost universal coverage. Microallocation decisions such as those involved when dialysis was scarce are particularly troubling because the disease or illness is life-threatening and the scarce resource offers the possibility of saving life. Here the question can even become, "Who shall live when not everyone can live?" Unlike contractual arrangements between patients and physicians, this question is not decided *by* the patient but *for* the patient by others.[17] In this section we investigate what principles of justice imply for microallocation, especially when they come into conflict with each other or with other principles and values.

We begin with a distinction between just procedures and just outcomes. Often we cannot guarantee a just outcome by any conceivable or feasible procedures, but we nevertheless remain concerned about the justice of the procedures themselves. As Rawls suggests, we may feel more secure in our judgments about just procedures than about just outcomes.[18] The common law tradition also stresses "natural justice," which tells us less about the content of a just decision than about approaches that are likely to yield just decisions. In order to obtain fair and impartial decisions, certain procedural rules are followed: no party may be condemned without a hearing, the parties are entitled to know the reason for the decision, no one may be a judge in his own case, etc. Concerns about procedural due process pervade the law and are relevant to the allocation of scarce resources from both legal and moral standpoints. Indeed, both procedures and outcomes need attention: Who should make the decisions? And what should the criteria be for the selection of recipients?

Two sets of rules and procedures are required. First it is necessary to formulate rules and procedures for determining the relevant pool of potential recipients, e.g., those eligible for kidney transplantation; then it is necessary to develop rules and procedures for final selection, e.g., those persons actually selected to receive a kidney. While these two sets of rules and procedures may overlap, it is useful to distinguish them and to consider them separately.

It is easier to secure agreement about rules of initial inclusion and exclusion because they involve minimum standards, e.g., age and medical acceptability, and appear to be more objective and more easily applied than rules of final selection. Nevertheless, they sometimes incorporate arbitrary distinctions and unfounded judgments, e.g., that only people above or below a certain age can benefit from a particular treatment. The criteria of inclusion and exclusion can be arranged in three basic categories, following a proposal by Nicholas Rescher: the constituency factor, the progress-of-science factor, and the prospect-of-success factor.[19] The constituency factor includes considerations such as clientele boundaries (e.g., veterans are served by veterans' hospitals), geographic boundaries (e.g., citizens of a state are served in a state-run hospital), and the ability to pay. It is appropriate to raise questions about all of these—particularly the last—from the standpoint of justice: exactly what factors constitute *relevant* similarities for purposes of determining the pool from which final selection can be made?

The prospect-of-success factor is operative at all stages, since a scarce medical resource should only be distributed to patients who have some reasonable chance of benefiting from it. To distribute otherwise would be an unjust use of resources. This prospect of success is usually analyzed in terms of "medical acceptability." While medical acceptability can only be formulated by experts in the area, the public has a strong interest in making sure that this expression does not incorporate covert and undefended moral and social standards. Some psychological factors may also be medically relevant; for example, some people are not able to adjust to the requirements of dialysis. But psychological criteria are more susceptible to covert value judgments and must be applied with great care. Perhaps one control on medical factors, including psychological ones, is to apply standards of medical acceptability as though the resource were unlimited. If physicians made scarcity irrelevant to their determination of the initial pool, they would exclude only those candidates who could not possibly benefit from the treatment.[20]

The second stage, which involves standards and procedures of final selection from the preliminary pool, is even more controversial. At this stage, three major approaches contend: (1) utilitarian principles of justice, (2) some form of chance or queuing that expresses equality of opportunity and equal access, and (3) some more or less objective standards. All these approaches have been employed at some medical institution or setting. For example, some dialysis centers considered social worth (sometimes in general terms, sometimes in such specific terms as value to one's family), some used queuing (a first-come, first-served system), and at least one used a lottery (a randomizing system). In effect, however, all centers used one form of queuing or the first-come, first-treated rule; they did not drop patients from dialysis or refuse a second or third transplant merely because someone of superior social worth subsequently appeared. Criteria such as age were also used, especially in establishing the pool for final selection during the early years. To take other examples, in North Africa during World War II the scarce resource of penicillin was distributed to U.S. soldiers suffering from venereal disease rather than to those suffering from battle wounds (on grounds of military need); and in England, when polio vaccine was scarce, it was distributed to children by a lottery.

One argument in favor of utilitarian selection is that medical institutions and personnel are "trustees" of society. Nicholas Rescher defends this criterion (though he does not defend an entirely utilitarian system):

In 'choosing to save' one life rather than another, 'the society,' through the mediation of the particular medical institution in question—which should certainly look upon itself as a trustee for the social interest—is clearly warranted in considering the likely pattern of future *services to be rendered* by the patient (adequate recovery assumed), considering his age, talent, training, and past record of performance. In its allocation . . . society 'invests' a scarce resource in one person as against another and is thus entitled to look to the probable prospective 'return' on its investment.[21]

It is unclear, however, that society's stake in medicine necessitates viewing selection as a means to broader social goals. Indeed, society may have a stake in protecting both the patient-physician relationship and the delivery of medical care from economic considerations of investment and return. It may value the relationship of "personal care," even when it is not socially productive. Were the physician to look through the patient to the society and attempt to realize society's goals, the relationship of personal care and trust could be radically altered.

Furthermore, there are different levels of responsibility in society so that not everyone has to act in the same way or even in terms of the same standards. The physician is not a policymaker. His or her primary responsibility is to the patient, and society has good reasons for insisting on the primacy of this responsibility of personal care. Physicians are to do all they can for their patients without counting society's resources and without taking into account the range of factors, e.g., statistical lives, that policymakers rightly should consider. As Howard Hiatt contends, it is not fair to ask the physician or other medical-care provider to set them [i.e., national priorities] in the context of his or her own medical practice. A physician or other provider must do all that is permitted on behalf of his patient. In that sense, the physician is or should be responsible, with his patient and the patient's family, for setting priorities for that patient's management, within the limits available. The patient and the physician want no less, and society should settle for no less.[22]

In contrast to those who affirm what George Kennan calls "the principle of the total ubiquity of responsibility," it is appropriate to structure social roles so that there is a division of responsibility. The obligations of the physician and the bureaucrat concerned with social goals are not identical. To whom and for what they are responsible depends, for example, on their positions, training, and the moral principles that structure their roles. Even if we regard medical personnel and institutions as, in some respects, trustees of society, we should not suppose that the physician's obligations are identical with those of the policymaker.[23]

Another approach uses objective criteria such as age, life expectancy, and number of dependents. This approach would escape some of the difficulties of application that plague utilitarian calculations, and it would avoid the comparative evaluations of persons that many critics of utilitarian selection find disagreeable. While these more objective criteria could be fairly applied, it is not clear that they could be adequately justified. Which of the following objective criteria, for example, could be justified: age, number of dependents, or sex? Such objective criteria seem arbitrarily selected and also tend to reduce persons to their socially-valued roles. Furthermore, they do not incorporate justice in the form of equality, equal access, and equal opportunity as well as the third approach, which uses chance or queuing. In a situation of scarcity, especially where selection may determine life or death, equality may require queuing, lottery, or randomization—whichever procedure is the most appropriate and feasible in the circumstances.[24] This conclusion was also reached by the Artificial Heart Assessment Panel of the National Heart and Lung Institute:

In the event artificial heart resources are in scarce supply, decisions as to the selection of candidates for implantation of the artificial heart should be made by physicians and medical institutions on the basis of medical criteria. If the pool of patients with equal medical needs exceeds supply, procedures should be devised for some form of random selection. Social worth criteria should not be used, and every effort should be exerted to minimize the possibility that social worth may implicitly be taken into account.[25]

Does this argument in support of the use of chance in microallocation—after judgments of medical acceptability have been made—necessarily exclude all utilitarian calculation? Utilitarian calculations are rarely justified in microallocation (in contrast to macroallocation where effectiveness and efficiency are central), but they should be employed under some circumstances. Some defenders of utilitarian selection invoke the model of *triage* to show that health care providers do and should make allocative decisions based on social worth. The paradigm case is triage in an emergency such as a school bus accident or earthquake. But, as we argued in Chapter 4, we must be cautious about generalizing from the emergency situation to ordinary medical practice.

Furthermore, triage decisions may take several different directions. In one type of situation, victims may be sorted out according to their medical needs: those who will die without immediate help; those whose treatment may be delayed without immediate danger; those with minor injuries; those for whom no treatment will be efficacious. Such a classification in terms of urgency of medical need establishes priorities of treatment that do not involve judgments about social worth. We can complicate this case by supposing that some of the injured persons are medical personnel whose injuries are minor. These persons may be given priority of treatment, so that they can be restored to help others. Again, in an outbreak of a disease, physicians may be inoculated first, in order to care for others.

These emergencies involve what Paul Ramsey calls a focused community with the clear and immediate need of survival. In such focused communities, some persons may be given priority over others because they can substantially contribute to the community, just as sailors on an overloaded craft in a storm may be given priority so that they can help save the others. In a focused community judgments about social worth are limited to the specific qualities and skills that are essential for the community's survival. Although these judgments are comparative, they do not attempt to assess the full worth of the person.[26]

The paradigm of triage suggests a way to legitimate certain presumably utilitarian exceptions within a larger system of chance or queuing. Advocates of departures from this system should appear before a lay review

board and should meet the following schematic burden of proof: patient
X would be given priority only if X's contribution is indispensable to
attaining (or preventing) socially significant state of affairs A, and only if
society so values (or fears) A that it would deny Y a second transplant or
would remove Z from dialysis in order to save X.[27] Perhaps the president
of the country in wartime would be given priority, but in few cases would
particular patients be truly indispensable to society. In those cases, we
should depart from the system of chance or queuing, even if reluctantly.

Another microallocation question involves some issues that also appear
in macroallocation decisions. In Case #20, a patient at a University
Hospital was kept alive for many months at a final cost of approximately
$250,000. His expenses had to be absorbed by the prepaid health program
in which he participated, and the resulting premium increases might have
been substantial had it not been for a reinsurance arrangement with Blue
Cross. In this case, there is no direct conflict between two identified
individuals for some scarce resource. Rather the question concerns how
much of the resources any particular patient should use. Such decisions
are complicated because in Case #20 no person at any point in the
decision procedure was ever in a position to know or evaluate how much
the total bill would be; instead, the decisions were incremental. Each step
was undertaken to respond to some immediate need, and no one could
appreciate how much the total process might consume, since no one could
predict what would happen next or how long the process would continue.

In the case of both macroallocation and microallocation, as well as the
other problems of justice discussed in this chapter, the agony of choice in
a situation of dilemma ought by now to be evident. Public policies
intended to provide just procedures cannot completely evade this context
of dilemma. The choices must be made, even if our choices in the light
of justice do not always eventuate in just outcomes and even if we choose
to use impersonal mechanisms, such as chance, in microallocation.

Notes

1. *Labyrinths* (New York: New Directions, 1962), pp. 30–35.
2. David Hume, *A Treatise of Human Nature,* ed. L. A. Selby-Bigge (Oxford University Press, 1888), pp. 490–500.
3. *The Totally Implantable Artificial Heart: A Report of the Artificial Heart*

Assessment Panel of the National Heart and Lung Institute (June 1973). DHEW Publication No. (NIH) 74–191.

4. Cf., e.g., Nicholas Rescher, *Distributive Justice* (Indianapolis: Bobbs-Merrill, 1966), Chapter 4.
5. See Ronald M. Green, "Health Care and Justice in Contract Perspective," in Robert M. Veatch and Roy Branson, eds., *Ethics and Health Policy* (Cambridge, Mass.: Ballinger, 1976), pp. 111–26.
6. Cf. Charles Fried, "Equality and Rights in Medical Care," *Hastings Center Report* 6 (February 1976): 29–34.
7. Audience Survey: Symposium on Death and Dying. Southeastern Dialysis and Transplantation Association Meetings. Miami, Florida. August, 1977 (unpublished).
8. W. K. Frankena, "Some Beliefs about Justice," *The Lindley Lecture,* University of Kansas (March 2, 1966), p. 10 (italics added).
9. *A Theory of Justice* (Cambridge: Harvard University Press, 1971), p. 74.
10. Both Thomas Nagel and Robert Nozick have provided theoretical reasons to show that, as Nagel puts it, ". . . yet one probably does deserve the punishments or rewards that flow from these undeserved qualities." From "Equal Treatment and Compensatory Discrimination," as reprinted in T. Beauchamp, ed., *Ethics and Public Policy* (Englewood Cliffs, N.J.: Prentice-Hall, 1975), p. 49, n 5. Nozick's far more radical challenge questions much of what we have argued above, but neither Nagel nor Nozick destroys the validity of the point we are making in this section. Cf. Nozick's *Anarchy, State, and Utopia* (New York: Basic Books, 1974), Chapter 7 and the first two sections of Chapter 8.
11. Rawls, *A Theory of Justice,* pp. 73f.
12. "The Idea of Equality," as reprinted in H. Bedau, *Justice and Equality* (Englewood Cliffs, N.J.: Prentice-Hall, 1971), p. 135.
13. For a discussion of some of the issues in macroallocation, see James Childress, "Priorities in the Allocation of Health Care Resources," in David H. Smith, ed., *No Rush to Judgment: Essays on Medical Ethics* (Bloomington, Ind.: Indiana University, The Poynter Center, 1977), pp. 128–48; Jay Katz and Alexander Morgan Capron, *Catastrophic Diseases: Who Decides What?* (New York: Russell Sage Foundation, 1975); and Paul Ramsey, *The Patient as Person* (New Haven: Yale University Press, 1970), Chapter 7.
14. Paul Starr, "The Politics of Therapeutic Nihilism," *The Hastings Center Report* 6 (October 1976): 26–30.
15. Gene Outka, "Social Justice and Equal Access to Health Care," *The Journal of Religious Ethics* (1974): 24.
16. Dan E. Beauchamp, "Public Health and Social Justice," *Inquiry* (March 1976): 4–6. Cf. also "Alcoholism as Blaming the Alcoholic," *The International Journal of Addictions* 11 (1976), especially pp. 42–49.
17. Much of the literature on microallocation decisions was stimulated by selection problems in kidney dialysis and transplantation. See James Childress,

"Who Shall Live When Not All Can Live?" *Soundings* 53 (1970): 339–55, reprinted in B-W, pp. 389–98; Katz and Capron, *Catastrophic Diseases: Who Decides What?;* Ramsey, *The Patient as Person;* Nicholas Rescher, "The Allocation of Exotic Medical Lifesaving Therapy," *Ethics* 79 (1969): 173–86, reprinted in B-W, pp. 378–89; and the literature mentioned in James Childress, "Rationing of Medical Treatment," *The Encyclopedia of Bioethics.*
18. Rawls, *A Theory of Justice.*
19. Rescher, "The Allocation of Exotic Medical Lifesaving Therapy," B-W, pp. 381–82.
20. See "Scarce Medical Resources," *Columbia Law Review* 69 (1969): 654, 656.
21. Rescher, "The Allocation of Exotic Medical Lifesaving Therapy," B-W, pp. 382–83.
22. Howard Hiatt, "Protecting the Medical Commons: Who is Responsible?" *The New England Journal of Medicine* (July 31, 1975): 235–41.
23. See Charles Fried, "Rights and Health Care—Beyond Equity and Efficiency," *The New England Journal of Medicine* (July 31, 1975): 241–45.
24. Other reasons for using some form of chance are presented in Childress, "Who Shall Live When Not All Can Live?" in B-W, 389–98 and "Rationing Medical Treatment," *The Encyclopedia of Bioethics.* Cf. also Ramsey, *The Patient as Person,* Chapter 7.
25. *The Totally Implantable Artificial Heart: A Report of the Artificial Heart Assessment Panel of the National Heart and Lung Institute,* p. 198.
26. Ramsey, *The Patient as Person,* pp. 257–58.
27. Cf. "Scarce Medical Resources," *Columbia Law Review,* p. 664.

7

The Professional and Patient Relationship

In addition to *distributive* justice, which was treated in the previous chapter, other interpretations of justice are also relevant to biomedical ethics. For instance, *commutative* justice focusses on the rights and duties of individuals in various relationships, especially those emerging from voluntary commitments and contracts.[1] Of special importance is the duty of fidelity. According to Paul Ramsey, the fundamental ethical question in biomedicine is: "What is the meaning of the faithfulness of one human being to another?"[2] While Ramsey interprets faithfulness along such theological lines as covenant-fidelity, it is commonly expressed in non-theological language in terms of duties of fidelity.

Because duties of fidelity arise from *voluntary* actions, such as making contracts, they cannot be used to explicate all the moral requirements in biomedicine, e.g., the duty of nonmaleficence. Nevertheless, they play a central role in biomedical ethics. In this chapter, we will explore the moral content and conflicts within relations between health care professionals and patients. Some of the moral rules and principles we will consider can be derived from the principles discussed in the previous four chapters. For example, the rule of confidentiality may be derived from the principles of autonomy, beneficence, and nonmaleficence. But in addition some moral principles and rules that will be discussed here may hinge on the terms of the relationship itself rather than on external principles.

Several moral conflicts emerge within these relationships. For example, the principle of veracity may require nondeception, yet the health care professional may determine that the use of a placebo would actually be in the patient's best interests. Other problems stem from a conflict of claims between patients and other individuals, or perhaps society itself. For example, it may be difficult, if not impossible, in some cases to respect the rule of confidentiality while also protecting other individuals and the society and in other cases to meet the needs of a particular patient while also satisfying the demands of a research protocol.

The principle of veracity

It is commonly agreed that we have a duty of veracity, i.e., a duty to tell the truth and not to lie or to deceive others. But as Henry Sidgwick observed many years ago, "it does not seem clearly agreed whether Veracity is an absolute and independent duty, or a special application of some higher principle."[3] Sidgwick's observation still holds. One contemporary philosopher, G. J. Warnock, has included the principle of veracity as an independent principle ranking with beneficence, nonmaleficence, and justice.[4] Others have held that the principle of veracity is derived from other principles, such as respect for persons or fidelity or utility. Whether the duty of veracity is independent or derived, it does express several other principles and values.

Three arguments for the duty of veracity are particularly applicable to the relationship between health care professionals and patients. The first argument holds that the duty of veracity is part of the respect we owe to persons. As Alan Donagan writes:

Relations between human beings are largely carried on by means of language; and much of what is communicated in language consists of expressions of opinion about what is the case. Unless it is required by a specific moral precept, nobody has a right to know another's opinion. The respect owed to other human beings includes respect for their liberty to withhold their thoughts when it is not their duty to divulge them; but, if anybody chooses to divulge his thoughts, the respect he owes to his audience requires that the thoughts he communicates must really be his. . . .[5]

Within biomedical contexts, respect for persons is commonly expressed through the principle of autonomy. Not to solicit *consent* for treatment from patients or for participation in research from subjects is to violate their autonomy and to fail to respect them as persons—as we saw in Chapter 3. But consent cannot express autonomy unless it is informed, and it therefore depends on communication and ultimately on truthtelling. Thus, a duty of veracity can be derived from a principle of respect for persons or autonomy.

Second, some philosophers, including W. D. Ross, argue that the duty of veracity is an expression of the duty of fidelity or promise-keeping.[6] When we use language to communicate with others, we implicitly promise that we will speak truthfully, that we will not lie by misrepresenting our opinions, and that we will not deceive our listeners. Our participation in society and our shared language engender a duty of veracity because of an implicit contract that is created. This contract generates the expectation that we will speak truthfully. Within biomedical contexts, it is sometimes possible also to point to a more specific though still implicit contract or promise. By entering into a relationship in the context of therapy or research, the patient or subject not only retains a general right to the truth but gains a special right to the truth regarding diagnosis, prognosis, procedures, etc.

Third, relationships of trust between human beings are necessary for fruitful interaction and cooperation. At the core of such relationships is confidence in and reliance upon others to respect the principle of veracity. This form of argument, commonly used by rule utilitarians, holds that lying can undermine relationships of trust and produce undesirable consequences. For example, relationships between health care professionals and their patients and between researchers and their subjects ultimately depend on trust. Lying thus fails to show respect for persons and their autonomy, violates implicit contracts, and also threatens relationships based on trust.[7]

Despite these arguments for the duty of veracity, the various codes of medical ethics tend to omit this duty. (See Appendix II.) The Hippocratic Oath does not impose it, nor does the Declaration of Geneva by the World Medical Association in 1948. According to the Principles of Medical Ethics of the AMA, the physician has discretion about what to tell his or her patients. There is no clear duty of veracity in these codes. In sharp contrast, one recent Patient's Bill of Rights (compare the American Hospital Association statement in Appendix II) holds that a patient has a right "to informed participation in all decisions involving his health care program," a right "to know what research and experimental protocols are being used" in the facility and what alternatives are available in the community, a right "to a clear, concise explanation of all proposed procedures in layman's terms, including the possibilities of any risk of mortality or serious side effects, problems related to recuperation, and probability of success," and a right "to know the identity and professional status of all those providing service."[8]

These differences between codes of medical ethics and the Patient's Bill of Rights in part reflect differences between physicians' and patients' perspectives—both of which are probably too limited. Physicians often think in terms of patients' needs and interests. This can lead them to a paternalistic stance rather than to an emphasis on patient autonomy. Patients, on the other hand, frequently think in terms of rights more so than in terms of needs and interests. These different perspectives are reflected in surveys of medical and lay views about telling the truth to cancer patients. According to one study, the majority (88 percent) of physicians tend not to disclose a diagnosis of cancer to their patients. According to another study, the majority of lay people (82 to 98 percent) indicate that they want to be told the truth if they have cancer.[9]

What does the principle of veracity entail and how much weight does it have? Like other duties in this volume, veracity is prima facie, not absolute. Nondisclosure, deception, and even lying can sometimes be justified when veracity conflicts with other duties. In many areas, but especially in disputes about veracity, moral debates involve the definition or description of the act as well as its justification. Let us consider "lying." We define "lying" as telling another person what one believes to be false in order to deceive him. So defined, "lying" would only be prima facie wrong and thus could be justified in some circumstances. If, however, "lying" is defined as intentionally withholding the truth from a person who has a right to it, then "lying" could be construed as absolutely wrong. The latter definition incorporates moral elements since it holds that the truth is due some persons but not others. It "resolves" moral dilemmas by redefining them, for some statements that would be described as lies according to our definition would not be lies according to this definition. In Chapter 2, we discussed Case #3 in terms of both definitions of lying.

Although lying has attracted more attention and discussion than other ways of departing from the principle of veracity, it is in fact only one species of deception. It is distinguished from other species because it involves statements and because it is intentional—one cannot accidentally tell a lie. Deception is broader and encompasses many acts other than lying. For example, when a physician gives his patient a placebo, he may or may not lie to the patient. In Case #5, the therapists intentionally deceived the patient for his own benefit, but they did not lie to him. The duty of veracity requires nondeception, as well as truth-telling, but non-lying deception probably does not threaten the relationship of trust as much as lying, because lying means that an agent asserts what he believes to be false in order to deceive another.

The duty not to lie to or otherwise deceive others is stronger than the duty to disclose information to others. The duty to disclose depends more on special relationships than does the duty not to lie to or deceive others. In a therapeutic relationship, for example, the patient entrusts his care to the therapist and has a right to information that the therapist would not be obligated to provide to total strangers. It is difficult to conceive of a positive duty to promote the truth by providing information apart from special relationships.

Both lies, as we have defined them, and other forms of deception are prima facie wrong and stand in need of justification; but they can some-times be justified. In Chapter 3, we considered some of the conditions that are necessary to justify deception and incomplete disclosure in research. Those conditions were so narrowly drawn that most biomedical and psychological research involving intentional deception would be unjusti-fied. Nevertheless, we held that some important low-risk research in-volving minor deception could be justified if the information that was not disclosed would have invalidated valuable research. We shall now consider some arguments for limited nondisclosure and deception in *therapeutic* settings.

The first argument for nondisclosure of some diagnoses and prognoses in the therapeutic setting represents what Sidgwick called "benevolent deception."[10] It holds that disclosure of a diagnosis of cancer, for ex-ample, would violate the duties of beneficence and nonmaleficence by causing the patient anxiety ("what you don't know can't hurt you"), by causing the patient to commit suicide, etc. One objection to this argument is based on the uncertainty of predicting consequences. Samuel Johnson made this point:

I deny the lawfulness of telling a lie to a sick man for fear of alarming him. You have no business with consequences; you are to tell the truth. Besides, you are not sure what effects your telling him that he is in danger may have. It may bring his distemper to a crisis, and that may cure him. Of all lying, I have the greatest abhorrence of this, because I believe it has been frequently practised on myself.[11]

Such an objection is especially applicable to act-utilitarian approaches to truth-telling. The more telling objections to "benevolent deception" stress violations of the principles of respect for persons and fidelity as well as the long-term threat to the relationship of trust between physicians and patients.

In Case #6, a radiologist did not warn his patients of the possibility of a fatal reaction to urography on the grounds that it would not benefit them to know and might be dangerous. He contended that if he had told the woman who died of the possible fatal reaction, she would have become upset. He would then have convinced her that the probability of benefit outweighed the slight chance of a fatal reaction. Thus, he argued, telling her would only have upset her and would not have changed the outcome. Even if such cases do not seriously threaten the relationship of trust, they involve violations of the principles of fidelity and autonomy. In particular, the radiologist denied the patient information necessary for informed consent and violated her right to make her own assessment of the risks and benefits. (Of course, not all possible information is necessary, as we argued in our discussion of informed consent and the reasonable-person standard in Chapter 3.)

Case #5 represents another instance of "benevolent deception." A retired army officer was having chronic pain after several abdominal operations. He had lost weight and was depressed, unkempt, and socially withdrawn. He was admitted to a psychiatric ward which had the clear expectation of reducing his reliance on Talwin to relieve his pain by substituting pain control. Nevertheless, the patient insisted that he needed his medication to control his pain. After group consultation, the therapists decided to withdraw the Talwin by gradually substituting saline, but without informing the patient. The substitution was effective, and although the patient was angry when he was told three weeks later, he asked that the saline be discontinued. He was able to control his pain and to resume relatively normal functions. The therapists justified this deceptive use of a placebo because of its "high probability of success." While it is tempting to justify the means by the ends, especially when they are successfully realized, alternative nondeceptive means might have worked. The prima facie duty of veracity dictates a search for available alternatives even if they sometimes require more time, energy, and money. Furthermore, on utilitarian grounds this deceptive use of a placebo may have long-term negative effects on the patient's self-image and may damage his trust in health care professionals.

A second argument for nondisclosure and deception is that health care professionals cannot know or cannot communicate the "whole truth," and if they could, many patients and subjects would not be able to comprehend and understand the "whole truth." Such an argument does not, however, undermine the duty of veracity, understood as the duty to be truthful, for this duty requires that health care professionals disclose as completely as possible what a reasonable patient would want to know and what particular patients want to know.[12]

A third argument for nondisclosure and deception is that some patients, particularly the very sick and the dying, do not really want to know the truth about their condition, despite what opinion surveys seem to reveal. According to this line of argument, neither the duty of fidelity nor the duty of respect for persons requires truth-telling, because patients indicate by various signals—if not by actual words—that they do not want to hear the truth. To the rejoinder that many and perhaps most patients appear to want disclosure of relevant information, proponents of this third argument for nondisclosure hold that the patients they have in mind *really* do not want to know even when they say they do. Claims about what patients really want are suspicious, and there is no moral alternative in such cases to respecting the autonomy of competent patients by acting on their expressed wishes and wants. Also, this third argument sets dangerous precedents for paternalistic actions, even if it is a correct view of patient wishes and wants in some cases.

In some instances, of course, patients genuinely do not want to know. For example, some patients with a high risk of developing Huntington's chorea, an incurable genetic disease, indicate that they would not be interested in a simple, safe, and accurate predictive test if one were developed. In one sample, twenty-three percent of the high-risk respondents indicated that they might not take such a test.[13] In other cases, patients who suspect that they have cancer explicitly ask not to be informed of the diagnosis and prognosis. What should health care professionals do when patients ask not to be given certain information? Some writers go so far as to argue that a patient has a *duty* to seek and appropriate the truth— not merely a *right* to the truth.[14] But to force unwanted information on a patient is generally to act paternalistically and to violate that patient's autonomy. To force a person to confront the truth seems to be an act of disrespect, though it might on occasion be justified—e.g., in cases of weak paternalism where a person acts from false beliefs. However, respect entails allowing persons to exercise the right not to know whenever they are adequately informed and are acting autonomously.

If the disclosure of information in part depends on a duty of fidelity, what responsibility does a health care professional have when a test undertaken for a specific purpose reveals information not specifically requested by the testee who might, however, be very interested in the information? In a case discussed by Robert Veatch,[15] a forty-one-year-old woman had unexpectedly become pregnant and was referred by her physician to the Human Genetics Unit in order to determine whether her fetus might have Down's syndrome (or mongolism). Because of her age she was considered to be at high risk of having a mongoloid child. The woman underwent amniocentesis, in which a sample of amniotic fluid surrounding the fetus was withdrawn by a needle for purposes of a biochemical or chromosomal analysis. The test showed that the fetus did not have Down's syndrome. There was no *extra* 21st chromosome. But the sex chromosomes were abnormal. They were XYY, rather than the normal patterns of XX for female or XY for male. There is considerable debate about the significance of the extra Y chromosome. Although some studies show that XYY males tend to commit more violent crimes, other studies reject those findings. What should the genetic counselor do? Would he fulfill his duty of fidelity and disclosure if he only reported that the fetus did not suffer from Down's syndrome? Or is he also morally required to report the other findings? Does the woman have a right to obtain this information even though she did not specifically request it? Does the fact that the correlation between the XYY chromosomes and antisocial behavior is not established make his disclosure even more risky since it (a) could lead to an abortion or (b) could be a self-fulfilling prophecy if the woman did not abort? Should the patient have the right to make her own decision about the significance of this information? If the duty of veracity is based on respect for persons and their autonomy, a strong case can be made for disclosure. However, there are cases in which nondisclosure might be preferable, and there are, of course, many ways of disclosing the truth with compassion and sensitivity.

In one type of situation, the AMA Principles of Medical Ethics (see

Appendix II) require disclosure of information in order to preserve trust between the public and the medical profession:

The medical profession should safeguard the public and itself against physicians deficient in moral character or professional competence. . . . They should expose, without hesitation, illegal or unethical conduct of fellow members of the profession. (Section 4)

Exposés by fellow physicians are, however, uncommon. On the basis of studies of professional ethics and competence, it is difficult to believe that all or most cases of deficiency in moral character or professional incompetence are disclosed to the proper bodies or to the public. The bond of loyalty to the profession, so accentuated in the tradition of medical ethics, makes such disclosures unlikely.

In addition to loyalty to colleagues, which may conflict with the duty to disclose information, the physician may also experience a conflict between the duty of confidentiality and the duty of veracity. Such a conflict is evident in Case #3, which we discussed in Chapter 2. After tests have shown that he is histocompatible, a father decides that he does not want to donate a kidney to his five-year-old daughter who needs a transplant. Because he fears that the truth might shatter his family, he asks the physician to tell the members of his family that he is not histocompatible. The physician then tells the family that "for medical reasons," the father should not donate a kidney. Although it is possible to analyze this case in utilitarian terms—maximizing good and minimizing harm—it is possible to argue that the father's relationship with the physician was confidential and that the duty to respect confidentiality outweighed the duty of veracity in this situation. Some would argue that the duty of confidentiality justifies nondisclosure (in this case) but does not justify a lie if the wife should press the physician for an explanation of "medical reasons." This problem leads us to a study of the rule of confidentiality in order that we might determine its basis, meaning, and limits.

The rule of confidentiality

Suppose the parents of a child suffering from a genetic disease insist that the physician not reveal this information to others in the family who may be at risk for having children with the same disease. Suppose, for example, that the child has Lesch-Nyhan syndrome, a disease involving uncontrollable self-mutilation. Because this disease is X-linked, the mother's sisters would be at risk. But the mother, let us suppose, dislikes her sisters, who live far away and never communicate. Furthermore, she feels the stigma of being a carrier of the disease and so wishes to conceal the information. In this case, her physician faces a conflict between his duty to respect the confidences of his patients and his general social responsibility. There is no way to avoid this conflict if his attempts to obtain the mother's permission to disclose this information should fail. The right and perhaps the duty to break therapeutic confidences under some circumstances indicate that the therapeutic role may sometimes have to yield to one's role as citizen and as protector of the interests of others.

There is widespread agreement, expressed in various ethical codes for health care professionals, that a rule of confidentiality should prevail in relationships with patients. The Hippocratic Oath urges secrecy regarding what "ought not to be spoken abroad," but does not limit secrecy to what is seen or heard in professional practice. The AMA Code holds that a "physician may not reveal the confidences entrusted to him in the course of medical attendance, or the deficiencies he may observe in the character of his patients, unless he is required to do so by law or unless it becomes necessary in order to protect the welfare of the individual or of the community" (Section 9). The World Medical Association International Code of Medical Ethics expressly holds that the physician owes his patient *"absolute secrecy* on all [information] which has been confided to him or which he knows because of the confidence entrusted to him" (emphasis added). Still, most codes and general theories hold that the rule of confidentiality is not absolute. In fact, it may be possible to specify several conditions under which confidentiality should not be maintained—e.g., some more specific variants of the conditions listed in the AMA Code. Before we turn to those conditions for justified breaches of confidentiality, we need to inquire into the basis of the rule and the warrants that support it.

Although we may find a person who betrays secrets despicable, it is not clear that he violates a general moral principle or rule against telling secrets. In most instances, he betrays other people who entered into certain relationships with him and counted on him to respect their confidences. His actions are despicable because he betrays the *trust* of other persons. Trust is confidence in and reliance upon others to respect certain principles and rules in their interactions. It is the expectation that others will respect boundaries, which often (but not always) are moral ones. Some of the limits set by professional codes, for example, are more matters of custom than of morality. But the patient may rely upon the health care professional to respect these customs and may rightly believe that their implicit contract has been violated if the professional fails to live up to these customary standards.

While the rule of confidentiality is based on custom, it also has moral warrants, some utilitarian and others deontological. Both the majority opinion and the dissenting opinion in the Tarasoff case (see Case #1) offer a utilitarian grounding for the rule of confidentiality—as discussed in Chapter 2. Their main disagreement, as we will see later, concerns the question of exceptions to the rule or conditions for overriding it in the psychotherapeutic relationship. According to Justice Clark's dissent, the psychiatrist does not have a duty to warn a potential victim about possible harm from a patient. Assurance of confidentiality is important because it enables people to seek help without the stigma that would result from public knowledge, because it encourages full disclosure that is essential for effective treatment, and because it is necessary for the maintenance of trust, "the very means by which treatment is effected." Justice Clark's line of argument is that psychiatry has an important social function in the reduction of violence and that it cannot fulfill that function without the rule of confidentiality in virtually absolute form. For the state to impose a duty to warn is to undermine the rule of confidentiality and thereby to diminish psychiatry's valuable social function.

A more deontological argument builds on the right of autonomy. One aspect of respecting autonomy is respect for a person's *privacy*. According to a landmark law review article in 1890 on the right of privacy, the individual has the right "of determining, ordinarily, to what extent his thoughts, sentiments, and emotions shall be communicated to others."[16] Whatever privacy includes, it involves personal control over information about oneself and over access to that information. Without such personal control, important human relationships such as love, friendship, and trust would be diminished. The image of concentric circles that some have proposed is useful.[17] The core self with its secrets is at the center, choosing to grant others access to that information in accord with the kinds of relationships it wants to establish. The outer circles represent less intense and less personal relationships that require less personal information. At stake is both the *amount* and the *kind* of information. As Charles Fried suggests, while we might not mind if a person knows a general fact about us, we might feel that our privacy has been invaded if he knows the details.[18] Similarly, we might not object if a good friend knows the nature of our illness, but we might protest that he has invaded our privacy if he observes us actually suffering from that illness.

We grant others access to information about ourselves as a part of such relationships as love, friendship, and trust. We may also have specific reasons for granting this information to some persons: when we wish to be treated by a physician, a psychiatrist, or other health care professionals, we may have to share personal information. Less may be required for the physician than for the psychiatrist or psychologist. For successful treatment by the latter, we must expose our innermost thoughts, feelings, emotions, dreams, and fantasies. We grant these health care professionals access to information about ourselves for our own diagnostic and therapeutic benefit. In general, we should retain control over access to that information, authorizing access when appropriate. For example, we might authorize a physician to grant an insurance company or a prospective employer access to the information.

Both utilitarian and deontological considerations thus can be invoked to support a rule of confidentiality. The harder questions, however, concern the stringency of the rule of confidentiality. Should it be viewed as merely a rule of thumb? Is it an absolute rule, as in the requirement of "absolute secrecy" in the International Code of Medical Ethics? Or should it be regarded merely as a rule asserting a prima facie duty? Some parts of the majority decision in the Tarasoff case (see Case #1) can be read as holding that the rule of confidentiality is only a rule of thumb. However, the decision as a whole indicates that maintaining confidentiality is a prima facie duty. Even the minority dissent does not claim that the rule is absolute. Disagreement occurs over the range of legitimate exceptions. In both opinions, an act is prima facie wrong insofar as it violates confidentiality, but the conditions under which it is actually wrong vary in the two opinions.

Our view follows from our discussion of rules in Chapter 2: the rule of confidentiality, which could be formulated as imposing duties on health care professionals or as creating rights for patients, states a prima facie duty. Anyone who thinks that a disclosure of confidential information is morally justified or even mandatory in some circumstances bears a burden of proof. While this approach requires a balancing of conflicting duties, it also establishes a structure of moral reasoning and justification. It is not enough to determine which act will respect the most duties or maximize the good, for the strong presumption against revealing confidences establishes the direction and burden of deliberation and justification.

Sometimes the health care professional has been viewed as having a "right" to violate confidences in some circumstances, but not as having a "duty" to do so. He is permitted, but not obliged, according to this view. Nevertheless, there are clear legal duties to divulge confidential information when necessary to report contagious diseases, gunshot wounds, child abuse, etc. The Court held in the Tarasoff case that psychiatrists have a "duty" to warn their patients' intended victims. The AMA Code holds that the physician should not violate the rule of confidentiality "unless he is required to do so by law or unless it becomes necessary in order to protect the welfare of the individual or of the community" (Section 9). Although some people interpret this statement as permitting but not requiring the physician to break confidences, we interpret it differently: one may not break a confidence except to fulfill another and more stringent duty— either a duty to obey the law, or a duty to protect the welfare of the patient or the community, e.g., a duty based on beneficence. There is no *right* to violate confidences in such cases unless there is also a *duty* to do so. The health care professional's breach of confidentiality thus cannot be justified unless it is necessary to meet a strong conflicting duty. This conclusion means that rules protecting confidences must sometimes give way to rules protecting other interests.

Before discussing duties that may justify violating the rule of confidentiality, we should note that some breaches of confidentiality are not violations of duties to the patient. For example, the company physician who informs his employers that an employee in a responsible position suffers from alcoholism may not actually violate a rule of confidentiality, for he may not be bound by this rule in the same way as a private physician. He could, for example, be under contract with the company and an employee's union to perform certain services, including the reporting of work-related information about patients. Nevertheless, both the company and the physician in such circumstances have the moral responsibility to insure that employee-patients actually understand at the outset that the traditional rule of confidentiality is not operative.

A distinction should be made between releasing information at the patient's *behest* and releasing it on the patient's *behalf without his consent.* Although the health care professional should generally release confidential information about a particular patient when the patient requests its release, the health care professional may encounter circumstances in which the patient refuses to authorize disclosures that would be in his best interest. When the patient authorizes disclosure of information—e.g., to his lawyer, to the court, to an insurance company, or to a family member— the health care professional does not violate the rule of confidentiality, which is designed to protect the patient's control over access to information about himself. Hereafter we shall be exclusively concerned with disclosures of confidential information without the patient's informed authorization.

What duties legitimately override the rule of confidentiality? While the AMA Code mentions both legal duties and actions necessary to protect patients or society, these two sets of conditions are not mutually exclusive. The law may lay down certain conditions for the protection of the individual and society or may simply allow general moral convictions to prevail. In either case, the law may not hold the health care professional accountable for a breach of confidentiality. Most instances of disclosing confidential information to protect *the patient* (rather than others) are not legally required. Some legal duties such as the requirement to report epileptic seizures to the division of motor vehicles (see Case #2) may be paternalistic in some dimensions and utilitarian in others. Even the legal requirement to report child abuse is not paternalistic. The health care professional has a legal duty to report child abuse in order to protect the child, and he has a duty of confidentiality only to the child, not to the parents, even if they are also his patients. His fiduciary relationship is with the child, whose interests he must protect.

Legal duties to break confidentiality in order to protect *others* pose a conflict of obligations for the health care professional. On the one hand, he is obligated to protect his patient; on the other hand, he is legally obligated to act to protect the society, even if he thinks the law is silly or unjust. There also is a *moral* obligation to obey the law, at least in a relatively just system,[19] but it is only a strong prima facie duty, not absolute. Sometimes it may be necessary for the health care professional to violate the duty to obey the law in order to fulfill his responsibility to his patient. Sometimes he may justifiably reason that he cannot adequately treat his patient over time if he obeys the law—e.g., in complicated circumstances where there is a legal duty to report venereal disease.

Violations of the rule of confidentiality where there is no legal duty to disclose information raise additional issues. First, it is easier to justify violations of confidentiality on grounds of the prevention of harm to others than on grounds of paternalism, especially for competent adults. The duty to report child abuse would be strong even in the absence of a statute because of the child's dependence and vulnerability. However, where competent adults are involved, breaches of confidentiality to protect the patient from himself usually involve a violation of autonomy, and therefore are difficult to justify. Suppose that a physician has to decide whether to disclose to a thirty-year-old woman's parents that their daughter's marriage is in trouble and that this is the cause of a "nervous condition" which has resulted in her hospitalization. She has asked him not to say anything to her parents, but he is convinced that her parents, who are also his patients, would help her recover. The alleged benefit to the patient is not of sufficient magnitude or probability to warrant overriding autonomy and the rule of confidentiality in these circumstances. If the physician's efforts to convince the woman that she should tell her parents fail, he should maintain confidentiality even if he believes it is not in the patient's best interest.

Second, if the duty to prevent harms is more stringent than the duty to provide benefits, it is easier to justify violations of confidentiality in order to prevent harms to patients or others than to justify violations on grounds of benefit to patients. But a clear distinction cannot always be drawn between producing benefits and preventing harms; and the duty to prevent a trivial harm may not be stronger than the duty to produce a major benefit. The type of harms and benefits may also make a relevant difference. If psychiatrists have a duty to warn intended victims of violence, is the line to be drawn at threats to physical existence and integrity, e.g., murder and rape? Or do we extend it to include threats to property?

Third, how *probable* must the benefit or harm be before a breach of confidentiality is justified? Is a remote chance of substantial harm to many people sufficient? In the Tarasoff case (#1 in Appendix I) the California Supreme Court focussed on society's interdependence: "In this risk-infested society we can hardly tolerate the further exposure to danger that would result from a concealed knowledge of the therapist that his patient was lethal."

Fourth, given the presumption against violating the rule of confidentiality and the significance of that rule, the health care professional should of course seek alternative and more acceptable ways of realizing a benefit or preventing a harm, short of disclosing confidential information (and violating other important moral principles and rules). Rarely is the breach of confidentiality justified if morally and legally acceptable alternatives exist. In one case, a physician had to determine whether to disclose a patient's homosexuality to his prospective wife, who was also the physician's patient. Although the physician chose to respect the rule of confidentiality, should he have tried to persuade the young man to tell his prospective wife? Or should he have discussed marriage and sexuality with the young woman so that she might have pressed her prospective fiance for more information? Since she was his patient, the physician had a stronger obligation to disclose information to her than he would have had if she had been a stranger, and this obligation makes his inaction less acceptable.[20]

Finally, most interesting cases of confidentiality involve uncertainty at the time the decision must be made. Uncertainty may occur on several different levels: basic information, diagnosis, prognosis, likelihood of an untoward event, etc. For example, in Case #2, the physician has to decide whether to inform the division of motor vehicles that his epileptic patient still suffers seizures, when this unconfirmed information came from a neighbor of the patient. In another case, a psychiatrist used hypnotic techniques to help a pilot recall suppressed information about his responsibility for the crash of a commercial plane. The information indicated that the pilot should not fly, at least temporarily. When the therapist was unable to convince the pilot that he should not fly until his problems were solved, what should he have done? How much certainty did he need for more vigorous action? Six months after returning to work, the pilot made an error of judgment that resulted in the crash of a transatlantic flight and the loss of many lives.[21] Suppose that a pilot of a commercial jet informs his physician that his forty-five-year-old mother was diagnosed as having Huntington's chorea. The physician has to determine whether to disclose to the airline this pilot's fifty percent risk of having the disease in the event the pilot fails to reveal it.[22] In these cases difficult matters of judgment are involved in determining the probability and magnitude of a harm (or benefit) that will justify the breach of confidentiality. There can be no simple formula for deciding such cases independent of the individual risk/benefit assessments themselves. (See Chapter 5.)

There is an important distinction between the probable effects of a disease (e.g., venereal disease) and the probable actions of an agent (e.g., a patient's threat to harm someone else). It may be easier to justify breaches of confidentiality to prevent a disease's negative effects than to prevent an agent's negative acts. Cases of doubt about whether an agent will do what he threatens to do may be harder to resolve than cases of doubt about the effects of a disease. The former cases, most of which emerge in psychiatric or psychotherapeutic relations, require more room for patient autonomy, but they do not indicate that a patient should never be committed for suicidal or homicidal tendencies. The Assembly of District Branches and the Board of Trustees of the American Psychiatric Association in 1973 annotated the principles of medical ethics for psychiatry and held (with special reference to court-ordered disclosures of confidences): "When the psychiatrist is in doubt, the right of the patient to confidentiality and, by extension, to unimpaired treatment, should be given priority."[23] An annotated AMA code (1971) appealed to a version of the Golden Rule as a test of the physician's responsibility to report contagious diseases. This test could also apply to various doubtful cases: "the physician should act as he would desire another to act toward one of his own family in like circumstances" (Section 9).

Conflicts among contractual and role obligations

In many cases, the health care professional has a duty of care because of an explicit or implicit contract with the patient. But in some cases, the therapeutic contract may actually be with a party other than the patient. The beneficiary need not hold one end of the chain of obligations and rights. For example, if someone promises John Doe to look after his children after his death, we would say that the promisor has an obligation to John Doe although the children are the primary beneficiaries.[24] When parents bring a child to a physician for treatment, the physician's primary responsibility is to the child, whose interests are paramount. Courts have rightly refused to allow Jehovah's Witnesses to reject medically necessary blood transfusions for their children, even though the courts have often allowed adult Jehovah's Witnesses to reject blood transfusions for themselves (as in Case #11; contrast Case #12). In some cases, parents may be charged with child neglect when they fail to seek or permit highly desirable medical treatment, even if it falls short of being necessary to save the child's life. Angela Holder has provided a summary of one such case: "A teenage boy suffered from a massive deformity of the face and neck. He was so grotesque he was excused from school attendance and was therefore illiterate. Surgery could correct the condition but could not be performed without blood transfusions. The mother objected on religious grounds to administration of blood and therefore would not consent to surgery. The court held that he was a 'neglected child' and ordered the surgery performed."[25]

In recent years there has been considerable moral debate about decisions regarding defective newborns who need surgery to sustain their lives. (See Cases #17 and #18.) In the much discussed Johns Hopkins Hospital case (#18), a mongoloid infant needed surgery for duodenal atresia. The parents refused to grant permission for the surgery, and the infant died of starvation after several days. In some cases, physicians or hospitals have gone to the courts to gain permission to provide the medical treatment refused by the parents. Such interventions are probably more common among physicians and hospitals in cases of refusal of treatment on *religious* grounds, partly because the health care professionals rarely share these belief systems. In cases where parents appeal to the best interests of the child and to familial interests, such as the prevention of disruption and strain on financial resources, physicians appear to be more willing to support the familial decision to refuse treatment. Of course, there may be major disagreements about what would be in the child's *interests,* or in the family's *interests,* but the point is that many physicians appear to be more comfortable with such judgments about interests than with refusals on religious grounds.[26] Our own view is that physicians have a primary responsibility to the patient, even if a third party establishes the initial contract. The physician ought to act in the patient's best interests, even when it is necessary to seek a court order to authorize surgery, a blood transfusion, or whatever. Other familial interests such as avoiding the depletion of financial resources should not be considered until a certain threshold is reached, viz., when significant patient interests would not be served by continued treatment or by a particular treatment.

The above examples focus on the conflict between the interests of the patient, the beneficiary, and the wishes of the contractor with the health care professional. In another major type of conflict it may be less clear exactly what the health care professional owes the "patient." Examples include a physician's contract to examine applicants for positions in a company or to determine whether applicants for insurance policies are good risks. In such cases, the health care professional may rightly not think of the person he examines as his patient. He has certain responsibilities of due care, but they may not be as comprehensive or as stringent as the responsibilities that obtain in the ordinary physician-patient relationship. They would include care in the examination so as not to injure the individual—e.g., by exposing him to excessive X rays. From a legal standpoint, the health care professional in some jurisdictions may not even have a duty to disclose the discovery of a disease to the examinee. For example, in one preemployment physical examination, X rays indicated that the woman who was subsequently hired had tuberculosis, but the physician and employer did not disclose these findings to her. After three years, the employee became ill with tuberculosis and was hospitalized for a prolonged period. In this case, the court held that the woman's only recourse was Workman's Compensation. The court did not allow her suit against her employer and the physician who examined her, on grounds that there was no established patient-physician relationship, and hence no duty to disclose the information to her.[27] From a moral standpoint both the employer and the physician had a duty to disclose this information in order to prevent harm to her; they did not merely have a duty to benefit her. Furthermore, one could argue that the employer and the physician had no right to withhold this information, because the woman had a moral right to it.

What does this moral duty of disclosure require in conflict situations where some institutional interests might be at stake? Suppose a company requires regular physical examinations of all employees by a company physician. The physician's contract requires him to inform the company about employees' health conditions that might bear on their work. If the company uses materials that might be hazardous to the employees, e.g., kepone or benzene, and the physician discovers symptoms of a disease that might be directly related to working conditions, what obligation does he have to report these findings to the employees as well as to the company? Does he have the same obligation if the employer expressly forbids such disclosures to employees? Health care professionals, we suggest, have a moral responsibility to oppose, avoid, and withdraw from contracts that would force them to withhold information of significant medical benefit to examinees.

In another type of situation, a health care professional may be under contract to, or otherwise obligated to, an institution to provide *care* for a group of individuals. In these cases, there can be no doubt that physicians, for example, owe "due care" to these individuals who are their "patients," despite the third-party contract or obligation. Examples include health care professionals in industries, prisons, and the armed services. In these settings, care of the patient may come into conflict with needs of the institution. The patient's needs generally should take precedence, but not always. Difficult cases may emerge, for example, on the battlefield. Triage in the battlefield setting may be different from triage in the peacetime emergency room. In the former setting the needs of the military may dictate that certain patients be given priority even when medical needs establish a different priority. In a celebrated example, when penicillin became available for use in North Africa in World War II, a difficult allocation decision had to be made because the supply was severely limited. Authorities decided to give the available penicillin to soldiers suffering from venereal disease rather than those who had been wounded on the battlefields. The former, they reasoned, could be restored to fighting capacity more easily and effectively than the latter. As we have seen in our discussion of justice and microallocation, it is not possible to generalize from the battlefield to ordinary medical practice. Even on the battlefield, however, medical needs should not be wholly subordinated to military needs. For example, conventions regarding the laws of war hold that the fallen enemy soldier with medical needs is to be given equal consideration along with one's own comrades.

In addition to allocation decisions that are contingent upon medical and institutional needs (Cf. Case #20, which we discussed in the section on microallocation), health care professionals in military and other institutions sometimes make judgments about "sickness" and "health" based on institutional values. In 1966 an Air Force newsletter reported that a twenty-six-year-old staff sergeant gunner who had been on active duty in Vietnam for seven months and had flown over one hundred missions developed a fear of flying because several of his acquaintances had died. The diagnosis was Gross Stress Reaction, "manifested by anxiety, tenseness, a fear of death expressed in the form of rationalizations, and inability to function. His problem was 'worked through' and insight . . . was gained to the extent that he was returned to full flying duty in less than six weeks."[28] This case raises numerous questions: Which medical and psychiatric labels, if any, are appropriate in such a case where the refusal could be seen as rational from the patient's standpoint but not from the military's? At what point should the psychotherapist refuse to engage in military or other service on the grounds that he cannot combine his responsibility to patients with institutional needs in that setting? Does the physician have an obligation to inquire into the justice of a particular war before engaging in it? Although there are borderline cases, such as the one in this Air Force Newsletter, in principle physicians and psychotherapists can function in the military and can render valuable service to wounded soldiers, even in an unjust war, without violating moral principles. Some actions, however, may violate canons of medical ethics and thus warrant disobedience to orders: e.g., an order for a physician to help torture a prisoner in order to gain information. An illustrative case occurred in the Vietnam War. Captain Howard B. Levy, a physician, refused to provide training in dermatology to Special Forces Aidmen on the grounds, in part, that it directed medicine to political rather than humanitarian ends. If this charge was correct, Captain Levy took a correct course of action.

Similarly, the two roles of research scientist and clinical practitioner may come into conflict. As an investigator, the physician acts to generate knowledge that can lead to progress in medicine that will ultimately benefit individual patients. As a clinical practitioner, he acts in the present patient's best interests. Both of these roles may function to "benefit the sick," but the scientific role aims to benefit statistical lives in the future, while the clinical role seeks to benefit particular patients now. Responsibility to future generations thus may come into conflict with "due care" for particular persons who are subjects as well as patients. The Declaration of Geneva of the World Medical Association affirms that "the health of my patient will be my first consideration." Yet, can this principle be affirmed under all conditions in the context of research involving patients as subjects? If not, should it be sacrificed or at least compromised in order to benefit more people in the future?

Controlled clinical trials are considered important and even necessary in order to make sure that an observed effect, e.g., reduced mortality from a particular disease, is really the result of a particular treatment rather than some other variable that the researcher might have missed, e.g., other conditions in the patient population. Among the controlled trials to determine the effectiveness and safety of treatments and procedures, the randomized clinical trial (RCT) is widely used. Instead of trying to match patients for variables so that some of the matched patients can receive A and some B, the RCT randomly assigns patients to different therapies or placebos. Randomization is used to keep variables other than the treatments under examination from distorting the study. It is often preferred to observational or retrospective studies on the grounds that its results have a higher degree of validity by virtue of its elimination of bias in assignment and reduction of extraneous variables. Thus, it appears to offer a sound inductive technique to validate knowledge.

Many questions can be raised about RCTs: Are they as essential as their proponents say? Can they be used without compromising acknowledged responsibilities to patients?[29] The increased probability of their results is only a matter of degree, and there might be reasons for preferring a less conclusive method if it would more fully respect our duties to current patients. Proponents of RCTs often argue, however, that RCTs do not violate moral duties to patients, because there is genuine doubt about the merits of existing therapies or of standard and new therapies. No patient will receive a treatment that is known to be less effective or more dangerous than another available alternative. Because current patients, in effect, are not asked to make any sacrifices, who could object to the use of RCTs? After all, they will in addition benefit future patients. It is, of course, possible that treatments rarely exhibit such perfect balance, especially if all the patient's circumstances are considered. Rarely would a physician be willing to determine by chance which treatment a patient receives except in the context of RCTs.

A vivid recent example (see Case #27) indicates some difficulties in the use of RCTs. A controlled, double-blind experiment on a new drug, adenine arabinoside (ara-A), indicated that it is an effective treatment for herpes simplex encephalitis. Of the ten people who were given the placebo, seven died. Of the eighteen who received ara-A, five died, seven recovered to lead reasonably normal lives, and six had serious brain or nerve damage. The ten who received the placebo also were given standard treatment, which mainly consists of palliative efforts. (No treatment prior to ara-A had been found to be effective.) Because ara-A had already been shown to be effective and nontoxic in other localized herpes simplex hominis infections, and because no other treatment prevented mortality and serious brain and nerve damage, moral questions arise about giving anyone the placebo. The experiment was stopped early, but it remains unclear whether it was necessary to have a placebo group instead of historical controls.

Even when there are no scientific or ethical grounds for opposing a particular randomized clinical trial—for example, of two treatments that are roughly equal in safety and efficacy—patients may have strong preferences for one or the other. Suppose that two surgical procedures for treating the same disease appear to have the same survival rate (say, an average of 15 years), and suppose we propose to test their effectiveness by an RCT. The patient might have a preference if treatment A has little risk of death during the operation but a high rate of death after ten years, while treatment B has a high risk of death during the operation or postoperative recovery but a low rate of death after recovery (say, for 30 years). A patient's age, family responsibilities, and other circumstances in life might lead him to prefer one over the other.[30] While a research institution could legitimately accept only patients who were willing to participate in certain research projects related to their own diseases, patients in other types of settings should be able to choose between treatments whenever both treatments are available.

Since patients commonly assume that decisions about their treatment are made in their best interests, and not in the interests of a research design, the physician-researcher should disclose all the alternatives to patient-subjects so that they can make an informed judgment about participation. One relevant item of information is the method of allocation to a particular treatment. Some contend that disclosure of such matters would cause distress that would be harmful to patients or would lead some patients to refuse to participate in the research. They also argue that disclosure of such matters is not necessary, since the patient does not need to know how the allocation is made between two treatments that appear to be equally effective and/or harmless. However, since the physician-researcher is a double agent, holding dual responsibilities, he has a fiduciary duty to inform his patient-subjects of everything that is relevant to their own decisions and, in particular, that might involve the physician-researcher in a conflict of interest.[31] The duty of disclosure persists throughout the period of the research and requires that the patient-subject be informed about developments that might be relevant to a decision to withdraw. (See the discussion on disclosure and informed consent in Chapter 3.)

Physician-researchers also face difficult questions about whether to stop an experiment before it has been completed, and even before there is enough information to have the preliminary data accepted. If a physician determines that his patient's condition is deteriorating and that the patient's interests dictate withdrawal from the research, he should be free to act on behalf of the patient, assuming, of course, that he does not act in opposition to the express wishes of the patient. Some research designs take advantage of emerging evidence to alter the protocol; some play the winner by utilizing what appear to be the best therapies until they fail. But in an RCT, particularly if it is a double-blind study, it may be difficult to determine whether the experiment as a whole should be stopped merely because some physician-researchers insist that they have enough evidence already. One proposal to handle the ethical conflict involves a differentiation of roles; it recommends an advisory committee to determine whether to continue or stop a trial. Such a committee "must consider the impact of its decision on the treatment of future patients. Although an individual physician may only be responsible for treating his current patients, the advisory committee must act as if the care of future patients rests in their hands, because their recommendations are likely to influence therapy for the many patients to follow."[32]

The proposal of a differentiation of roles by using an advisory committee may be procedurally sound, but it fails to resolve the ethical questions. Instead, it relocates them. Even if occupants of different roles represent different interests, e.g., the physicians represent current patients' interests, while the scientists and the advisory committee represent future patients' interests, it is still necessary to determine when it is legitimate to impose certain risks on current patients in order to benefit future ones. It must be determined whether medical knowledge and scientific progress with their undisputed benefits are optional or mandatory, whether the increased probabilities of the knowledge gained by randomized clinical trials are worth the moral costs, and whether the benefits outweigh the burdens. When the physician charged with the care of particular patients is convinced that their interests are being sacrificed for the benefit of others, he should not surrender his judgment to the advisory committee. He should remain a patient advocate. In other cases, an institutional review board may determine that the research fails to offer patient-subjects adequate protection from harm, and it should demand revisions in the research protocol and possibly should refuse to allow the research.

Some hold that the researcher-physician's commitment to the welfare of his patients offers the best protection, even in a research project authorized by an institutional review board. Others, however, contend that we should differentiate roles so that physicians do not use their own patients in research. Their point is not that a person cannot be both an investigator and a clinician, but that a person should not assume both roles for the same patient-subject.[33] A similar argument supports not allowing the physician who is going to transplant a kidney from A to B to determine when A is dead. Proposals for procedures will depend in part on conceptions of human nature and convictions about the importance of reducing conflicts of interests. In many cases role-differentiation may obviate some of the moral conflicts. Nevertheless, answers to procedural questions will not be satisfactory unless we also have answers to more substantive questions. What is at stake is not merely who can and should protect patients' interests, but how much weight should be given to the interests of current patients and how much to future patients. Our view is that medical knowledge and scientific progress are important but often are optional. Generally the broader duty of beneficence is less stringent than the duty to "benefit the sick," who already have a special relationship with health care professionals. This conclusion should not be construed to subvert research. Rather, we should promote research methods that will enable us to pursue knowledge while simultaneously protecting the interests of current patients.

Notes

1. See Aristotle, *Nichomachean Ethics,* Book 5.
2. Paul Ramsey, *The Patient as Person* (New Haven, Conn.: Yale University Press, 1970), xii.
3. Sidgwick, *The Methods of Ethics,* 7th ed. (London: Macmillan, 1907), p. 315.
4. G. J. Warnock, *The Object of Morality* (London: Methuen and Co., 1971), pp. 85–86.
5. Donagan, *The Theory of Morality* (Chicago: University of Chicago Press, 1977), p. 88. See also Charles Fried, *Right and Wrong* (Cambridge, Mass.: Harvard University Press, 1978), Chapter 3.

6. See Ross, *The Right and the Good* (Oxford: Clarendon Press, 1930), Chapter 2.

7. Sissela Bok stresses the harm of lies to the one lied to, to the liar, and to social trust. See *Lying: Moral Choice in Public and Private Life* (New York: Pantheon Books, 1978), pp. 188 et passim. For discussions of utilitarianism and veracity, see David Lewis, "Utilitarianism and Truthfulness," *Australasian Journal of Philosophy* 50 (May 1972): 17–19, and Peter Singer, "Is Act-Utilitarianism Self-Defeating?" *Philosophical Review* 81 (1972): 94–104. See also Arnold Isenberg, "Deontology and the Ethics of Lying," *Philosophy and Phenomenological Research* 24 (1964): 465–80, and Roderick M. Chisholm and Thomas D. Feehan, "The Intent to Deceive," *The Journal of Philosophy* 74 (March 1977): 143–59.

8. See George J. Annas, *The Rights of Hospital Patients: The Basic ACLU Guide to a Hospital Patient's Rights* (New York: Avon Books, 1976). For a discussion of the duty of veracity in various codes, see Sissela Bok, "Truth-telling," *The Encyclopedia of Bioethics*.

9. See Donald Oken, "What to Tell Cancer Patients," *Journal of the American Medical Association* 175 (April 1, 1961): 1120–28; W. D. Kelly and S. R. Friesen, "Do Cancer Patients Want to Be Told?" *Surgery* 27 (June 1950): 822–26; and the discussion in Veatch, *Death, Dying and the Biological Revolution* (New Haven, Conn.: Yale University Press, 1976), Chapter 6.

10. See Sissela Bok's discussion of similar arguments in *Lying,* Chapter 15.

11. Boswell, *Life of Johnson,* vol. 4, p. 306, as quoted in Alan Donagan, *The Theory of Morality,* p. 89.

12. See Bok, *Lying* (Chapter 1) for a discussion of the distinction between truth and truthfulness.

13. See "Huntington's Disease: Some Prefer Not to Know," *Medical World News* 15 (April 5, 1974).

14. See Veatch, *Death, Dying, and the Biological Revolution,* Chapter 6.

15. Robert Veatch, *Case Studies in Medical Ethics* (Cambridge, Mass.: Harvard University Press, 1977), pp. 137–39.

16. Samuel Warren and Louis Brandeis, "The Right of Privacy," *Harvard Law Review* 4 (1890): 193.

17. See Alan Westin, *Privacy and Freedom* (New York: Atheneum, 1967).

18. See Charles Fried, *An Anatomy of Values* (Cambridge, Mass.: Harvard University Press, 1970), p. 141.

19. See James F. Childress, *Civil Disobedience and Political Obligation* (New Haven, Conn.: Yale University Press, 1971), and John Rawls, *A Theory of Justice* (Cambridge, Mass.: Harvard University Press, 1971), Chapter 6.

20. Harvey Kuschner, Daniel Callahan, Eric J. Cassell, and Robert M. Veatch, "The Homosexual Husband and Physician Confidentiality," *The Hastings Center Report* 7 (April 1977): 15–17.

21. Bernard B. Raginsky, "Hypnotic Recall of Aircrash Cause," *The International Journal of Clinical and Experimental Hypnosis* 17 (1969): 1–19.

22. Aubrey Milunsky, *The Prevention of Genetic Disease and Mental Retardation* (Philadelphia: W. B. Saunders, 1975), p. 75.

23. "The Principles of Medical Ethics with Annotations Especially Applicable to Psychiatry," *American Journal of Psychiatry* 130 (September 1973): 1063.

24. See H. L. A. Hart's discussion in "Are There Any Natural Rights?" *Philosophical Review* 64 (1955): 175–91.

25. Summary of *In re Sampson,* 317 NYS 2d, NY 1970, by Angela Holder, *Medical Malpractice Law* (New York: John Wiley and Sons, 1975), p. 17.

26. See, for example, Anthony Shaw, "Dilemmas of 'Informed Consent' in Children," *The New England Journal of Medicine* 289 (October 25, 1973): 885–90.

27. Holder, *Medical Malpractice Law,* p. 19. A summary of *Lotspeich v. Chance Vought Aircraft Corporation,* 369 SW 2d Tex (1963).

28. *PACAF Surgeon's Newsletter* 7 (December 1966): 5, reprinted in *The Hastings Center Report* 6 (February 1976): 20 (with commentary); see also, Veatch, *Case Studies in Medical Ethics,* pp. 245–50. For further discussion of the physician in the military, see Robert M. Goldwyn and Victor W. Sidel, "The Physician and War," *Ethical Issues in Medicine: The Role of the Physician in Today's Society,* ed. E. Fuller Torrey (Boston: Little, Brown and Co., 1968), pp. 325–46.

29. A thorough and helpful study of randomized clinical trials appears in Charles Fried, *Medical Experimentation: Personal Integrity and Social Policy* (New York: American Elsevier, 1974). For other criticisms, see Milton C. Weinstein, "Allocation of Subjects in Medical Experiments," *The New England Journal of Medicine* 291 (December 12, 1974): 1278–85. For defenses of RCTs, see David P. Byar et al., "Randomized Clinical Trials: Perspectives on Some Recent Ideas," *The New England Journal of Medicine* 295 (July 8, 1976): 74–80, and several writings by Thomas Chalmers, including Thomas C. Chalmers et al., "Controlled Studies in Clinical Cancer Research," *The New England Journal of Medicine* 287 (July 13, 1972): 75–78, and L. W. Shaw and T. C. Chalmers, "Ethics in Cooperative Clinical Trials," *Annals of the New York Academy of Science* 169 (1970): 487–95.

30. See Weinstein, "Allocation of Subjects in Medical Experiments," p. 1280.

31. See Fried, *Medical Experimentation,* p. 71.

32. Byar et al., "Randomized Clinical Trials: Perspectives on Some Recent Ideas," p. 78. These authors are commenting on a proposal by Thomas C. Chalmers et al., "Controlled Studies in Clinical Cancer Research," pp. 75–8.

33. See Fried, *Medical Experimentation,* pp. 160–61.

8

Ideals, Virtues, and Integrity

Throughout this book we have concentrated on acts and policies in the light of various principles and rules which determine obligations and rights. In this final chapter, we will examine some further aspects of morality that also shape what people, including health care professionals, ought to do and be. These other aspects are ideals, virtues, and integrity.

Ideals

At the end of Camus' *The Plague,* Dr. Rieux determines to make a record of those who fought the pestilence; it would be a record of "what had to be done . . . despite their personal afflictions, by all who, while unable to be *saints* but refusing to bow down to pestilences, strive their utmost to be *healers.*"[1] These healers were heroes, not saints. According to J. O. Urmson, saints and heroes may either (a) do their duty where most people would not do it, or (b) go beyond their duty where most people would not. In the first category (a), *saints* do their duty in situations in which most people fail because of inclination, desire, or self-interest, while *heroes* do their duty in situations in which most people succumb to fear and to the desire for self-preservation. Urmson thus distinguishes between saints and heroes primarily in terms of the forces they resist but others yield to: the saint resists inclination, desire, and self-interest; the hero resists fear and the desire for self-preservation.[2]

Some features that Urmson does not emphasize are also important. Saintliness requires regular fulfillment of duty over time; it demands consistency and constancy of conduct. A final judgment about one's saintliness cannot be made until one's record is complete. Furthermore, the agent's motives in fulfilling the duty may be very important; one who craves public recognition by fulfillment of duty is not considered a saint. By contrast, an agent may be a hero by virtue of a brief acceptance of considerable risk while fulfilling his duty. The contrast between a saint and a hero may be illustrated this way: a physician who works several years in a poverty area for long hours at low pay may be a *saint,* although we probably would not apply that honorific title unless we thought he also fulfilled his other duties, e.g., his familial duties. But however a physician may conduct himself in other settings, he may be a *hero* by overcoming his fear about losing his life in order to remain even several days in a plague-stricken city.

In addition to these "minor saints and heroes" (for Urmson, those who do their duty where others would not), there are (b) major saints and heroes who go beyond their duties. Saint Francis is an example of a major saint, while a soldier falling on a hand grenade to save his comrades is an example of a major hero. Physicians and scientists engaging in self-experimentation have also been major heroes. For example, Daniel Carrion injected in his arm blood from a patient's verruga peruana (an unusual disease marked by many vascular eruptions of the skin and mucous membranes as well as fever and severe rheumatic pains) only to discover that it had given him a fatal disease (Oroya fever). Similarly, Werner Forssman performed the first heart catheterization on himself, walking to the radiological room with the catheter sticking in his heart.[3]

It is important to note that these major heroes, who voluntarily took on certain risks for moral ends, may not have considered their actions to be morally optional. Indeed, many heroes (and saints) would explain their conduct in the language of "ought" and even of necessity: "I had to act in this way." Not all moral "oughts," it seems, can be reduced to duties or obligations. Although the physician who heroically goes beyond his duty may say that he only did what he had to do, others would not be able to reproach him if he did not act in this way. No one could tell him that this act is his duty; no one could blame him if he failed to do it—if, for example, he decided to turn around after reaching the airport on his way to the plague-stricken city.

By comparison to ordinary duties, saintly and heroic actions conform to ideals. They transcend our duties and indicate higher possibilities, but we do not expect many persons to realize them. Indeed, they mark out optional but praiseworthy conduct. With the addition of this sort of conduct, we have at least four categories of action: (a) actions that are right and obligatory (e.g., truth-telling); (b) actions that are wrong and prohibited (e.g., murder); (c) actions that are permissible in that they are not wrong; (d) actions that are morally optional but also supererogatory, meritorious, and praiseworthy. For most of this book, we have concentrated on (a) and (b); in this section we are concerned with (d). Actions that go beyond our duties may merit praise, but failure to perform them will not deserve blame.

The distinction between guilt and shame may cast some additional light on these issues. The moral notions of guilt and shame come from different parts of morality. As John Rawls puts it, "in general, guilt, resentment, and indignation invoke the concept of right, whereas shame, contempt, and derision appeal to the concept of goodness."[4] If someone feels *guilty* for what he has done, he invokes a moral standard of right and wrong, expects others to feel resentment and indignation at his actions, and can relieve his feelings of guilt by acts of reparation or by forgiveness. Thus, if a physician lies to a patient, he violates a moral principle and can expect the patient to be resentful and others to be indignant. He can overcome his feeling of guilt either by apologizing and trying to make it up to the patient or by receiving the patient's forgiveness. If, however, a person feels *shame,* he invokes an ideal (e.g., self-control under trying situations, going the second mile, turning the other cheek, and self-sacrifice), expects others to feel contempt for his shortcomings, and can overcome the feeling of shame for his failure by improving in the future. If, for example, a physician volunteers to undertake a risky mission in a plague-stricken city but turns back at the airport, he may feel shame because he has not been able to live up to his ideal, and others may be contemptuous because he could not meet his own self-imposed standards. He can overcome his shame by a closer approximation of his ideals in the future. Of course, some acts may involve both guilt and shame because they violate standards of both rightness and goodness.

In asserting that some heroic actions are morally praiseworthy, we do not suggest that all heroic actions are, on balance, praiseworthy. Many factors must be considered in the evaluation of a person and his acts. If, for example, we think that a physician went to the plague-stricken city because of his desire to get away from his family or to gain public recognition or to have a set of experiences that could be the basis for a book, we are not likely to praise him for what he did. Motives, the reasons for doing something, affect our judgment of the person and what he did. Furthermore, people who take risks in accord with higher, but optional, ideals sometimes do not merit our moral praise, because they also neglect certain duties in the process. On balance we might criticize them for their failure to live up to their duties rather than praise them for their heroic deeds. For example, imagine that a physician volunteers to take the grave risk of serving in a plague-stricken city that has attracted the world's sympathy. Suppose there is no other physician in his small town, and his departure leaves his patients bereft of medical services. Should his voluntary heroic action be praised, or should it be condemned?

Similar issues emerge in medical practice and research when physicians and others, including the courts and the society at large, have to decide how to respond to offers of heroic actions that go beyond ordinary duties. Such issues are especially poignant when physicians must determine whether to accept a person's offer of an organ for transplantation. Although a person's pursuit of an ideal of self-giving or assumption of risks for the sake of others may be praiseworthy, the action is justified in medical practice and research only if informed and voluntary. Here several questions arise: does the prospective donor really understand the risks and benefits? What sort of information, if any, is relevant to a decision if the person understands little about the risks and benefits? Are the risks unreasonable? For purposes of discussion we can consider two distinct cases: an offer from a family member and an offer from a stranger.

Following Urmson, we have so far excluded cases of "natural affection" that involve assumptions of risk or sacrifice for relatives or friends (e.g., a mother going back into a burning house to rescue her child), but they are important. Suppose a mother offers to donate a kidney to her child. If there is a good match and the mother has no physical or psychological conditions that would make her donation too risky, her offer will probably be accepted. When pressed, she may indicate that she did not really calculate the probable benefits and risks but decided to be a donor even before hearing all the medical information about risks and benefits. She may even insist that she had no other choice. This does not mean, as some claim, that she did not give *informed* consent. Even when a donor decides almost immediately upon learning that a family member needs a transplant, he or she may be acting from a sense of moral obligation and thus may have all the morally relevant information.[5] We also should make sure that the donor is not being unduly influenced by familial or other pressures into making a decision against his or her wishes. (See Chapter 3.)

There are some risks, however, that we might hesitate to allow individuals to take even when we are certain that their decision is informed and voluntary. Would we, for example, be willing to remove a woman's only kidney for transplantation to her son if she has given her informed and voluntary consent? Our decision might vary according to the factual circumstances—for example, whether the mother will probably die shortly because of some other illness and whether she could probably do as well on dialysis. If, however, we consider a mother's informed and voluntary decision to give her heart to her son, we would have moral grounds for refusing to accept and act on her offer. In this case, we face not the risk but the certainty of death. Even if the mother feels that her action is a moral sacrifice that she ought to make for her son, we can accept her right to her views, thus respecting her autonomy, but we should not accept her offer. In these circumstances we should not make ourselves accomplices in her effort to be faithful to her conception of what she ought to be and do.

Let us now consider heroic actions by strangers. As a rule, the medical profession is suspicious of the living unrelated donor, the person who volunteers to donate an organ to a stranger. By the late 1960s there were only approximately 60 living unrelated donors who were not also spouses of the recipients or who had not undergone a nephrectomy for other reasons. Since that time there have been few, if any, transplants of kidneys from living unrelated donors.[6] Some studies show that people in general do not think that the gift of an organ to a stranger is unreasonable. They call into question the medical profession's reluctance to use living unrelated donors.[7] In part this issue turns on the nature of a reasonable risk. It is not at all clear that the donation of a kidney to a stranger involves so much risk to the donor that questions should be raised about his or her competence. While some opponents of a policy of donation to strangers argue that volunteers are emotionally unstable, proponents of a more permissive policy argue that self-giving enhances the donor's self-esteem and thus is not irrational from the standpoint of

risk-benefit analysis. In some circumstances, e.g., where the donor has a
medical condition that would make the donation very dangerous, medical
practitioners could violate their duty to do no harm by being accomplices
to risk-taking. Furthermore, if the donor's act would increase certain risks
for others, we would have grounds for refusing the gift—for example, if a
woman with three small children wanted to donate her kidney to a
stranger. Similar questions and answers apply to nontherapeutic research
involving human subjects.

For purposes of discussion we have stressed dramatic instances of
heroic action. But, as Urmson stresses, there are many different ways to
go beyond or to exceed one's duty without being heroic, let alone saintly.
For example, a physician could be more understanding or patient without
being saintly or heroic. Often, of course, it is not clear just how we should
characterize our duty, whether in medical practice or elsewhere, and it is
thus not clear what would go beyond the limits of duty. What is the
physician's duty to his patients: to spend a certain amount of time and
energy on their behalf? to perform certain acts? to accomplish certain
ends? If the duty is to spend a certain amount of time, the physician can
go beyond that duty by increasing his hours of work. If it is to perform
certain tasks such as surgery, he can exceed it by displaying certain
attitudes, e.g., gentleness. On some definitions of the physician's responsibilities, such attitudes would not exceed duty but would simply
enable the physician to fulfill his duty more completely or perhaps at a
higher level. But not every act or attitude that is desirable or praiseworthy
is part of the physician's duty to his patients.

Virtues and character

In our discussions of right and wrong, duties and obligations, as well as
ideals, we have emphasized acts rather than agents. But in addition to our
judgments about right and wrong acts, obligatory and permissible acts,
praiseworthy and blameworthy acts, we make judgments about *moral
goodness and badness.* We make judgments of moral value about persons,
traits of character, dispositions, motives, and intentions. We talk about
good and bad people, about good and bad motives, about virtues and
vices. In short, we look not only at doing but at being, not only at duties
and obligations but also at virtues, not only at conduct but also at

character. We consider the moral worth of agents as well as the worth of their acts. Without these additional themes, our view of the moral life, in medical practice and elsewhere, would be truncated.

Both deontological and utilitarian theories address the same question: what ought I to do? While they offer different answers to this question, theirs is a family quarrel, for they share a fairly uniform conception of the moral life: people confront dilemmas, problems, and situations which they have difficulty resolving, and the task of ethics is to deal with these problems. But several contemporary philosophers and theologians have argued that we, like the classical tradition represented by Plato and Aristotle, ought to ask first of all: Who should I be? Whereas many ethical theories find some inspiration in legal analogies and perspectives, the proponents of an agent ethics, or an ethics of virtue, use an aesthetic analogy. Judgments about persons, motives, etc., tend to be closer to aesthetic judgments, while judgments about acts tend to be more akin to legal assessments.[8]

We do not agree with those (a) who try to drive a wedge between an ethics of duty and an ethics of virtue or between acts and agents, or (b) who try to make the ethics of virtue primary. Especially troubling is the view that if persons, such as health care professionals or researchers have good motives and are virtuous, their acts will be acceptable. Henry Beecher, who exposed some of the moral problems in research involving human subjects, insisted that it is important to get the subjects' informed consent; but he held that a "more reliable safeguard is provided by the presence of an intelligent, informed, conscientious, compassionate, responsible researcher."[9] While we do expect morally good persons to perceive and do what is morally right, we also know from experience that persons of good moral character and motives sometimes fail to discern what is right. Furthermore, such persons are often the first to recognize that they do not know what ought to be done. Hence, a discussion of the morality of acts remains important and, indeed, indispensable. We make assessments of ourselves and others in part by reference to what we and they do. Yet we do not merely sum up a physician's acts in determining whether he is a morally good physician. A person who can never be counted on to tell the truth would hardly be said to be virtuous or to have the virtue of veracity, but not everyone who tells a lie is to be considered a liar—if the latter is taken as a trait of character. While much depends on the definition of a lie, as we have seen, some lies may be justified; and we do not call a person who tells only justified lies a liar. A physician who deceives his patient by giving a placebo (see Case #5) may not be called a liar even if we are convinced that his act was wrong. If someone tells what we consider to be an unjustified lie, we may dismiss it by saying that it was "out of character" for him to tell that lie. By this attribution we mean that he can generally be counted on to tell the truth, to exemplify the virtue of veracity, even though he did not tell the truth in that situation. When, however, we determine that telling a lie is "in character," we appropriately consider that person a liar. Our appraisal of the agent, then, depends on whether we think that the act in question displays his character. Even several right or wrong acts will not necessarily lead us to declare that someone has a good or a bad character. Much depends on the particular circumstances, the person's previous acts, etc.

Which traits of character should be cultivated by persons in general and which by health care professionals in particular? The virtues that one emphasizes will depend on one's general moral theory: there will be a correlation between virtues, on the one hand, and duties and ideals, on the other. There will also be a correlation between wrong acts and vices. If a theory recognizes a duty of promise-keeping, it will also recognize the virtue of faithfulness; if it affirms a duty of beneficence, it will affirm the virtue of benevolence. Since rule utilitarianism and rule deontology recognize many of the same standards of right and wrong, they also emphasize many of the same virtues. Specifically, for medical practice, the important virtues are correlated with the duties and ideals of the profession. Virtues are settled habits and dispositions to do what we ought to do (where "ought" judgments encompass both ordinary duties and ideals).

Professional codes, including the "Ethical Principles of the American Medical Association," not only stress duties but also call for the cultivation of certain virtues. Insisting that "the prime objective" of the medical profession is to render service to humanity (reward or financial gain being a "subordinate consideration"), the AMA code insists that the physician must be "an upright man," "pure in character and . . . diligent and conscientious in caring for the sick." It also endorses the virtues that Hippocrates commended: modesty, sobriety, patience, promptness, and piety. Over the years, the AMA code has put less and less emphasis on the virtues. Indeed, the remaining references are limited, perfunctory, and marginal to the code. Reflecting on these developments, Jonsen and

Hellegers lament this turn of events and claim that "these exhortations to virtue constitute the heart of code ethics," thus making these codes more than mere rules of etiquette.[10] This general claim is debatable, but Jonsen and Hellegers go on to argue that in addition to the general virtues the good person should possess, there are virtues that are appropriate to particular roles: just as the soldier should possess courage and the judge fairness, the physician should be trustworthy. But Jonsen and Hellegers' position needs clarification, for trustworthiness is itself a summary term that depends on several general and specific virtues. A person is worthy of trust and a physician is worthy of trust only if he or she has certain other virtues, i.e., habits and dispositions to perform certain acts. It is thus inappropriate to talk about a "virtue of trustworthiness," parallel to the soldier's courage or the judge's fairness. We consider physicians and others worthy of trust if we can rely upon them to act in multiple ways required by moral principles and rules. For one to be trustworthy, then, one must display several different virtues.

While many virtues such as modesty, patience, promptness, and fearlessness have had a place in medical codes, the most important moral virtues correlate with the major principles and rules of ethics as applied to medical practice. These include, but are not limited to, veracity, benevolence (including nonmalevolence), respect for persons (particularly their autonomy), and justice. Obviously, these virtues are not peculiar to medical practitioners, but are important for all human beings in their interactions. Within particular settings, however, one might specify the virtue of benevolence in different ways. For example, in medical practice, terms such as compassion, understanding, and caring would be stressed.[11]

Among the virtues that we have considered, it is possible to distinguish primary virtues—traditionally called cardinal virtues—from secondary virtues. These primary virtues, correlated with fundamental principles, include benevolence, justice, nonmalevolence, and respect for autonomy, while secondary virtues are correlated with derived principles and rules. Furthermore, some virtues can be correlated with ideals, e.g., charitableness. In addition to these virtues that correlate with principles, rules, and ideals, some virtues such as courage, conscientiousness, and integrity, which are general and abstract, apply across the whole moral life.[12] In the next section, we will consider conscientiousness and integrity both as virtues and as reasons for action.

Integrity and conscience

Conscientiousness and integrity are important virtues. Often agents appeal directly to their conscience and to their integrity to interpret and justify their acts in medical practice and scientific research. What is the function of appeals to conscience and integrity? How much weight should we give them? How should others respond to them?

In Case #28, George, who is unemployed, believes that he cannot accept a position because of his moral scruples about research on chemical and biological warfare. Yet he needs this position so that his wife can stop working and they can restore family stability and better meet their children's needs. Furthermore, the other candidate for the position would uncritically pursue the research if he took the position. Thus, George has a chance to help his family and perhaps to prevent a fanatic from getting this position. What should he do, given his commitments and attitudes?

As in George's dilemma, the claims of conscience often require nonparticipation in what the agent takes to be morally wrong. For instance, according to the International Code of Nursing Ethics of 1953 (omitted from the 1973 code in Appendix II), "the nurse is under an obligation to carry out the physician's orders intelligently and loyally and *to refuse to participate in unethical procedures.*" Furthermore, the nurse should expose the "incompetence or unethical conduct of associates" but "only to the proper authority." Suppose a nurse thinks that the doctor's orders to turn off a respirator for a young patient are unethical. On the one hand, she may think that the doctor's orders are so unethical that she must not only refuse to implement them but must also expose them to the proper authority. On the other hand, she may think that her cooperation in the doctor's orders would involve her in a moral wrong although she is not convinced that others would act wrongly in disconnecting the machine. Thus, she does not feel compelled to expose the matter to others. In effect, the nurse says to the physician: "I see that the arguments you give are sufficient for you to feel that you are doing the right thing by switching off the machine. I don't doubt that you are acting according to your conscience, but my conscience tells me differently."[13]

Similarly, a gynecologist may be conscientiously opposed to performing an abortion procedure although he does not necessarily call into question the conscientious convictions of others. He may not even be opposed to a liberal abortion law, but he draws the line at his own conduct or material cooperation in abortion procedures. In Case #29, for example, a Roman Catholic gynecologist believed that he should leave Britain in order to practice medicine in accord with his conscience, as influenced by religious training and belief.

The language of conscience takes interesting forms. While testifying before the House Committee on Un-American Activities, Arthur Miller refused to answer a question: "I am trying to, and I will, protect my sense of myself . . . my conscience will not permit me to use the name of another person." A physician who refuses to perform amniocentesis for a woman who wants to determine the sex of her child so that she can abort if it is a boy may say, "I couldn't live with myself if I did that." We have many expressions which reflect this moral perspective: "A person has to answer to himself." "I would hate myself in the morning." "I could not look myself in the mirror." Or, as several kidney donors have exclaimed, "I had to do it. I couldn't have backed out, not that I had the feeling of being trapped, because the doctors offered to get me out. I just had to do it."[14] These various statements from ordinary discourse express our frequent appeal to conscience, which includes the fear of loss of integrity and wholeness if the agent acts in certain ways.

But what precisely is this phenomenon called conscience?[15] In general, conscience is a mode of consciousness and thought about one's own acts and their value or disvalue. It is often *retrospective*. In being conscious of and thinking about his past acts, an agent's conscience comes into play. It appears primarily as a *bad conscience,* in the form of feelings of guilt, shame, and disunity when one believes one's own acts wrong or bad. Hannah Arendt, however, insists that "only good people are ever bothered by a bad conscience, whereas it is a very rare phenomenon among real criminals. A good conscience does not exist except as the absence of a bad one."[16] Most often the good conscience is described by nouns such as "peace," "wholeness," and "integrity," or by adjectives such as "quiet," "clear," and "easy."

When a person appeals to his conscience or describes his act as conscientious, he makes both a hypothetical and a prospective claim. He claims that if he were to commit the act in question, he would violate his conscience. This violation would result not only in such unpleasant feelings as guilt and shame but also in a fundamental loss of integrity, wholeness, and harmony in the self. He thus makes a prediction about what would happen to him if he were to commit such an act, a prediction based on the imaginative projection of concrete courses of action in the light of his moral standards.

Conscience is also personal; it is an agent's consciousness of and reflection on his own acts in relation to his standards of judgment. It is a first-person claim, deriving from standards that he may or may not also apply to the conduct of others. When Socrates affirmed that "it is better to suffer wrong than to do wrong," he meant, as Hannah Arendt puts it, that "it was better *for him,* just as it was better for him 'to be in disagreement with multitudes than, being one, to be in disagreement with [himself].'"[17] Perhaps George in the case previously discussed would have raised moral questions about anyone's participation in research on chemical and biological warfare, and perhaps the gynecologist in Case #29 would have held that it is morally wrong for others and not only himself to perform abortions. But it would have been odd and even absurd for either of them to say, "My conscience indicates that you should not do that." In judging others or advising them about their conduct, I may consult my conscience by imagining what I would think and feel if I were to act in a certain way. I may then say that someone else ought not to engage in that conduct, but I *cannot logically* justify this admonition by saying "I would have a guilty conscience if he did that." Perhaps I would have a guilty conscience if I failed to advise him and to try to stop him, but my reasons for *his* abstention from that conduct must involve more than an appeal to my conscience. They must invoke the moral values, principles, and rules that are determinative for my conscience. My integrity, however, is not violated if someone acts in ways that I find morally unacceptable.

A person's appeal to his conscience usually involves an appeal to moral standards, but conscience cannot itself be the sole justificatory standard. Conscience is the mode of consciousness that results from reflection on and judgment about one's past, present, or future conduct in relation to those standards. Thus, to appeal to conscience is not necessarily to presuppose that moral rightness and wrongness are determined by the need for moral integrity or a good conscience, as though these could serve, in effect, as the source or ground of obligation. As Thomas Nagel suggests, "If by committing murder one sacrifices one's moral purity or integrity, that can only be because there is *already* something wrong with murder. The general reason against committing murder cannot therefore be merely that it makes one an immoral person."[18]

But if conscience emerges only subsequent to moral judgments, we face some puzzles: what does it mean to consult conscience and to have a conflict of conscience? When a person consults his conscience, he examines his moral convictions to determine what he really thinks and feels, reconsidering principles and rules and determining their weight and relevance to the situation at hand. When he consults his conscience, it will only give him one answer: do what you believe you ought to do. The appeal to conscience is thus only one step in the reexamination of one's moral convictions and is not morally sufficient.

A "conflict of conscience" appears when a person faces two conflicting moral demands, neither of which can be met without a partial rejection of the other. He faces a conflict of conscience because he has a firm judgment, rightly or wrongly, that both courses of action are required. George's conscience may direct him both to refuse the position because it involves immoral research on chemical and biological warfare and to accept the position because it will prevent the research from falling into the hands of zealots and will also benefit his family. Perhaps he has misconstrued his situation and the relevant moral standards, and the only way out is to reconsider them. An apparent "conflict of conscience" may be the situation of a "doubtful conscience," unsure about the relevant standards and their weight. Perhaps, however, he faces a genuine moral tragedy. For example, if an agent holds certain beliefs about the fetus, he may feel that it is wrong either to kill the fetus or to allow the mother to die.

When the agent is clear on moral grounds that he ought or ought not to do something, his appeal to conscience usually reflects several features of his situation. First, he is convinced, as we have seen, that the ethical standards at stake are so *important* and *fundamental* that their violation would lead to a loss of integrity and wholeness. Second, this appeal to conscience usually asserts a personal *sanction* rather than an authority. The dictate of conscience is formal: "do what you believe to be right, and avoid what you believe to be wrong, *or else*." The "or else" is the threat of the loss of integrity, wholeness, and peace. Third, he claims that he will not be able to forget the deed; hence, its performance will continue to disrupt the self. Fourth, he cannot deny that the deed is his own. He cannot shift the responsibility for the act to someone else. For example,

he cannot as a military doctor plead "superior orders," for even if others
do not hold him responsible, he has to answer to himself. When Captain
Howard B. Levy, a military physician, refused to obey his commander's
order to establish and operate a program for Special Forces Aid Men in
dermatology in 1966, he argued that to obey the order would implicate
him in the war crimes that the Special Forces committed in Vietnam and
would for him as a physician be a violation of medical ethics.[19] Such an
appellant to conscience insists that he will not only be unable to forget the
deed but that he will remember it as his own and as his responsibility. Of
course, a person who makes these claims about himself and his acts may
be a victim of self-deception, for he might be able to forget his act or to
shift the responsibility to someone else. Perhaps he will even come to
consider the act justified. Nevertheless, at this point in time his conscience
will not allow him to act.

Even those who proclaim "Let your conscience be your guide" do not
usually hold that conscience is an infallible guide. Traditionally, theologians who have held that it is always culpable to act against conscience
have also recognized the possibility of an "erroneous conscience." As Alan
Donagan summarizes the tradition,

Christian moral theologians were not content with allowing the inculpability of
impermissible actions done at the behest of conscience; they also ruled that an
action done against conscience is always culpable. A man is not merely held
inculpable if he does something impermissible in accordance with his conscience,
he is held culpable if he does not. The reason is simple. In acting against
conscience, a violation of the moral law must be intended; and such intentions are
always culpable, even though, because of the agent's erroneous conscience, nothing
materially wrong is done.[20]

Agents have to determine not only how they will act in light of their
consciences but how they will respond to the consciences of others, including their colleagues, subordinates, and patients. Since people act
culpably when they intentionally violate their consciences, it is prima facie
morally wrong to force them to act against their consciences. It is only
prima facie wrong, because it may sometimes be justified and even
necessary to protect the innocent, as, for example, when a person is
inoculated against his moral convictions in order to protect others in the
community.

Coercion of conscience may occur in many different ways. For instance, the state may coerce an individual through the threat of imprison-

ment, or a hospital administrator may threaten an employee who is conscientiously opposed to abortions with dismissal or with no increase in salary. But it is not necessary for our purposes to draw out the distinctions between these different agents and modes of coercion. In general, a society (this term will cover governmental and nongovernmental—including medical—institutions and personnel) is better and more desirable insofar as it respects and protects consciences. At the very least, it should operate with a presumption in favor of noninterference with and protection of consciences.

An agent's conscience may set him or her in opposition to what others take to be *positive* or *negative duties*. For example, an agent's conscience may lead him to repudiate what others take to be the positive or affirmative duties of serving in the military, of accepting a life-saving blood transfusion, and of being inoculated. But it may lead him to violate what others take to be negative duties, such as refraining from certain actions, e.g., providing an FDA-banned drug to his patients. Individuals and the society bear a heavy burden of proof in arguing that coercion of conscience is really necessary to protect others, to preserve fairness, etc. In some cases, the society may be able to protect an individual's conscience by pursuing its end in other ways. In some cases, it can provide other forms of service for the objector, e.g., the objector to abortions. Occasionally, it may be able to protect the individual's conscience by performing the act in question. For example, for some Jehovah's Witnesses the prohibition against taking blood means that they cannot consent to blood transfusions but that court-ordered transfusions would not be their responsibility. In the Georgetown College Case (#12), Judge J. Skelly Wright granted the Georgetown University Hospital the right to give blood transfusions to a woman, although she and her husband refused to consent to transfusions which were necessary because she had lost two thirds of her body's blood supply from a ruptured ulcer. He determined that neither she nor her husband wanted her death but that they could not consent to the blood transfusions. By granting a court order, he thought he could protect their consciences and also save her life.[21] But this removal of responsibility by the actions of medical practitioners and the state will not work for all conscientious refusers of blood transfusions or other medical treatments. Many consciences impose strict liability. For example, some Jehovah's Witnesses may hold that blood transfusions contaminate the recipients even if the responsibility belongs to the medical practitioners and the state.

Although we agree with the court decision in Case #11—to allow a woman to refuse a blood transfusion while not allowing her to refuse it for an infant—we still have to ask what responsibility the hospital and the state have toward the child, who now may be considered an abomination by its family.

In general, many of the issues of conscience appeared in slightly different form in our discussion of autonomy, for the right of self-determination includes the right of conscientious action. The principles and rules for justified interferences with autonomy are thus also applicable to conscientious action.

When we encounter serious moral disagreements, or conflicts of consciences, we often fall back on procedures, e.g., in hospitals, and on what MacIntyre calls "secondary virtues."[22] These secondary virtues concern *how* we act, while primary virtues concern *what* is done. Among the secondary virtues are sincerity and conscientiousness. As John Rawls notes, "In times of social doubt and loss of faith in long established values, there is a tendency to fall back on the virtues of integrity: truthfulness and sincerity, lucidity, and commitment, or, as some say, authenticity."[23] Mutual trust in situations of serious moral conflict—for example, when a nurse feels that a physician is acting unethically—may depend on the willingness of all parties to preserve the secondary virtues and to abide by procedures. In addition, conscientiousness implies a willingness to consider and reconsider one's position and to analyze and appraise the various arguments for and against one's moral conclusion.

Notes

1. Albert Camus, *The Plague,* trans. from the French by Stuart Gilbert (New York: Random House, Vintage Books, 1972), p. 287. (Italics added.)
2. J. O. Urmson, "Saints and Heroes," *Essays in Moral Philosophy,* ed. A. I. Melden (Seattle: University of Washington Press, 1958), pp. 198–216. Another valuable analysis of these and related issues is Joel Feinberg, "Supererogation and Rules," *Ethics* 71 (1961): 276–88. It should be noted that the words "saint," "saintly," "hero," and "heroic" are not always moral evaluative words. They are evaluative words in other contexts than a moral one; e.g., religious or military or athletic.
3. Jay Katz, ed., *Experimentation with Human Beings* (New York: Russell Sage Foundation, 1972), pp. 136–40.
4. John Rawls, *A Theory of Justice,* p. 484; cf. David A. J. Richards, *A Theory of Reasons for Action* (Oxford: Clarendon Press, 1971); and Herbert Morris,

ed., *Shame and Guilt* (Belmont, Calif.: Wadsworth Press, 1971). Our analysis in this paragraph draws from Rawls's account.

5. See Carl H. Fellner and John R. Marshall, "Kidney Donors—The Myth of Informed Consent," *American Journal of Psychiatry* 126 (March 1970): 1245–51. On p. 1250, they write: "all relevant data are immediately available to him [i.e., the renal donor]." See also, Robert M. Eisendrath et al., "Psychologic Considerations in the Selection of Kidney Transplant Donors," *Surgery, Gynecology and Obstetrics* 129 (August 1969): 243–48.

6. Carl H. Fellner, "Organ Donation: For Whose Sake?" *Annals of Internal Medicine* 79 (October 1973): 590.

7. See Carl H. Fellner and Shalom H. Schwartz, "Altruism in Disrepute," *The New England Journal of Medicine* 284 (March 18, 1971): 582–85.

8. See Edmund Pincoffs, "Quandary Ethics," *Mind* 80 (1971): 552–71; Lawrence C. Becker, "The Neglect of Virtue," *Ethics* 85 (January 1975): 110–22; Iris Murdoch, *The Sovereignty of Good* (New York: Schocken Books, 1971); and Stanley Hauerwas, *Vision and Virtue: Essays in Christian Ethical Reflection* (Notre Dame, Ind.: University of Notre Dame Press, 1977).

9. H. K. Beecher, "Ethics and Clinical Research," *The New England Journal of Medicine* 274 (1966): 1354–60.

10. Albert R. Jonsen and André E. Hellegers, "Conceptual Foundations for an Ethics of Medical Care," *Ethics of Health Care: Papers of the Conference on Health Care and Changing Values,* November 27–29, 1973, ed. Laurence R. Tancredi (Washington, D.C.: National Academy of Sciences, 1974), pp. 3–20; see Paul Ramsey, "Commentary," in the same volume, pp. 21–29, for a critique.

11. See Stanley Hauerwas, "Care," *Encyclopedia of Bioethics,* ed. Warren T. Reich (New York: Free Press, 1978) and Milton Mayeroff, *On Caring* (New York: Harper and Row, Perennial Library Edition, 1972).

12. This paragraph is influenced by William Frankena, *Ethics,* especially p. 64. Frankena has two cardinal virtues, benevolence and justice, parallel to his two basic moral principles, beneficence and justice. We cannot here touch on many interesting questions relating to the virtues, for example, whether they are to be considered as integrated and unified. See, for further discussion, Stanley Hauerwas, *Vision and Virtue* and *Character and the Christian Life: A Study in Theological Ethics* (San Antonio: Trinity University Press, 1975); P. T. Geach, *The Virtues* (Cambridge: Cambridge University Press, 1977); and David B. Harned, *Faith and Virtue* (Philadelphia: United Church Press, 1973).

13. A. V. Campbell, *Moral Dilemmas in Medicine,* 2nd ed. (Edinburgh: Churchill Livingstone, 1975), p. 25.

14. Carl H. Fellner, "Organ Donation: For Whose Sake?" *Annals of Internal Medicine* 79 (October 1973): 591.

15. For a fuller discussion of these points, see James F. Childress, "Appeals to Conscience," *Ethics* (forthcoming) from which many of these points are drawn.

16. Hannah Arendt, "Thinking and Moral Considerations: A Lecture," *Social Research* 38 (Autumn 1971): 418.
17. Hannah Arendt, *Crises of the Republic* (New York: Harcourt, Brace, Jovanovich, 1972), p. 62. See Plato, *Gorgias,* 482 and 489.
18. Thomas Nagel, "War and Massacre," *Philosophy and Public Affairs* 1 (Winter 1972): 132.
19. See Robert M. Veatch's discussion of this case, *Case Studies in Medical Ethics* (Cambridge, Mass.: Harvard University Press, 1977), pp. 61–64. Veatch draws an excessively sharp distinction between professional and human ethics.
20. Alan Donagan, *The Theory of Morality* (Chicago: University of Chicago Press, 1977), pp. 131–38.
21. *Application of President and Directors of Georgetown College,* 331F. 2d 1000 (D.C. Cir.), certiorari denied, 377 U.S. 978 (1964). See excerpts in Samuel Gorovitz et al., eds., *Moral Problems in Medicine* (Englewood Cliffs, N.J.: Prentice-Hall, 1976), pp. 230–32.
22. Alasdair MacIntyre, *Secularization and Moral Change* (London: Oxford University Press, 1967), p. 24.
23. John Rawls, *A Theory of Justice,* p. 519.

Appendix I

Cases

Case #1

Facts in the case

October 27, 1969, Prosenjit Poddar killed Tatiana Tarasoff. Plaintiffs, Tatiana's parents, allege that two months earlier Poddar confided his intention to kill Tatiana to Dr. Lawrence Moore, a psychologist employed by the Cowell Memorial Hospital at the University of California at Berkeley. They allege that on Moore's request, the campus police briefly detained Poddar, but released him when he appeared rational. They further claim that Dr. Harvey Powelson, Moore's superior, then directed that no further action be taken to detain Poddar. No one warned plaintiffs of Tatiana's peril.

Plaintiffs, Tatiana's mother and father, . . . [allege] that on August 20, 1969, Poddar was a voluntary outpatient receiving therapy at Cowell Memorial Hospital. Poddar informed Moore, his therapist, that he was going to kill an unnamed girl, readily identifiable as Tatiana, when she returned home from spending the summer in Brazil. Moore, with the concurrence of Dr. Gold, who had initially examined Poddar, and Dr. Yandell, assistant to the director of the department of psychiatry, decided that Poddar should be committed for observation in a mental hospital. Moore orally notified Officers Atkinson and Teel of the campus police that he would request commitment. He then sent a letter to Police Chief

William Beall requesting the assistance of the police department in securing Poddar's confinement.

Officers Atkinson, Brownrigg, and Halleran took Poddar into custody,
but, satisfied that Poddar was rational, released him on his promise to
stay away from Tatiana. Powelson, director of the department of psychiatry at Cowell Memorial Hospital, then asked the police to return
Moore's letter, directed that all copies of the letter and notes that Moore
had taken as therapist be destroyed, and "ordered no action to place
Prosenjit Poddar in 72-hour treatment and evaluation facility."

Plaintiffs' second cause of action, entitled "Failure to Warn of a Dangerous Patient," . . . adds the assertion that defendants negligently permitted Poddar to be released from police custody without "notifying the
parents of Tatiana Tarasoff that their daughter was in grave danger from
Posenjit Poddar." Poddar persuaded Tatiana's brother to share an apart-
ment with him near Tatiana's residence; shortly after her return from
Brazil, Poddar went to her residence and killed her.

Majority opinion in the case   TOBRINER, Justice.

We shall explain that defendant therapists cannot escape liability merely
because Tatiana herself was not their patient. When a therapist determines, or pursuant to the standards of his profession should determine,
that his patient presents a serious danger of violence to another, he incurs
an obligation to use reasonable care to protect the intended victim against
such danger. The discharge of this duty may require the therapist to take
one or more of various steps, depending upon the nature of the case. Thus
it may call for him to warn the intended victim or others likely to apprise
the victim of the danger, to notify the police, or to take whatever other
steps are reasonably necessary under the circumstances. . . .

In each instance the adequacy of the therapist's conduct must be
measured against the traditional negligence standard of the rendition of
reasonable care under the circumstances. . . . In sum, the therapist owes
a legal duty not only to his patient, but also to his patient's would-be
victim and is subject in both respects to scrutiny by judge and jury. . . .
Some of the alternatives open to the therapist, such as warning the victim,
will not result in the drastic consequences of depriving the patient of his
liberty. Weighing the uncertain and conjectural character of the alleged
damage done the patient by such a warning against the peril to the
victim's life, we conclude that professional inaccuracy in predicting vio-

lence cannot negate the therapist's duty to protect the threatened victim. . . .

We recognize the public interest in supporting effective treatment of mental illness and in protecting the rights of patients to privacy. . . , and the consequent public importance of safeguarding the confidential character of psychotherapeutic communication. Against this interest, however, we must weigh the public interest in safety from violent assault.

The revelation of a communication under the above circumstances is not a breach of trust or a violation of professional ethics; as stated in the Principles of Medical Ethics of the American Medical Association (1957), section 9: "A physician may not reveal the confidence entrusted to him in the course of medical *attendance . . . unless he is required to do so by law or unless it becomes necessary in order to protect the welfare of the individual or of the community."* (Emphasis added.) We conclude that the public policy favoring protection of the confidential character of patient-psychotherapist communications must yield to the extent to which disclosure is essential to avert danger to others. The protective privilege ends where the public peril begins. . . .

Minority opinion in the case   CLARK, Justice (dissenting).
Until today's majority opinion, both legal and medical authorities have agreed that confidentiality is essential to effectively treat the mentally ill, and that imposing a duty on doctors to disclose patient threats to potential victims would greatly impair treatment. . . .

Policy generally determines duty. Principal policy considerations include foreseeability of harm, certainty of the plaintiff's injury, proximity of the defendant's conduct to the plaintiff's injury, moral blame attributable to defendant's conduct, prevention of future harm, burden on the defendant, and consequences to the community.

Overwhelming policy considerations weigh against imposing a duty on psychotherapists to warn a potential victim against harm. While offering virtually no benefit to society, such a duty will frustrate psychiatric treatment, invade fundamental patient rights and increase violence.

The importance of psychiatric treatment and its need for confidentiality have been recognized by this court. "It is clearly recognized that the very practice of psychiatry vitally depends upon the reputation in the community that the psychiatrist will not tell. . . ."

Assurance of confidentiality is important for three reasons.

Deterrence from treatment

First, without substantial assurance of confidentiality, those requiring treatment will be deterred from seeking assistance. It remains an unfortunate fact in our society that people seeking psychiatric guidance tend to become stigmatized. Apprehension of such stigma—apparently increased by the propensity of people considering treatment to see themselves in the worst possible light—creates a well-recognized reluctance to seek aid. This reluctance is alleviated by the psychiatrist's assurance of confidentiality.

Full disclosure

Second, the guarantee of confidentiality is essential in eliciting the full disclosure necessary for effective treatment. The psychiatric patient approaches treatment with conscious and unconscious inhibitions against revealing his innermost thoughts. . . .

Successful treatment

Third, even if the patient fully discloses his thoughts, assurance that the confidential relationship will not be breached is necessary to maintain his trust in his psychiatrist—the very means by which treatment is effected. . . .

Given the importance of confidentiality to the practice of psychiatry, it becomes clear the duty to warn imposed by the majority will cripple the use and effectiveness of psychiatry. Many people, potentially violent—yet susceptible to treatment—will be deterred from seeking it; those seeking it will be inhibited from making revelations necessary to effective treatment; and, forcing the pyschiatrist to violate the patient's trust will destroy the interpersonal relationship by which treatment is effected.

Violence and civil commitment

By imposing a duty to warn, the majority contributes to the danger to society of violence by the mentally ill and greatly increases the risk of civil commitment—the total deprivation of liberty—of those who should not be confined. The impairment of treatment and risk of improper commitment resulting from the new duty to warn will not be limited to a few patients but will extend to a large number of the mentally ill. Although under existing psychiatric procedures only a relatively few receiving treatment will ever present a risk of violence, the number making threats is huge, and it is the latter group—not just the former—whose treatment will be impaired and whose risk of commitment will be increased.

[This case is adapted from *Tarasoff v. Regents of the University of California,* California Supreme Court (17 California Reports, 3rd Series, 425. Decided July 1, 1976.) The language is that of the court. The "facts" and "majority opinion" are written by Justice Tobriner. The "dissenting opinion" is written by Justice Clark. The comments are brief excerpts from each opinion.]

Case #2

The law of a particular state in the United States requires a physician to report to the Department of Public Health any condition that causes lapses of consciousness. The Department then relays this information to the Division of Motor Vehicles, which commences action to cancel the patient's driving privileges. Patient X, who had been treated earlier for epilepsy, reports his seizures are now under control. Having his wife's confirmation that he has not lost consciousness in the past year and his physician's confirmation that he is under medical supervision, the Division of Motor Vehicles returns his license. Later the physician receives a telephone call from someone who claims to be the patient's neighbor. This caller insists that the patient still has seizures which he refuses to report and that the wife is too terrified of the husband to notify the physician or anyone else. The neighbor refuses to identify herself and refuses to inform the Division of Motor Vehicles.

[This case was prepared by Dr. James Laster, Chief, Department of Neurology, Permanente Medical Group, Santa Clara, California.]

Case #3

A five-year-old girl had been a patient in a medical center for three years because of progressive renal failure secondary to glomerulonephritis. She had been on chronic renal dialysis, and the possibility of a renal transplantation was considered. The effectiveness of this procedure in her case was questionable. On the other hand, it was the feeling of the professional staff that there was a clear possibility that a transplanted kidney would not undergo the same disease process. After discussion with the parents, it was decided to proceed with plans for transplantation. Tissue typing was performed on the patient; it was noted that she would be difficult to match. Two siblings, age two and four, were thought to be too young to serve as donors. The girl's mother turned out not to be histocompatible. The father, however, was found to be quite compatible with his daughter. He underwent an arteriogram, and it was discovered that he had anatomically favorable circulation for transplantation. The nephrologist met alone with the father, and gave him these results. He informed the father that the prognosis for his daughter was quite uncertain. After some thought, the girl's father decided that he did not wish to donate a kidney to his daughter. He admitted that he did not have the courage, and that, particularly in view of the uncertain prognosis, the very slight possibility of a cadaver kidney, and the degree of suffering his daughter had already sustained, he would prefer not to donate. The father asked the physician to tell everyone else in the family that he was not histocompatible. He was afraid that if they knew the truth, they would accuse him of allowing his daughter to die. He felt that this would "wreck the family." The physician felt very uncomfortable about this request. However, he agreed to tell the man's wife that "for medical reasons" the father should not donate a kidney.

[This case is reprinted by permission from Melvin D. Levine, Lee Scott, and William J. Curran, "Ethics Rounds in a Children's Medical Center: Evaluation of a Hospital-Based Program for Continuing Education in Medical Ethics," *Pediatrics* 60 (August 1977): 205.]

Case #4

Laud Humphreys, a sociologist, recognized that the public and the law-enforcement authorities hold highly simplistic stereotyped beliefs about men who commit impersonal sexual acts with one another in public restrooms. "Tearoom sex," as fellatio in public restrooms is called, accounts for the majority of homosexual arrests in the United States. Humphreys decided that it would be of considerable social importance for society to gain more objective understanding of who these men are and what motivates them to seek quick, impersonal sexual gratification.

For his Ph.D. dissertation at Washington University, Humphreys set out to answer this question by means of participant observation and structured interview: He stationed himself in "tearooms" and offered to serve as "watchqueen"—the individual who keeps watch and coughs when a police car stops nearby or a stranger approaches. He played that role faithfully while observing hundreds of acts of fellatio. He was able to gain the confidence of some of the men he observed, disclose his role as scientist, and persuade them to tell him about the rest of their lives and about their motives. Those who were willing to talk openly with him tended to be among the better-educated members of the "tearoom trade." To avoid bias, Humphreys secretly followed some of the other men he observed and recorded the license numbers of their cars. A year later and carefully disguised, Humphreys appeared at their homes claiming to be a health-service interviewer and interviewed them about their marital status, race, job, and so on.

Humphreys' findings destroy many stereotypes. Fifty-four percent of his subjects were married and living with their wives, and superficial analysis would suggest that they were exemplary citizens who had exemplary marriages. Thirty-eight percent of Humphreys' subjects clearly were neither bisexual nor homosexual. They were men whose marriages were marked with tension; most of the 38 percent were Catholic or their wives were, and since the birth of their last child conjugal relations had been rare. Their alternative source of sex had to be quick, inexpensive, and impersonal. It could not entail any kind of involvement that would threaten their already shaky marriage and jeopardize their most important asset—their standing as father of their children. They wanted only some form of orgasm-producing action that was less lonely than masturbation and less involving than a love relationship. Of the other 62 percent of Humphreys' subjects, 24 percent were clearly bisexual, happily married, well educated, economically quite successful, and exemplary members of their community. Another 24 percent were single and were covert homosexuals. Only 14 percent of Humphreys' subjects corresponded to society's stereotype of homosexuality. That is, only 14 percent were members of the gay community and were interested primarily in personal homosexual relationships (Humphreys, 1970).

Informal inquiry (Knerr, 1977) indicated that Humphreys' research has helped persuade police departments to stop using their resources on arrest for this victimless crime. Many would count this as a social benefit.

There were also social costs. The research occurred in the middle 1960s before institutional review boards were in existence. The dissertation proposal was reviewed only by Humphreys' Ph.D. committee. Only after the research had been completed did the other members of the Sociology Department learn of it. A furor arose when some of those other members of the department objected that Humphreys' research had unethically invaded the privacy and threatened the social standing of the subjects, and petitioned the president of Washington University to rescind Humphreys' Ph.D. degree. The turmoil resulted in numerous other unfortunate events, including a fist fight among faculty members and the exodus of about half of the department members to positions at other universities.

There was considerable public outrage as well. Journalist Nicholas von Hoffman, who was given some details of the case by one of the angered members of the Sociology Department, wrote an article about Humphreys' research and offered the following condemnation of social scientists: "We're so preoccupied with defending our privacy against insurance investigators, dope sleuths, counterespionage men, divorce detectives and credit checkers, that we overlook the social scientists behind the hunting blinds who're also peeping into what we thought were our most private and secret lives. But they are there, studying us, taking notes, getting to know us, as indifferent as everybody else to the feeling that to be a complete human involves having an aspect of ourselves that's unknown." (von Hoffman, 1970).

[This case was prepared by Dr. Joan Sieber, Visiting Research Scholar, The Kennedy Institute, 1977–78, and Professor of Psychology, California State University, Hayward. The relevant materials include:
Humphreys, L., *Tearoom Trade: Impersonal Sex in Public Places* (Chicago: Aldine Publishing Co., 1970).
Knerr, C., "What To Do Before and After the Subpoena Arrives," in Joan Sieber, ed., *Ethical Decision Making in Social Science Research* (in preparation).
von Hoffman, Nicholas, "Sociological Snoopers," *The Washington Post* B1, Col. 1 and B9, Col. 5 (January 30, 1970).]

Case #5

A sixty-five-year-old retired army officer who had had several abdominal operations for gallstones, postoperative adhesions, and bowel obstructions, was admitted to a psychiatric ward because of chronic abdominal pain, loss of weight, and social withdrawal. Although he had had a productive military, teaching, and research career, he was now somewhat depressed and unkempt, and had poor hygiene. Furthermore, he and his wife had curtailed their social activities because he could not control his pain without assuming awkward and embarrassing postures. He relied on six self-administered injections each day of Talwin (pentazocine) which he believed to be essential to control his pain. Having used this nonaddictive medication for more than two years, he had so much tissue and muscle damage that he had difficulty finding injection sites. His goal for therapy was to "get more out of life in spite of my pain."

In this psychiatric ward, which included individual behavior therapy programs, daily group therapy, ward government, social activities, etc., the staff ignored pain behaviors in order to avoid reinforcing them. Their positive procedures included relaxation techniques, covert imagery, and cognitive relabelling. Although the patient had voluntarily admitted himself to this ward, where adjustment in medication was a clear expectation, he refused to allow direct modification of his Talwin dosage levels on the grounds that his experience showed that the level of medication was indispensable to control his pain. After considerable discussion with colleagues, the therapists decided to withdraw the Talwin over time, without the patient's knowledge, by diluting it with increasing proportions of normal saline. Although the patient experienced nausea, diarrhea, and cramps, he thought that these withdrawal symptoms were actually the result of Elavil (amitriptyline), which the therapists had introduced to relieve the withdrawal symptoms. While the therapists did not use Elavil to deceive the patient, it served that purpose because he blamed it for his discomfort. The staff had informed the patient that his medication regime would be modified, but had not given him the details.

After three weeks of saline injections, the therapists explained what had been done. At first the patient was incredulous and angry, but he asked that the saline be discontinued and the self-control techniques continued. When he was discharged three weeks later, he reported that he experienced some abdominal pain but that he could control it more effectively with the self-control techniques than previously with the Talwin. A follow-up six months later showed that he was still using the relaxation techniques and had resumed social activities and part-time teaching.

The therapists justified this deceptive use of a placebo on grounds of its effectiveness: "We felt ethically obliged to use a treatment that had a high probability of success. To withhold the procedure may have protected some standard of openness but may not have been in his [the patient's] best interests. We saw no option without ethical problems. Although it is precarious to justify the means by the end, we felt more obliged to use a procedure designed to help the patient achieve a personally and medically desirable goal."

[Based on the description of an actual case provided by Philip Levendusky and Loren Pankratz, "Self-Control Techniques as an Alternative to Pain Medication," *Journal of Abnormal Psychology* 84 (1975): 165–68. This case is discussed in detail in several articles in the same issue.]

Case #6

A woman had a fatal reaction during urography. The radiologist indicated that he did not warn this patient (or any other patients) of a possible fatal reaction to urography because it would not do any good. "I could have told her," he said, "that there was a chance she might have a reaction and even die. After calming her down I would then have told her that she had seen two urologists in the past week and both of them had told her she needed urography. I have done 6,000 to 8,000 urograms in the past 13 years and no one has ever had a fatal reaction. We have been doing urograms at this hospital for at least 25 years and no one has ever had a fatal reaction. Because the indications for urography were great and the chances for a reaction were remote I am sure I would have convinced Mrs. E . . . to have the procedures. She would have then had the reaction and died and the fact that I warned her would have done Mrs. E . . . absolutely no good." According to the American College of Radiology, "our responsibility is to our patients and to do what is best for our patients medically. Informing patients of risks and possible death from urography may not be in the best interest of the patient and . . . it may be dangerous."

[Robert W. Allen, "Informed Consent: A Medical Decision," *Radiology* 119 (April 1976): 233–34.]

Case #7

The problem of involuntary commitment is illustrated by the case of Mrs. Catherine Lake, a woman who suffered from chronic brain syndrome with arteriosclerosis. As a result, she had periods of confusion and mild loss of memory, interspersed with times of mental alertness and rationality. She often wandered away from her home, and her hospitalization occurred as a result of this wandering. During her third hospitalization, she petitioned for release on grounds of unlawful deprivation of liberty.

A psychiatrist who testified at her hearing claimed that she was unable to remember when her sister, her son, and her husband had died. She also showed paranoid tendencies, believing that government agencies had taken her pension away from her. However, the psychiatrist was concerned mainly about Mrs. Lake's wandering, which presented a risk of harm to herself. But she showed no tendency to harm others, nor to harm herself intentionally. Her commitment was based solely on the need for supervision because of her confused and defenseless state.

Mrs. Lake also testified at her hearing. She appeared to be fully rational, and stated that she understood her condition and the risks involved in her living outside the hospital. But she preferred to accept these risks rather than endure continued hospitalization.

The District Court, supported by the U.S. Court of Appeals, denied her petition. The court found that Mrs. Lake's family lacked the means to provide needed supervision for her. They claimed that she was "a danger to herself in that she has a tendency to wander about the streets, and is not competent to care for herself." The legal basis for her involuntary commitment was a statute providing for hospitalization of a person who "is mentally ill, and because of that illness, is likely to injure himself or others if allowed to remain at liberty." The court declared that "injure" ought to be construed broadly enough to include Mrs. Lake's situation.

However, about six months later, the Court of Appeals agreed to consider a rehearing of the case, identifying several crucial issues: How should "likely to injure himself" be interpreted? Is one who is "likely to injure himself" also automatically incompetent to choose between risk and hospitalization? Must the court consider community resources other than commitment to a mental hospital? Is equal protection denied by commitment of a person like Mrs. Lake, who would be released if her family had the means to care for her?

The case was finally returned to the District Court for an inquiry into alternative courses of treatment. The court was asked to consider whether Mrs. Lake could be released if she agreed to carry an identification card, to accept public health nursing care, to live in a foster home, or under other similar conditions. Judge Bazelon, presiding officer of the Court of Appeals, instructed the District Court that the burden of finding alternatives ought to be on the court, not on Mrs. Lake, since she lacked access to the necessary information. Bazelon referred to the position of the Department of Health, Education, and Welfare, which mandates provision of a wide spectrum of services so that the interests of both the mentally ill person and the public will be served. He also espoused the view of the National Council on the Aging, which recommends that "care and services be provided so as to be most satisfying to the person concerned." In line with this view, Bazelon ordered that "every effort should be made to find a course of treatment which appellant might be willing to accept."

[This case was prepared by Carol Tauer, based on material in Jay Katz, Joseph Goldstein, and Alan M. Dershowitz, *Psychoanalysis, Psychiatry, and Law* (New York: Free Press, 1967), pp. 552–54, 710–13. For subsequent details concerning this case, see *Lake* v. *Cameron*, 267 F. Supp. 155 (D. D.C. 1967).]

Case #8

P.Z., now twenty-seven years old, is an involuntary mental patient at Lakeland State Hospital where he was committed in June 1971, after amputating his right hand. He had been previously committed to Lakeland for eight months in 1966 (after perforating his right eardrum) and for 18 months in 1969 (after removing his right eye). In all, P.Z. has spent approximately eight years in hospitals undergoing medical treatment, e.g., treatment for meningitis following the perforation of his eardrum, and for psychiatric care of a custodial and involuntary nature.

For a variety of reasons, P.Z. now wishes to leave the hospital, but his family is strongly opposed. P.Z.'s father, a factory foreman whose job is in some jeopardy due to recession layoffs, points out that the family is already in debt more than $30,000 for the medical care necessitated by P.Z.'s penchant for self-mutilation. Neither P.Z.'s parents nor his siblings can control his self-destructive outbursts at home; indeed, they are very frightened that he will turn upon them as well. P.Z., on the other hand, maintains that he has been confined long enough, that he is not dangerous, and that, in any event, there is "no treatment for me in the hospital." He states repeatedly that "I believe in God and in brotherly love" and that "One man must sacrifice himself to God for the good of all men." P.Z. believes that he is the only one whom God has selected for that sacrifice and maintains that he enucleated his right eye and amputated his right hand upon "direct orders from God," and that he and God thereby established a "covenant." P.Z. now wants release from the hospital in order to "carry God's love to His children"; he emphasizes his commitment to this work by stating: "I would cut off my right foot if God told me to."

What rights does P.Z. have to determine where and how he shall live, and what mental competence does he have to assert such rights? Alternatively, what rights may be asserted by his family, or by society, to restrain, isolate, or "contain" him? If others have the right ultimately to restrain P.Z., must they also provide him with treatment beyond mere containment? If so, is custodial treatment sufficient? May society compel P.Z. to undergo more drastic, irreversible treatments, with or without his consent?

[This case was prepared by P. Browning Hoffman, M.D. for presentation in the series of Medicine and Society Conferences at the University of Virginia School of Medicine and is used by permission.]

Case #9

Two sisters, sixty-eight and seventy years of age, and their husbands were searching for a schizophrenic daughter who had disappeared after her discharge from a psychiatric hospital. While their car waited for a stoplight, a nearby construction machine hit a gasoline line. The spraying gas exploded, leveling a city block and igniting the car.

The sisters arrived in our burn center two hours later. The younger sister had 91 percent full-thickness, 92 percent total-body burn, with moderate smoke inhalation; the older had 94.5 percent full-thickness, 95.5 percent total-body burn, with severe smoke inhalation. The burn team agreed that survival was unprecedented in both cases. Both women were alert and interviewed separately.

The younger sister asked about death directly, looking intently into the physician's eyes. When he answered, she replied matter-of-factly, "Well, I never dreamed that life would end like this, but since we all have to go sometime, I'd like to go quietly and comfortably, I don't know what to do about my daughter. . . ."

After she was made comfortable, the nurse obtained a description of the missing daughter and possible whereabouts. The social worker alerted the police to look for her, and telephoned relatives, informing them of the accident as gently as could be conveyed by telephone. The husbands were located at another burn unit. An attempt was made to arrange a final spousal conversation, but both husbands were intubated.

Meanwhile, the older sister doubted whether her injuries were as serious as reported. "I feel so good, wouldn't I be hurting horribly if I were going to die?" The effect of full-thickness burns on nerve endings was explained. The physician reiterated that we wished to do what she thought was best for her. She hedged, "What did my sister say? I'll go along with her decision." Since the patient seemed unsure of her decision, she was offered full therapy in the room with her sister. She then refused the therapy adamantly, but denied that she was dying.

The sisters' beds were placed next to each other so that they could see and touch each other easily. They discussed funeral arrangements and then joked, in the next breath, about the damage done to their hair. The hospital chaplain prayed with them. By active listening, he was able to convey to the older sister that her husband was not to blame for the accident as she had thought. "It's good to go out not cursing him after all our years together," she said. The younger sister died several hours later, after her sister lapsed into a coma; the older sister died the next day. The daughter was not located.

[This case is reprinted by permission from Sharon H. Imbus, R.N., M.Sc., and Bruce E. Zawacki, M.D., "Autonomy for Burn Patients When Survival Is Unprecedented," in *The New England Journal of Medicine* 297 (August 11, 1977): 309.]

Case #10

A sixty-year-old male, with no living relatives or family, underwent a routine physical examination in preparation for a brief but much anticipated trip to Australia. During the examination, the physician discovered that the man suffered from a terminal case of cancer. The physician had treated the man for many years and knew that he suffered prolonged and serious depression whenever informed of serious health problems. The depression always had serious side effects: the man suffered migraine headaches and so worried about himself that he could not exercise rational control over his deliberations and decisions. At times in the past he had expressed a desire to kill himself, but psychiatric examinations always showed that he both lacked resolution and suffered powerful guilt whenever he actually attempted to think out how he might take his own life. He had strong beliefs about the immorality of suicide.

One week after the routine physical examination, the patient asked his physician a series of questions about his health. One of his questions was "Did you discover anything in the examination that might indicate a serious problem either now or in the future?" The physician believed that his patient would not suffer from the cancer at all while in Australia and answered the question by saying, "The examination shows that you have never been in better physical condition." The physician had good evidence to indicate that no treatment would be effective against the cancer and had consulted with two specialists, who corroborated his hypothesis. The physician worried about telling such a bald lie to his patient but firmly believed that it was a justified lie.

[This hypothetical case was prepared especially for this volume.]

Case #11

Janet P., a practicing Jehovah's Witness, had refused to sign a consent for blood infusions before the delivery of her daughter. Physicians determined that the newborn infant needed transfusions to prevent retardation and possible death. When the parents refused permission for these transfusions, a hearing was conducted at the Columbia Hospital for Women to decide whether the newborn infant should be given transfusions over the parents' objections. Superior Court Judge Tim Murphy ordered a guardian appointed to sign the necessary releases, and the baby was given the transfusions. During the hearing, Janet P. began hemorrhaging, and attending physicians said she needed an emergency hysterectomy to stem the bleeding. Her husband, also a Jehovah's Witness, approved the hysterectomy but not infusions of blood. This time Judge Murphy declined to order transfusions for the mother, basing his decision on an earlier

D.C. Court of Appeals Ruling. Janet P. bled to death a few hours later. Her baby survived.

[This case is based on a news report by Martha M. Hamilton in *The Washington Post*, November 14, 1974. It was prepared by James J. McCartney.]

Case #12

Mrs. Jones was brought to the hospital by her husband for emergency care, having lost two thirds of her body's blood supply from a ruptured ulcer. She had no personal physician, and relied solely on the hospital staff. She was a total hospital responsibility. It appeared that the patient, age twenty-five, mother of a seven-month-old child, and her husband were both Jehovah's Witnesses, the teachings of which sect, according to their interpretation, prohibited the injection of blood into the body. When death without blood became imminent, the hospital sought the advice of counsel, who applied to the District Court in the name of the hospital for permission to administer blood. Judge Tamm of the District Court denied the application, and counsel immediately applied to me [Judge J. Skelly Wright], as a member of the Court of Appeals, for an appropriate writ.

I called the hospital by telephone and spoke with Dr. Westura, Chief Medical Resident, who confirmed the representations made by counsel. I thereupon proceeded with counsel to the hospital, where I spoke to Mr. Jones, the husband of the patient. He advised me that, on religious grounds, he would not approve a blood transfusion for his wife. He said, however, that if the court ordered the transfusion, the responsibility was not his. I advised Mr. Jones to obtain counsel immediately. He thereupon went to the telephone and returned in ten or fifteen minutes to advise that he had taken the matter up with his church and that he had decided that he did not want counsel.

I asked permission of Mr. Jones to see his wife. This he readily granted. Prior to going into the patient's room, I again conferred with Dr. Westura and several other doctors assigned to the case. All confirmed that the patient would die without blood and that there was a better than fifty percent chance of saving her life with it. Unanimously they strongly recommended it. I then went inside the patient's room. Her appearance confirmed the urgency which had been represented to me. I tried to communicate with her, advising her again as to what the doctors had said. The only audible reply I could hear was "Against my will." It was obvious that the woman was not in a mental condition to make a decision. I was reluctant to press her because of the seriousness of her condition and because I felt that to suggest repeatedly the imminence of death without blood might place a strain on her religious convictions. I asked her whether she would oppose the blood transfusion if the court allowed it. She indicated, as best I could make out, that it would not then be her responsibility. . . .

I . . . signed the order allowing the hospital to administer such transfusions as the doctors should determine were necessary to save her life. . . .

[This case is taken from *Application of the President and Directors of Georgetown College*, 331 F. 2d 1000 (D.C. Cir.), certiorari denied, 377 U.S. 978 (1964).]

Case #13

A sixty-eight-year-old man with end-stage renal disease secondary to chronic glomerulonephritis had been on maintenance hemodialysis for ten years. At the initiation of dialysis, he was supervising his own accounting firm and continued in this role until he retired at age sixty-five. The patient smoked for many years and had developed progressive pulmonary failure over the past four years. Despite intensive treatment of his lung disease, there was no improvement in pulmonary function. Significant hypoxia (pO_2 = 48 mm Hg) could not be treated with oxygen therapy because the patient continued to smoke. The patient had a myocardial infarction two years ago, and since that time his dialysis was complicated by severe hypotension from decreased cardiac output. His predialysis blood pressure was usually 30/60 mm Hg. Over the past year he developed intermittent psychotic behavior. Despite intensive inpatient psychiatric care for six months, there was no mental improvement. The psychiatric diagnosis was chronic, psychotic, organic brain syndrome due to cerebral arteriosclerosis, hypoxia, and decreased cardiac output with aggravation by the emotional stresses of chronic hemodialysis. Two psychiatrists concluded that the patient was competent. Because of the cumulative effect of multiple organ failures, the patient's general condition could be noted to progressively deteriorate. For three months he was so debilitated that he would crawl down the hall because he didn't have the strength to walk. The nephrologist informed the family that the patient would probably expire in three to four months.

On some days during the past year, the patient seemed mentally clear and would privately request his physician and nurses to discontinue dialysis because he was so miserable; however, on other occasions, and particularly in the presence of his youngest son (age thirty years), he expressed a desire to continue dialysis. On many occasions the patient was agitated and confused from his organic brain syndrome and, on these occasions, he would hit nursing personnel with his fists. He had damaged dialysis equipment and frightened other patients by throwing large objects. In order to protect other patients and personnel, the nephrologist ordered sedation to the point of immobility (and incidental noncommunicativeness). The nephrologist recommended to the oldest son that dialysis be discontinued. Because his mother was dead, he wanted to discuss the matter with his younger brother and sister and his father's one brother and two sisters.

Multiple medical conferences were held to explain the situation to the patient and his family. After weeks of family deliberation, the oldest son indicated that he, his sister, his uncle, and both aunts wanted to stop dialysis because of the magnitude and the prolongation of suffering. They pointed out that the patient had once been a respected and proud man. The youngest son, who would get the proceeds of a life insurance policy if his father lived for three more months, was opposed and indicated he would sue the physician and hospital if dialysis was discontinued.

[This case was written from a case history at St. Francis Hospital, Honolulu, by Dr. Arnold W. Siemsen, Institute of Renal Diseases, St. Francis Hospital.]

Case #14

A doctor aged sixty-eight was admitted to an overseas hospital after a barium meal had shown a large carcinoma of the stomach. He had retired from practice five years earlier, after severe myocardial infarction had left his exercise tolerance considerably reduced. The early symptoms of the carcinoma were mistakenly thought to be due to myocardial ischaemia. By the time the possibility of carcinoma was first considered, the disease was already far-advanced; laparotomy showed extensive metastatic involvement of the abdominal lymph nodes and liver. Palliative gastrectomy was performed with the object of preventing perforation of the primary tumor into the peritoneal cavity, which appeared to the surgeon to be imminent. Histological examination showed the growth to be an anaplastic primary adenocarcinoma. There was clinical and radiological evidence of secondary deposits in the lower thoracic and lumbar vertebrae.

The patient was told of the findings and fully understood their import. In spite of increasingly large doses of pethidine, and of morphine at night, he suffered constantly with severe abdominal pain and pain resulting from compression of spinal nerves by tumor deposits.

On the tenth day after the gastrectomy the patient collapsed with classic manifestations of massive pulmonary embolism. Pulmonary embolectomy was successfully performed in the ward by a registrar. When the patient had recovered sufficiently he expressed his appreciation of the good intentions and skill of his young colleague. At the same time, he asked that if he had a further cardiovascular collapse no steps should be taken to prolong his life, for the pain of his cancer was now more than he would needlessly continue to endure. He himself wrote a note to this effect in his case records, and the staff of the hospital knew his feelings.

His wish notwithstanding, when the patient collapsed again, two weeks after the embolectomy—this time with acute myocardial infarction and cardiac arrest—he was revived by the hospital's emergency resuscitation team. His heart stopped on four further occasions during that night and each time was restarted artificially. The body then recovered sufficiently to linger for three more weeks, but in a decerebrate state, punctuated by episodes of projectile vomiting accompanied by generalized convulsions. Intravenous nourishment was carefully combined with blood transfusion and measures necessary to maintain electrolyte and fluid balance. In addition, antibacterial and antifungal antibiotics were given as prophylaxis against infection, particularly pneumonia complicating the tracheotomy that had been performed to ensure a clear airway. On the last day of his illness, preparations were being made for the work of the failing respiratory centre to be given over to an artificial respirator, but the heart finally stopped before this endeavor could be realized.

[This case is reprinted by permission from W. St. C. Symmers, Sr., "Not Allowed to Die," *British Medical Journal* 1 (1968): 442.]

Case #15

By 1976, sixty-seven-year-old Joseph Saikewicz had lived in state institutions for over forty years. His I.Q. was ten, and his mental age was approximately two years and eight months. He could communicate only by gestures and grunts, and he responded only to gestures or physical contacts. He appeared to be unaware of dangers and became disoriented when removed from familiar surroundings.

His health was generally good until April, 1976, when he was diagnosed as having acute myeloblastic monocytic leukemia, which is inevitably fatal. In approximately 30 to 50 percent of cases of this type of leukemia, chemotherapy can bring about temporary remission which usually lasts between two and thirteen months. The results are poorer for patients older than sixty. In addition, chemotherapy often has serious side effects including anemia and infections.

At the petition of the Belchertown State School, where Saikewicz was located, the Probate Court appointed a guardian ad litem with authority to make the necessary decisions concerning the patient's care and treatment. The guardian ad litem noted that Saikewicz's illness was incurable, that chemotherapy had significant adverse side effects and discomfort, and that Saikewicz could not understand the treatment or the resulting pain. For all these reasons he concluded "that not treating Mr. Saikewicz would be in his best interests." The Supreme Judicial Court of Massachusetts upheld this decision on July 9, 1976 (although its opinion was not issued until November 28, 1977). Mr. Saikewicz died on September 4, 1976.

[This case is drawn from *Superintendent of Belchertown* v. *Saikewicz,* Mass. 370 N.E. 2d 417 (1977).]

Case #16

Baby girl Betsy Novick had immediately apparent physical malformations when she was born. A diagnosis of Seckel or "bird-headed" dwarfism was made. She had, in addition to low birth weight and length, large eyes, a large, beaklike nose, narrow face, receding lower jaw, strabismus, and a club foot. Seckel dwarfism, an autosomal recessive genetic disease, had affected Mr. Novick's brother as well. Life expectancy is good, but a much simplified gross cerebral structure is related to mental retardation. It was apparent that institutionalization would be necessary. The Novick's were of modest means and the vivid memory of the devastating impact of Mr. Novick's brother immediately convinced him that the child could not be cared for at home.

The Novick's lived in the state that has the lowest per capita income spent on institutions for the retarded. Although court action promised some marginal improvements in the institutions, they promised to be bleak, understaffed, custodial institutions for the foreseeable future. The fact that Betsy had rather peculiarly repulsive features led the parents to fear that she would receive particularly poor care, yet they saw no alternative.

In the next two months Betsy developed a persistent pyloric stenosis, a narrowing of the pylorus between the stomach and intestines causing projectile vomiting that did not respond to phenobarbital, atropine, or special diet. If not surgically treated, death by starvation would result. The parents, at first stunned by the additional severe medical problem, considered the alternatives. They envisioned the virtually certain, severe burden and suffering to be placed on the child in any institutions conceivably available in the next decade or two. They decided that it was a burden the child should not bear, even though in principle they knew society should be providing better support for them. They decided against the surgery. The child died after two weeks of deterioration.

[This case was prepared by Robert M. Veatch of the Hastings Center and is used by permission.]

Case #17

H. R. was a two-day-old male infant for whom pediatric surgical consultation was requested because of vomiting of feedings and large quantities of green fluid.

The infant was born to a forty-five-year-old woman who had two normal teenagers and had thought she was through menopause and safely out of range of pregnancy. Both parents were in good health and the pregnancy had been uneventful. The baby had unmistakable stigmata of Down's syndrome, promptly confirmed by chromosome karyotyping which identified a trisomy of chromosome 21. In addition he had a grade 3/6 heart murmur but no cyanosis or signs of congestive heart failure.

Roentgenographic examination confirmed the clinical impression of duodenal obstruction which could only be relieved by surgery. The parents, both well educated, had expressed their intention to institutionalize the baby prior to the diagnosis of intestinal obstruction. When asked by the physician caring for the baby if they would give consent for operative intervention, the father said, "I have no alternative, do I?" There was no reply, and the father signed the consent form. The surgery was successful, and ten days later the infant was on his way to the state institution.

[This case was prepared by Anthony Shaw, M.D. for presentation in the series of Medicine and Society Conferences at the University of Virginia School of Medicine and is used by permission.]

Case #18

THE FAMILY SETTING
Mother, 34 years old, hospital nurse.
Father, 35 years old, lawyer.
Two normal children in the family.

In late fall of 1963, Mr. and Mrs. _____ gave birth to a premature baby boy. Soon after birth, the child was diagnosed as a "mongoloid" (Down's syndrome) with the added complication of an intestinal blockage (duodenal atresia). The latter could be corrected with an operation of quite nominal risk. Without the operation the child could not be fed and would die.

At the time of birth Mrs. _____ overheard the doctor express his belief that the child was a mongol. She immediately indicated she did not want the child. The next day, in consultation with a physician, she maintained this position, refusing to give permission for the corrective operation on the intestinal block. Her husband supported her in this position, saying that his wife knew more about these things (i.e., mongoloid children) than he. The reason the mother gave for her position—"It would be unfair to the other children of the household to raise them with a mongoloid."

The physician explained to the parents that the degree of mental retardation cannot be predicted at birth—running from very low mentality to borderline subnormal. As he said: "Mongolism, it should be stressed, is one of the milder forms of mental retardation. That is, mongols' I.Q.s are generally in the 50-80 range, and sometimes a little higher. That is, they're almost always trainable. They can hold simple jobs. And they're famous for being happy children. They're perennially happy and usually a great joy." Without other complications, they can anticipate a long life.

Given the parents' decision, the hospital staff did not seek a court order to override the decision. The child was put in a side room and, over an 11-day period, allowed to starve to death.

Following this episode, the parents undertook genetic counseling (chromosome studies) with regard to future possible pregnancies.

[This case, frequently referred to as the Johns Hopkins Hospital case, is reprinted by permission from James M. Gustafson, "Mongolism, Parental Desires, and the Right to Life," *Perspectives in Biology and Medicine* 17 (Summer 1973): 529–30, published by the University of Chicago Press.]

Case #19

An eight-year-old white boy was recently brought to the Birth Defects Treatment Center for recommendations about future care. He was the third child of middle-class parents and was born and treated elsewhere. At birth he was found to have a large meningomyelocele with a neurologic deficit below T_{12}. The parents were told that he would die. He was given routine care, did not develop meningitis, and remained at the local hospital until five and a half months of age when he was transferred to a state institution for chronic care. At ten months of age, because of progressive enlargement of the head which made nursing care difficult, he was transferred to another hospital where a ventriculoatrial shunt was placed, and the back was repaired. The child was returned to the state institution.

By two and a half years he was using two-word sentences, but was found to have cortical blindness. Over the next several years he had multiple orthopedic procedures, including replacement of dislocated hips, tendon achilles lengthening, osteotomies and repair of fractures. He was always returned to the institution. At six years of age he was found to have severe hydronephrosis, and an ileal loop was performed.

At eight years of age he is in a school for the blind and has an I.Q. of 80. He goes home to his parents on weekends, but they have established little rapport with him. It is difficult for him to sit because of the marked paralytic kyphosis, which also interferes with the ileal stoma so that a collecting device cannot be kept in place. . . . His hips have redis-located; the hydronephrosis is of moderate degree. The family is receiving psychiatric help to cope with this child when he is home. The child needs a spinal fusion to allow him to sit without obstructing his loop and revision of the ileal stoma to permit adequate drainage.

[This case is reprinted by permission from John M. Freeman, M.D., "The Shortsighted Treatment of Myelomeningocele: A Long-Term Case Report" in *Pediatrics* 53 (March 1974): 311–13.]

Case #20

In October, 1976, Mr. Stanley Wilks, a forty-three-year-old civilian mathematician for the Army, became seriously ill with what was to be diagnosed as idiopathic hemorrhagic pancreatitis. Treatment for this disease lies mainly in managing complications while waiting for the inflammation to subside. Mr. Wilks required multiple operations, and his condition deteriorated until it forced his physicians to paralyze him with curare in order to manage his failing respirations and to preserve his caloric reserve. He was burning up more than 5,000 calories a day, more than double the normal 2,000, and was losing weight rapidly even with intensive intravenous feedings. Although this procedure was intended to last only a few days, Mr. Wilks remained paralyzed on a respirator for a long period, two and a half months, before he regained the strength to breathe on his own. At that point, he appeared to be on the way to recovery. However, he developed an overwhelming abdominal infection in July, 1977, and died a few days later, still in the hospital. Until the last few days, at no time did he or his family wish to discontinue therapy and at no time was the prognosis for recovery considered to be hopeless.

The bill for his hospitalization was approximately $250,000 which would have been borne by the prepaid health maintenance program to which Mr. Wilks belonged had it not been for a re-insurance arrangement with Blue Cross.

[This case was prepared by Dr. Joanne Lynn and James J. McCartney. See also *The Washington Post,* April 19, 1977, pp. A1 & A6.]

Case #21

State Bill 529 calls for the establishment of community-based homes for the care and education of the mentally retarded. The bill provides one home for every fifteen persons presently institutionalized in four state institutions for the mentally retarded at a cost of $55.8 million. The estimated costs for the new care for the present population of 7,600 will be $70 million a year.

The bill was introduced by Representative John Sheehan who spoke in favor of it. He painted a dismal picture of antiquated institutions bereft of basic human necessities or amenities. Thousands of human beings, many unclothed, spend their lives huddled in dark, drab rooms, where they are supervised by an overworked staff, many of whom have no professional training. Sheehan, who has the support of the parents' organization, the State Department of Mental Health, the local ACLU, and the religious leadership, concluded his case by pleading, "Justice requires that we extend this token contribution to these citizens, burdened by physical and psychological suffering, and by the degradation of our society's past inhumanity to its fellow humans."

Representative James Hudson and Dr. Robert Simmons, while emphasizing their concern for care of the retarded, spoke in opposition to the bill. Representative Hudson, noting that he was the elected representative of all the citizens in his district, argued that he had an obligation to examine the alternative uses for the $14 million in additional funds called for by the bill. But first, he pointed out that the new total sum of $70 million equalled 1.5 percent of the state's budget, a budget raised by all its citizens, while the institutionalized population equalled only one-tenth of one percent of the state's population. The proposed increase of $14 million could buy hot lunches for all the state's school children; it could also provide job training for productive members of society. Hudson argued that the fairest thing to do would be to spread the money evenly among those who would be productive. "Our task as legislators," he concluded, "must be to serve the greatest good of the greatest number."

Dr. Simmons, as a physician, argued that the money could be used more efficiently in providing health care for three groups: normal or more nearly normal children (thousands of whom could be reached for every mentally retarded child), those potentially engaged in productive labor, and pregnant women. He showed that much mental retardation can be eliminated through prenatal diagnosis which he estimated to cost $200 per case for Down's syndrome compared to $60,000 for each institutionalized child. Even allowing that some of the institutionalized retarded might be gainfully employed if they were in high-quality, community-based homes, the savings from spending the funds on detection rather than on more expensive forms of institutionalized care are enormous.

The legislative committee must now make its decision on the bill.

[This case, written by Robert M. Veatch, appeared as Case #529 in "Who Has First Claim on Health Care Resources?" *The Hastings Center Report* (August 1975): 13 and is used by permission.]

Case #22

Thomas Merriam was Director of Budget Planning at the National Institutes of Health and chief advisor to the Assistant Secretary on the congressional message on the 1976 fiscal year NIH budget. He was under a great deal of pressure from Dr. Alan Sanders, Director of the National Institute of Arthritis, Metabolism, and Digestive Diseases, to increase the budget for research on arthritis.

Dr. Sanders argued that in 1974 3,377,000 persons in the United States suffered from arthritis severe enough that their activity was limited. There were almost 4 million hospital days attributable to arthritis and 57 million days of bed disability. There was anger in Dr. Sanders' voice during the meeting Merriam had with the Institute director. It was as if he could not get anyone to take arthritis seriously. He claimed that because there were virtually no deaths attributable to arthritis, the government policy analysts were grossly underemphasizing the disease that produced the second largest number of persons with limitation of activity in the United States. The suffering was enormous, yet the planners were using formulas that calculated number of days of life likely to be added for research dollar invested. This meant that arthritis would receive virtually no funding if Merriam and his associates relied exclusively on the formula.

Sanders claimed that the National Cancer Institute and the Heart and Lung Institute were getting more money than they could use because of the excessive emphasis on death prevention rather than suffering prevention. Sanders conceded that cancer and heart disease also produce some disability. The cancer institute was less the target of his attack since the cancer budget was not part of the NIH planning, it being separated out by the Nixon administration as part of the war on cancer. He emphasized the inequity between the heart institute and the funds for arthritis. The number of persons with limitation of activity is about the same in the two cases (3.9 million for heart disease compared with 3.4 million for arthritis). Yet the heart institute budget was $290,511,000, while the arthritis portion of Sanders' institute's budget was only $14,076,000. Expressed in days of disability, there were 93 million days for heart disease and 57 million for arthritis. How, Sanders asked, can that difference justify the much larger difference in the budgets?

Merriam was frustrated after his conversation with Sanders. He wanted an objective, statistically certain way of allocating the research funds between a condition like heart disease that produces some disability, but is the primary cause of death, and a condition like arthritis that is also a serious debilitator, but causes no death. He considered his options:

1. Use cost/benefit ratios to maximize the number of days of life added per dollar invested.
2. Use cost/benefit analysis to calculate the dollars lost to the economy from work lost from the two conditions, and use that ratio to propose funds for the two programs.
3. Use cost/benefit analysis to calculate both costs of the diseases and costs of the potential research, and use dollars most efficiently.
4. Survey people asking them how they would like their money to be spent, and allocate the funds by calculating the average apportionment.
5. Allocate funds in proportion to the number of people suffering from the two conditions regardless of deaths, costs of treatment, costs of research, or any other variables.
6. Ask experts working on research in the two areas what the likelihood of a breakthrough might be, and use those estimates as a basis for allocating funds.

7. Turn the matter over to the politicians to decide what the priorities
   ought to be.

Merriam needed a principle for dealing with Dr. Sanders' complaint.
What should he do?

[This case is based on actual data, but does not reflect actions or positions taken
by actual employees of the National Institutes of Health during the period
described in this case. It is Case 570: *Arthritis and Heart Disease: Where Should
Research Funds Go?* prepared by Robert M. Veatch of the Hastings Center and is
used by permission.]

Case #23

The totally implantable artificial heart is a blood pump constructed of
synthetic materials, driven by a motor and a power source, all of which
are totally and permanently implanted within the body in place of the
natural heart. Such a device is now being developed at the National Heart
and Lung Institute, and, through NIH contracts, in various research
centers and corporations. The first phase of its development, the design,
engineering, and testing of components, is substantially complete, and
preparations are being made for extensive animal experimentation. Three
alternative power systems are being contemplated: an electric motor
powered by a biological fuel cell, an electric motor powered by rechargeable batteries, or a nuclear engine powered by 53 grams of Plutonium 238.
The pump must be made of materials which are compatible with blood
and are sufficiently durable to meet work demands. The power system
must be responsive to physiological needs of the body. Candidates for this
artificial heart would be persons whose own diseased heart is incapable of
cardiac output sufficient to sustain life. The diseased natural heart would
be totally removed and replaced by the artificial pump, controls, and
power source. It has been estimated that between 17,000 and 50,000
patients annually might benefit from such a device. The total costs for
medical care, hospitalization, the device itself, and the energy source will
be in the order of $15,000 to $25,000, and probably more for the nuclear-
powered heart. (Later estimates are that the costs will run $50,000 to
$75,000/implantation.)

[This case was prepared by James J. McCartney. It is based on two published reports, Albert R. Jonsen, "The Totally Implantable Artificial Heart," *The Hastings Center Report* 3 (November 1973): 1 and *The Totally Implantable Artificial Heart: A Report of the Artificial Heart Assessment Panel of the National Heart and Lung Institute.* DHEW Publication No. (NIH) 74–191, June 1973.]

Case #24

Mrs. J.W., a sixty-year-old hotel maid, was admitted to a county hospital in May complaining of "failing health, loss of weight, and stomach troubles." The patient lived alone, had two daughters and eight grandchildren, and was covered by a Blue Cross-Blue Shield insurance plan offered by her employer. She had a small savings and looked forward to continued independent life, supported by this, Social Security, and a small pension.

Initial history, examination, and routine lab tests were not helpful, showing only a history of active tuberculosis and a present mild anemia. She had lost approximately 50 of her 180 pounds over six months. Her abdominal complaints were variable and rather vague, but tended to be a persistent "ache" in the midabdomen and intermittent constipation or diarrhea. Chest X ray showed multiple healed lesions of tuberculosis and a small hazy density in the right upper lobe. Initially the diagnosis was suspected to be cancer of the colon with a metastasis to the lung. However, all of the usual diagnostic examinations failed to confirm this or any other diagnosis. A gallium scan showed a vague area of increased uptake in the right loin, signifying some sort of inflammation at this site. Eventually, even bone marrow examination and bronchoscopy (passing a flexible tube through the airways to see lesions and obtain tissue) were done, again without yield. The physicians were aware that there were treatable and even curable possibilities for diagnosis remaining. Definite diagnosis was probably available by surgery, although the choice of operating upon the technically difficult lung lesion or the ill-defined abdominal problem would be very difficult. The physicians presented the patient with one last diagnostic option. A nearby private hospital had "computerized axial tomography" which could take very precise pictures of the body as if in cross section (a CAT scan). Although the likelihood that this would be helpful for her problem was not known, since the machine had only been available for a few years, it held out the possibility of some decisive information, either as to diagnosis or as to other diagnostic maneuvers. However, her insurance would not pay the cost of this procedure and she would have to pay at least $500. (The county hospital's application for the machine had been turned down by the Regional Health Planning Authority.) She was greatly afraid to spend so large a part of her liquid assets, but she was much more indisposed to undergo surgery and decided upon the CAT scan. It disclosed definite evidence of an invasive carcinoma of the midportion of the pancreas, which was confirmed by percutaneous needle biopsy. The patient was informed of the diagnosis and the very dismal prognosis under any therapy, and she chose to have only palliative and supportive therapy as they became necessary. She used her remaining savings to help her family and died in the home of one of her daughters six months later.

[This case was prepared by Dr. Joanne Lynn.]

Case #25

A forty-year-old widow with chronic glomerulonephritis has been on maintenance hemodialysis for ten years. Over the past two years she has been progressively deteriorating from multiple complications which have included severe renal osteodystrophy, inability to obtain adequate blood access, and malnutrition from intermittent depression. Peritoneal dialysis cannot be accomplished because of multiple abdominal surgical procedures with adhesions. Her physician has recommended transplantation because he feels she will not survive over four to six months on dialysis.

The patient has four children (ages eleven to fourteen years) and wants a transplant to allow her to live and provide for the future well-being of her children.

The patient's forty-four-year-old brother is a farmer with eight children. He refused to donate or be tissue typed. The patient has a forty-two-year-old sister who was willing to donate but was not tissue typed because she has been an insulin-requiring diabetic for ten years.

The patient also has a thirty-five-year-old mentally retarded brother who has been institutionalized since age eight. This brother is an A match with four antigens being identified. He is so severely retarded that he cannot comprehend or understand any of the risks of nephrectomy. He is able to take care of his own personal needs and ambulate with guidance. He neither recognizes his own family members nor interacts with medical staff. The patient would regularly drive 300 miles to see her brother four times per year until twelve years ago, when her own personal and family needs reduced the frequency to one to two times per year. She has not seen her brother for three years, because of her own medical illnesses. At the present time she feels she has a duty to her brother but there is no particular closeness.

Her fourteen-year-old daughter would like to donate a kidney, even though she is a 2-antigen mismatch. The daughter has demonstrated a perceptive, thorough, and reasonably unemotional grasp of her mother's situation and needs, and of the seriousness of her own potential donation. ABO blood types for the retarded brother and the daughter are compatible.

The patient's older brother and sister feel the donor should be the younger, mentally retarded brother. The diabetic sister is the legal guardian of the retarded brother. Both parents are dead. She has been on the cadaveric transplant waiting list for two years.

The following statements are reasonable projections based on known data:

	2-yr. kidney survival	2-yr. patient survival
Retarded brother to patient	70%	85%
Minor child to patient	60%	75%
Cadaveric to patient	40%	65%

[This case was written from a case history at St. Francis Hospital, Honolulu, by Dr. Arnold W. Siemsen, Institute of Renal Diseases, St. Francis Hospital.]

Case #26

The Willowbrook State School is an institution for mentally retarded children on Staten Island, New York. The population of Willowbrook increased from 200 in 1949 to over 6,000 in 1963. Hepatitis was first noticed among residents of Willowbrook in 1949, and in 1954 Dr. Saul Krugman and his associates, Dr. Joan Giles, Dr. Jack Hammond et al., began to study the disease there. Of the 5,200 residents at Willowbrook during one part of their study, 3,800 were severely retarded with I.Q.'s of less than 20. In addition, at least 3,000 of the children were not toilet-trained. Since infectious hepatitis is transmitted via the intestinal-oral route, and since susceptible children were constantly being admitted to the institution, there was a persistent and continuing endemic situation of contagious hepatitis. In fact, virtually all susceptible children became infected within the first six to twelve months of residence at the institution. This strain of hepatitis, however, was especially mild in the three to ten age range.

In an attempt to develop an effective prophylactic agent, Krugman and his associates did a number of different studies, some of which involved artificially exposing children to the Willowbrook strain of hepatitis infection. Of the 10,000 admissions to Willowbrook since 1956, approximately 750–800 children were admitted to Krugman's special hepatitis unit. These study groups included only children whose parents gave written consent. Originally, information was conveyed to individual parents by letter or personal interview. In later studies the group technique, i.e., discussing the project in detail with a group of prospective consenting parents, was employed. Children who were wards of the state or children without parents were never included in the studies.

Studies were carried out in a special unit with optimum isolation facilities to protect the children from other infectious diseases. Even when overcrowding forced the institution to stop further admissions for awhile in 1964, room was available in this special unit for children whose parents 'volunteered' them for this project. One direct benefit of the study to the children themselves was that, in addition to being protected from other infectious diseases, they also frequently developed immunity from hepatitis itself after contraction of the mild form administered by Krugman. These studies were reviewed and sanctioned by various local, state, and federal agencies.

[This case was prepared by James J. McCartney.]

Case #27

On August 11, 1977, Whitley et al. reported in the *New England Journal of Medicine* that a new drug, adenine arabinoside (ara-A) had been tested and found to be highly useful in the treatment and cure of biopsy-proved herpes simplex encephalitis, a disease considered fatal to approximately seventy percent of those who contract it. This collaborative study, supported by the National Institute of Allergy and Infectious Disease, was a controlled, double-blind experiment with ten of the twenty-eight patients treated receiving a placebo instead of the experimental drug.

This same drug, ara-A, within its apparent antiviral dose range, was found previously by Ch'ien and others to have produced no demonstrable hepatic, renal, or hematologic toxicity. In the current study, of the eighteen patients treated with ara-A for ten days, five died. Of the thirteen survivors, seven recovered to lead reasonably normal lives, while the other six have serious brain or nerve damage, possibly because the drug treatment was started too late. Of the ten given the placebo, seven died while only two recovered to lead reasonably normal lives. The experiment was eventually stopped and all patients were treated with ara-A.

[This case was prepared by James J. McCartney on the basis of information in *The New England Journal of Medicine* 297 (August 11, 1977): 289–94 and *Journal of Infectious Disease* 128 (1973): 658–63.]

Case #28

Having recently completed his Ph.D. degree in chemistry, George has not been able to find a job. His family has suffered from his failure since they are short of money, his wife has had to take a full-time job, and the small children have been subjected to considerable strain, uncertainty, and instability. An established chemist can get George a position in a laboratory that pursues research in chemical and biological warfare. Despite his perilous financial and familial circumstances, George feels that he cannot accept this position because of his conscientious opposition to chemical and biological warfare. The older chemist notes that while he is not enthusiastic about this project, the research will continue whatever George decides. Furthermore, if George does not take the position it will be offered to another young man who would probably pursue the research with alacrity and promptitude. Indeed, the older chemist confides, his concern about this other candidate's nationalistic fervor and uncritical zeal for research in chemical and biological warfare in part led him to recommend George. George's wife is puzzled and hurt by George's reaction since she sees nothing wrong with such research. She is mainly concerned about the instability of their family and their children's problems.

[Adapted from Bernard Williams, "A Critique of Utilitarianism," in J.J.C. Smart and Bernard Williams, *Utilitarianism For and Against* (Cambridge: Cambridge University Press, 1973), pp. 97–98.]

Case #29

The 1967 Abortion Act in Britain included a conscientious objection clause, similar to the federal and many state conscience clauses in the United States. It indicated that no doctor or nurse is required to participate in abortion procedures if he or she is conscientiously opposed to such procedures on religious or ethical grounds. Nevertheless, some report that institutions and individuals make it very difficult for conscientious objectors to abortions to gain certain appointments, etc. As one conscientious objector to abortion reports: "It was indeed a surprise to be informed by an eminent professor, after a hospital interview, that as a Roman Catholic gynaecologist 'there is no place for you to practise within the National Health Service.' One had always assumed . . . that the British 'system' is based on fair play and, above all, respect for the individual conscience. It soon became quite obvious that in order to stay in the specialty in Britain I would have had to change a conscientiously held abhorrence to the direct taking of human life. I chose to leave country, home, and family in order to practise medicine in full freedom of conscience."

[This case is adapted from R. Walley, "A Question of Conscience," *British Medical Journal* (June 12, 1976): 1456.]

Codes of Ethics

The Hippocratic Oath
World Medical Association, Declaration of Geneva
American Medical Association, Principles of Medical Ethics
World Health Organization, Constitution
American Hospital Association, A Patient's Bill of Rights
The Nuremberg Code
World Medical Association, Declaration of Helsinki
Department of Health, Education, and Welfare, Regulations on the
    Protection of Human Subjects
International Council of Nurses, Code for Nurses

The Hippocratic Oath

I swear by Apollo Physician and Asclepius and Hygieia and Panaceia and all the gods and goddesses, making them my witnesses, that I will fulfil according to my ability and judgment this oath and this covenant:

To hold him who has taught me this art as equal to my parents and to live my life in partnership with him, and if he is in need of money to give him a share of mine, and to regard his offspring as equal to my brothers in male lineage and to teach them this art—if they desire to learn it—without fee and covenant; to give a share of precepts and oral instruction and all the other learning to my sons and to the sons of him who has instructed me and to pupils who have signed the covenant and have taken an oath according to the medical law, but to no one else.

I will apply dietetic measures for the benefit of the sick according to my ability and judgment; I will keep them from harm and injustice.

I will neither give a deadly drug to anybody if asked for it, nor will I make a suggestion to this effect. Similarly I will not give to a woman an abortive remedy. In purity and holiness I will guard my life and my art.

I will not use the knife, not even on sufferers from stone, but will withdraw in favor of such men as are engaged in this work.

Whatever houses I may visit, I will come for the benefit of the sick, remaining free of all intentional injustice, of all mischief and in particular of sexual relations with both female and male persons, be they free or slaves.

What I may see or hear in the course of the treatment or even outside of the treatment in regard to the life of men, which on no account one must spread abroad, I will keep to myself holding such things shameful to be spoken about.

If I fulfil this oath and do not violate it, may it be granted to me to enjoy life and art, being honored with fame among all men for all time to come; if I transgress it and swear falsely, may the opposite of all this be my lot.

[Reprinted by permission of the publisher from Ludwig Edelstein, *Ancient Medicine,* edited by Oswei Temkin and C. Lillian Temkin (Baltimore: Johns Hopkins University Press, 1967).]

The World Medical Association Declaration of Geneva

Physician's Oath

At the time of being admitted as a member of the medical profession:

I solemnly pledge myself to consecrate my life to the service of humanity;

I will give to my teachers the respect and gratitude which is their due;

I will practice my profession with conscience and dignity; the health of my patient will be my first consideration;

I will maintain by all the means in my power, the honor and the noble traditions of the medical profession; my colleagues will be my brothers;

I will not permit considerations of religion, nationality, race, party politics or social standing to intervene between my duty and my patient;

I will maintain the utmost respect for human life from the time of conception, even under threat, I will not use my medical knowledge contrary to the laws of humanity;

I make these promises solemnly, freely and upon my honor.

[Adopted by the General Assembly of the World Medical Association, Geneva, Switzerland, September 1948 and amended by the 22nd World Medical Assembly, Sydney, Australia, August 1968. Reprinted by permission.]

The American Medical Association Principles of Medical Ethics

Preamble

These principles are intended to aid physicians individually and collectively in maintaining a high level of ethical conduct. They are not laws but standards by which a physician may determine the propriety of his conduct in his relationship with patients, with colleagues, with members of allied professions, and with the public.

Section 1
The principal objective of the medical profession is to render service to humanity with full respect for the dignity of man. Physicians should merit the confidence of patients entrusted to their care, rendering to each a full measure of service and devotion.

Section 2
Physicians should strive continually to improve medical knowledge and skill, and should make available to their patients and colleagues the benefits of their professional attainments.

Section 3
A physician should practice a method of healing founded on a scientific basis; and he should not voluntarily associate professionally with anyone who violates this principle.

Section 4
The medical profession should safeguard the public and itself against physicians deficient in moral character or professional competence. Physicians should observe all laws, uphold the dignity and honor of the profession and accept its self-imposed disciplines. They should expose, without hesitation, illegal or unethical conduct of fellow members of the profession.

Section 5
A physician may choose whom he will serve. In an emergency, however, he should render service to the best of his ability. Having undertaken the care of a patient, he may not neglect him; and unless he has been discharged he may discontinue his services only after giving adequate notice. He should not solicit patients.

Section 6
A physician should not dispose of his services under terms or conditions which tend to interfere with or impair the free and complete exercise of his medical judgment and skill or tend to cause a deterioration of the quality of medical care.

Section 7
In the practice of medicine a physician should limit the source of his professional income to medical services actually rendered by him, or under his supervision, to his patients. His fee should be commensurate with the services rendered and the patient's ability to pay. He should neither pay nor receive a commission for referral of patients. Drugs, remedies or appliances may be dispensed or supplied by the physician provided it is in the best interests of the patient.

Section 8
A physician should seek consultation upon request; in doubtful or difficult cases; or whenever it appears that the quality of medical service may be enhanced thereby.

Section 9
A physician may not reveal the confidences entrusted to him in the course
of medical attendance, or the deficiencies he may observe in the character
of patients, unless he is required to do so by law or unless it becomes
necessary in order to protect the welfare of the individual or of the
community.

Section 10
The honored ideals of the medical profession imply that the responsibilities of the physician extend not only to the individual, but also to
society where these responsibilities deserve his interest and participation
in activities which have the purpose of improving both the health and the
well-being of the individual and the community.

[Adopted by the American Medical Association in 1957 and reprinted with
permission.]

Constitution of the World Health Organization

The States Parties to this Constitution declare, in conformity with the
Charter of the United Nations, that the following principles are basic to
the happiness, harmonious relations and security of all peoples:

Health is a state of complete physical, mental and social well-being and not merely
the absence of disease or infirmity.

The enjoyment of the highest attainable standard of health is one of the fundamental rights of every human being without distinction of race, religion, political
belief, economic or social condition.

The health of all peoples is fundamental to the attainment of peace and security
and is dependent upon the fullest co-operation of individuals and States.

The achievement of any State in the promotion and protection of health is of
value to all.

Unequal development in different countries in the promotion of health and
control of disease, especially communicable disease, is a common danger.

Healthy development of the child is of basic importance; the ability to live
harmoniously in a changing total environment is essential to such development.

The extension to all peoples of the benefits of medical, psychological and related
knowledge is essential to the fullest attainment of health.

Informed opinion and active co-operation on the part of the public are of the utmost importance in the improvement of the health of the people.

Governments have a responsibility for the health of their peoples which can be fulfilled only by the provision of adequate health and social measures.

Accepting these principles, and for the purpose of co-operation among themselves and with others to promote and protect the health of all peoples, the Contracting Parties agree to the present Constitution and hereby establish the World Health Organization as a specialized agency within the terms of Article 57 of the Charter of the United Nations.

[Reprinted from *World Health Organization: Basic Documents,* 26th ed. (Geneva: World Health Organization, 1976), p. 1.]

American Hospital Association
A Patient's Bill of Rights

The American Hospital Association presents a Patient's Bill of Rights with the expectation that observance of these rights will contribute to more effective patient care and greater satisfaction for the patient, his physician, and the hospital organization. Further, the Association presents these rights in the expectation that they will be supported by the hospital on behalf of its patients, as an integral part of the healing process. It is recognized that a personal relationship between the physician and the patient is essential for the provision of proper medical care. The traditional physician-patient relationship takes on a new dimension when care is rendered within an organizational structure. Legal precedent has established that the institution itself also has a responsibility to the patient. It is in recognition of these factors that these rights are affirmed.

1. The patient has the right to considerate and respectful care.

2. The patient has the right to obtain from his physician complete current information concerning his diagnosis, treatment, and prognosis in terms the patient can be reasonably expected to understand. When it is not medically advisable to give such information to the patient, the information should be made available to an appropriate person in his behalf. He has the right to know, by name, the physician responsible for coordinating his care.

3. The patient has the right to receive from his physician information necessary to give informed consent prior to the start of any procedure and/or treatment. Except in emergencies, such information for informed consent should include but not necessarily be limited to the specific procedure and/or treatment, the medically significant risks involved, and the probable duration of incapacitation. Where medically significant alternatives for care or treatment exist, or when the patient requests information concerning medical alternatives, the patient has the right to such information. The patient also has the right to know the name of the person responsible for the procedures and/or treatment.

4. The patient has the right to refuse treatment to the extent permitted by law and to be informed of the medical consequences of his action.

5. The patient has the right to every consideration of his privacy concerning his own medical care program. Case discussion, consultation, examination, and treatment are confidential and should be conducted discreetly. Those not directly involved in his care must have the permission of the patient to be present.

6. The patient has the right to expect that all communications and records pertaining to his care should be treated as confidential.

7. The patient has the right to expect that within its capacity a hospital must make reasonable response to the request of a patient for services. The hospital must provide evaluation, service, and/or referral as indicated by the urgency of the case. When medically permissible, a patient may be transferred to another facility only after he has received complete information and explanation concerning the needs for and alternatives to such a transfer. The institution to which the patient is to be transferred must first have accepted the patient for transfer.

8. The patient has the right to obtain information as to any relationship of his hospital to other health care and educational institutions insofar as his care is concerned. The patient has the right to obtain information as to the existence of any professional relationships among individuals, by name, who are treating him.

9. The patient has the right to be advised if the hospital proposes to engage in or perform human experimentation affecting his care or treat-

ment. The patient has the right to refuse to participate in such research projects.

10. The patient has the right to expect reasonable continuity of care. He has the right to know in advance what appointment times and physicians are available and where. The patient has the right to expect that the hospital will provide a mechanism whereby he is informed by his physician or a delegate of the physician of the patient's continuing health care requirements following discharge.

11. The patient has the right to examine and receive an explanation of his bill regardless of source of payment.

12. The patient has the right to know what hospital rules and regulations apply to his conduct as a patient.

No catalog of rights can guarantee for the patient the kind of treatment he has a right to expect. A hospital has many functions to perform, including the prevention and treatment of disease, the education of both health professionals and patients, and the conduct of clinical research. All these activities must be conducted with an overriding concern for the patient, and, above all, the recognition of his dignity as a human being. Success in achieving this recognition assures success in the defense of the rights of the patient.

[Approved by the American Hospital Association House of Delegates, February 6, 1973, and reprinted by permission of the American Hospital Association.]

The Nuremberg Code

The great weight of the evidence before us is to the effect that certain types of medical experiments on human beings, when kept within reasonably well-defined bounds, conform to the ethics of the medical profession generally. The protagonists of the practice of human experimentation justify their views on the basis that such experiments yield results for the good of society that are unprocurable by other methods or means of study. All agree, however, that certain basic principles must be observed in order to satisfy moral, ethical and legal concepts:

1. The voluntary consent of the human subject is absolutely essential.

This means that the person involved should have legal capacity to give consent; should be so situated as to be able to exercise free power of choice, without the intervention of any element of force, fraud, deceit, duress, over-reaching, or other ulterior form of constraint or coercion; and should have sufficient knowledge and comprehension of the elements of the subject matter involved as to enable him to make an understanding and enlightened decision. This latter element requires that before the acceptance of an affirmative decision by the experimental subject there should be made known to him the nature, duration, and purpose of the experiment; the method and means by which it is to be conducted; all inconveniences and hazards reasonably to be expected; and the effects upon his health or person which may possibly come from his participation in the experiment.

The duty and responsibility for ascertaining the quality of the consent rests upon each individual who initiates, directs or engages in the experiment. It is a personal duty and responsibility which may not be delegated to another with impunity.

2. The experiment should be such as to yield fruitful results for the good of society, unprocurable by other methods or means of study, and not random and unnecessary in nature.

3. The experiment should be so designed and based on the results of animal experimentation and a knowledge of the natural history of the disease or other problem under study that the anticipated results will justify the performance of the experiment.

4. The experiment should be so conducted as to avoid all unnecessary physical and mental suffering and injury.

5. No experiment should be conducted where there is an *a priori* reason to believe that death or disabling injury will occur; except, perhaps, in those experiments where the experimental physicians also serve as subjects.

6. The degree of risk to be taken should never exceed that determined by the humanitarian importance of the problem to be solved by the experiment.

7. Proper preparations should be made and adequate facilities provided to protect the experimental subject against even remote possibilities of injury, disability, or death.

8. The experiment should be conducted only by scientifically qualified persons. The highest degree of skill and care should be required through

all stages of the experiment of those who conduct or engage in the experiment.

9. During the course of the experiment the human subject should be at liberty to bring the experiment to an end if he has reached the physical or mental state where continuation of the experiment seems to him to be impossible.

10. During the course of the experiment the scientist in charge must be prepared to terminate the experiment at any stage, if he has probable cause to believe, in the exercise of the good faith, superior skill and careful judgment required of him that a continuation of the experiment is likely to result in injury, disability, or death to the experimental subject.

[Reprinted from *Trials of War Criminals before the Nuernberg Military Tribunals under Control Council Law No. 10*, vol. 2 (Washington, D.C.: U.S. Government Printing Office, 1949), pp. 181–82.]

The World Medical Association Declaration of Helsinki

Introduction

It is the mission of the medical doctor to safeguard the health of the people. His or her knowledge and conscience are dedicated to the fulfillment of this mission.

The Declaration of Geneva of the World Medical Association binds the doctor with the words, "The health of my patient will be my first consideration," and the International Code of Medical Ethics declares that, "Any act or advice which could weaken physical or mental resistance of a human being may be used only in his interest."

The purpose of biomedical research involving human subjects must be to improve diagnostic, therapeutic and prophylactic procedures and the understanding of the aetiology and pathogenesis of disease.

In current medical practice most diagnostic, therapeutic or prophylactic procedures involve hazards. This applies *a fortiori* to biomedical research.

Medical progress is based on research which ultimately must rest in part on experimentation involving human subjects.

In the field of biomedical research a fundamental distinction must be recognized between medical research in which the aim is essentially diagnostic or therapeutic for a patient, and medical research, the essential object of which is purely scientific and without direct diagnostic or therapeutic value to the person subjected to the research.

Special caution must be exercised in the conduct of research which may affect the environment, and the welfare of animals used for research must be respected.

Because it is essential that the results of laboratory experiments be applied to human beings to further scientific knowledge and to help suffering humanity, The World Medical Association has prepared the following recommendations as a guide to every doctor in biomedical research involving human subjects. They should be kept under review in the future. It must be stressed that the standards as drafted are only a guide to physicians all over the world. Doctors are not relieved from criminal, civil and ethical responsibilities under the laws of their own countries.

I. Basic principles

1. Biomedical research involving human subjects must conform to generally accepted scientific principles and should be based on adequately performed laboratory and animal experimentation and on a thorough knowledge of the scientific literature.

2. The design and performance of each experimental procedure involving human subjects should be clearly formulated in an experimental protocol which should be transmitted to a specially appointed independent committee for consideration, comment and guidance.

3. Biomedical research involving human subjects should be conducted only by scientifically qualified persons and under the supervision of a clinically competent medical person. The responsibility for the human subject must always rest with a medically qualified person and never rest on the subject of the research, even though the subject has given his or her consent.

4. Biomedical research involving human subjects cannot legitimately be carried out unless the importance of the objective is in proportion to the inherent risk to the subject.

5. Every biomedical research project involving human subjects should be preceded by careful assessment of predictable risks in comparison with foreseeable benefits to the subject or to others. Concern for the interests of the subject must always prevail over the interests of science and society.

6. The right of the research subject to safeguard his or her integrity must always be respected. Every precaution should be taken to respect the privacy of the subject and to minimize the impact of the study on the subject's physical and mental integrity and on the personality of the subject.

7. Doctors should abstain from engaging in research projects involving human subjects unless they are satisfied that the hazards involved are believed to be predictable. Doctors should cease any investigation if the hazards are found to outweigh the potential benefits.

8. In publication of the results of his or her research, the doctor is obliged to preserve the accuracy of the results. Reports of experimentation not in accordance with the principles laid down in this Declaration should not be accepted for publication.

9. In any research on human beings, each potential subject must be adequately informed of the aims, methods, anticipated benefits and potential hazards of the study and the discomfort it may entail. He or she should be informed that he or she is at liberty to abstain from participation in the study and that he or she is free to withdraw his or her consent to participation at any time. The doctor should then obtain the subject's freely-given informed consent, preferably in writing.

10. When obtaining informed consent for the research project the doctor should be particularly cautious if the subject is in a dependent relationship to him or her or may consent under duress. In that case the informed consent should be obtained by a doctor who is not engaged in the investigation and who is completely independent of this official relationship.

11. In case of legal incompetence, informed consent should be obtained from the legal guardian in accordance with national legislation. Where physical or mental incapacity makes it impossible to obtain informed consent, or when the subject is a minor, permission from the responsible

relative replaces that of the subject in accordance with national legislation.

12. The research protocol should always contain a statement of the ethical considerations involved and should indicate that the principles enunciated in the present Declaration are complied with.

II. Medical research combined with professional care (clinical research)

1. In the treatment of the sick person, the doctor must be free to use a new diagnostic and therapeutic measure, if in his or her judgment it offers hope of saving life, reestablishing health or alleviating suffering.

2. The potential benefits, hazards and discomfort of a new method should be weighed against the advantages of the best current diagnostic and therapeutic methods.

3. In any medical study, every patient—including those of a control group, if any—should be assured of the best proven diagnostic and therapeutic method.

4. The refusal of the patient to participate in a study must never interfere with the doctor-patient relationship.

5. If the doctor considers it essential not to obtain informed consent, the specific reasons for this proposal should be stated in the experimental protocol for transmission to the independent committee (1, 2).

6. The doctor can combine medical research with professional care, the objective being the acquisition of new medical knowledge, only to the extent that medical research is justified by its potential diagnostic or therapeutic value for the patient.

III. Non-therapeutic biomedical research involving human subjects (non-clinical biomedical research)

1. In the purely scientific application of medical research carried out on a human being, it is the duty of the doctor to remain the protector of the life and health of that person on whom biomedical research is being carried out.

2. The subjects should be volunteers—either healthy persons or patients for whom the experimental design is not related to the patient's illness.

3. The investigator or the investigating team should discontinue the research if in his/her or their judgment it may, if continued, be harmful to the individual.

4. In research on man, the interest of science and society should never take precedence over considerations related to the wellbeing of the subject.

[Adopted by the 18th World Medical Assembly, Helsinki, Finland, 1964, and as revised by the 29th World Medical Assembly, Tokyo, Japan, 1975. Reprinted by permission.]

Department of Health, Education, and Welfare Regulations on the Protection of Human Subjects

§ 46.101 Applicability.

(a) The regulations in this part are applicable to all Department of Health, Education, and Welfare grants and contracts supporting research, development, and related activities in which human subjects are involved.

(b) The Secretary may, from time to time, determine in advance whether specific programs, methods, or procedures to which this part is applicable place subjects at risk, as defined in §46.103(b). Such determinations will be published as notices in the FEDERAL REGISTER and will be included in an appendix to this part.

§ 46.102 Policy.

(a) Safeguarding the rights and welfare of subjects at risk in activities supported under grants and contracts from DHEW is primarily the responsibility of the institution which receives or is accountable to DHEW for the funds awarded for the support of the activity. In order to provide for the adequate discharge of this institutional responsibility, it is the policy of DHEW that no activity involving human subjects to be supported by DHEW grants or contracts shall be undertaken unless an Institutional Review Board has reviewed and approved such activity, and the institution has submitted to DHEW a certification of such review and approval, in accordance with the requirements of this part.

(b) This review shall determine whether these subjects will be placed at risk, and, if risk is involved, whether:

(1) The risks to the subject are so outweighed by the sum of the benefit to the subject and the importance of the knowledge to be gained as to warrant a decision to allow the subject to accept these risks;

(2) The rights and welfare of any such subjects will be adequately protected; and

(3) Legally effective informed consent will be obtained by adequate and appropriate methods in accordance with the provisions of this part.

(c) Unless the activity is covered by subpart B of this part, if it involves as subjects women who could become pregnant, the Board shall also determine as part of its review that adequate and appropriate steps will be taken to avoid involvement of women who are in fact pregnant (as evidenced by any of the presumptive signs of pregnancy, such as missed menses, or by a medically acceptable pregnancy test), when such activity would involve risk to a fetus.

(d) Where the Board finds risk is involved under paragraph (b) of this section, it shall review the conduct of the activity at timely intervals.

(e) No grant or contract involving human subjects at risk shall be made to an individual unless he is affiliated with or sponsored by an institution which can and does assume responsibility for the subjects involved. [40 FR 11854, Mar. 13, 1975. Redesignated and amended at 40 FR 33528, Aug. 8, 1975.]

§ 46.103 Definitions.

(a) "Institution" means any public or private institution or agency (including Federal, State, and local government agencies).

(b) "Subject at risk" means any individual who may be exposed to the possibility of injury, including physical, psychological, or social injury, as a consequence of participation as a subject in any research, development, or related activity which departs from the application of those established and accepted methods necessary to meet his needs, or which increases the ordinary risks of daily life, including the recognized risks inherent in a chosen occupation or field of service.

(c) "Informed consent" means the knowing consent of an individual or his legally authorized representative, so situated as to be able to exercise free power of choice without undue inducement or any element of force, fraud, deceit, duress, or other form of constraint or coercion. The basic elements of information necessary to such consent include:

(1) A fair explanation of the procedures to be followed, and their purposes, including identification of any procedures which are experimental;

(2) A description of any attendant discomforts and risks reasonably to be expected;

(3) A description of any benefits reasonably to be expected;

(4) A disclosure of any appropriate alternative procedures that might be advantageous for the subject;

(5) An offer to answer any inquiries concerning the procedures; and

(6) An instruction that the person is free to withdraw his consent and to discontinue participation in the project or activity at any time without prejudice to the subject.

(d) "Secretary" means the Secretary of Health, Education, and Welfare or any other officer or employee of the Department of Health, Education, and Welfare to whom authority has been delegated.

(e) "DHEW" means the Department of Health, Education, and Welfare.

(f) "Approved assurance" means a document that fulfills the requirements of this part and is approved by the Secretary.

(g) "Certification" means the official institutional notification to DHEW in accordance with the requirements of this part that a project or activity involving human subjects at risk has been reviewed and approved by the institution in accordance with the "approved assurance" on file at DHEW.

(h) "Legally authorized representative" means an individual or judicial or other body authorized under applicable law to consent on behalf of a prospective subject to such subject's participation in the particular activity or procedure.

[Code of Federal Regulations, Title 45, U.S. Code, Part 46, revised as of January 11, 1978.]

International Council of Nurses
Code for Nurses: Ethical Concepts Applied to Nursing

The fundamental responsibility of the nurse is fourfold: to promote health, to prevent illness, to restore health and to alleviate suffering.

The need for nursing is universal. Inherent in nursing is respect for life, dignity and rights of man. It is unrestricted by considerations of nationality, race, creed, color, age, sex, politics or social status.

Nurses render health services to the individual, the family and the community and coordinate their services with those of related groups.

Nurses and People

The nurse's primary responsibility is to those people who require nursing care.

The nurse, in providing care, promotes an environment in which the values, customs and spiritual beliefs of the individual are respected.

The nurse holds in confidence personal information and uses judgment in sharing this information.

Nurses and Practice

The nurse carries personal responsibility for nursing practice and for maintaining competence by continual learning.

The nurse maintains the highest standards of nursing care possible within the reality of a specific situation.

The nurse uses judgment in relation to individual competence when accepting and delegating responsibilities.

The nurse when acting in a professional capacity should at all times maintain standards of personal conduct which reflect credit upon the profession.

Nurses and Society

The nurse shares with other citizens the responsibility for initiating and supporting action to meet the health and social needs of the public.

Nurses and Co-Workers

The nurse sustains a cooperative relationship with co-workers in nursing and other fields.

The nurse takes appropriate action to safeguard the individual when his care is endangered by a co-worker or any other person.

Nurses and the Profession

The nurse plays the major role in determining and implementing desirable standards of nursing practice and nursing education.

The nurse is active in developing a core of professional knowledge.

The nurse, acting through the professional organization, participates in establishing and maintaining equitable social and economic working conditions in nursing.

[Adopted by the International Council of Nurses, May 1973 and reprinted by permission.]

Bibliography of Suggested Readings

Original Texts (Ethical Theory):

Feinberg, Joel. *Social Philosophy.* Englewood Cliffs, N.J.: Prentice-Hall, 1973.

Frankena, William K. *Ethics.* 2nd Edition. Englewood Cliffs, N.J.: Prentice-Hall, 1973.

Hudson, W. D. *Modern Moral Philosophy.* Garden City, N.Y.: Doubleday Anchor, 1970.

MacIntyre, Alasdair. *A Short History of Ethics.* New York: Macmillan, 1966.

Mackie, J. L. *Ethics: Inventing Right and Wrong.* Harmondsworth, Eng.: Penguin Books, 1977.

Rawls, John. *A Theory of Justice.* Cambridge, Mass.: Harvard University Press, 1971.

Taylor, Paul. *Principles of Ethics: An Introduction.* Encino, Calif.: Dickenson Publishing Co., 1975.

Original Texts (Biomedical Ethics):

Brody, Howard. *Ethical Decisions in Medicine.* Boston: Little, Brown and Company, 1976.

Campbell, Alastair V. *Moral Dilemmas in Medicine.* 2nd ed. Edinburgh: Churchill-Livingston, 1975.

Fletcher, Joseph. *Morals and Medicine.* Boston: Beacon Press, 1960.

Fried, Charles. *Medical Experimentation: Personal Integrity and Social Policy.* New York: American Elsevier Publishing Co., 1974.

Ramsey, Paul. *Ethics at the Edges of Life.* New Haven: Yale University Press, 1978.

———. *The Patient as Person.* New Haven: Yale University Press, 1970.

Veatch, Robert. *Death, Dying, and the Biological Revolution: Our Last Quest for Responsibility.* New Haven: Yale University Press, 1976.

Anthologies:

Beauchamp, Tom L. and Walters, LeRoy, eds. *Contemporary Issues in Bioethics.* Encino, Calif.: Dickenson Publishing Co., 1978.

Gorovitz, Samuel et al., eds. *Moral Problems in Medicine.* Englewood Cliffs, N.J.: Prentice-Hall, 1976.

Humber, James M. and Almeder, Robert F., eds. *Biomedical Ethics and the Law.* New York: Plenum Press, 1976.

Hunt, Robert and Arras, John, eds. *Ethical Issues in Modern Medicine.* Palo Alto, Calif.: Mayfield Publishing Co., 1977.

Katz, Jay, comp. *Experimentation with Human Beings: The Authority of the Investigator, Subject, Professions and State in the Human Experimentation Process.* New York: Russell Sage Foundation, 1972.

Reiser, Stanley Joel, Dyck, Arthur J., and Curran, William J., eds. *Ethics in Medicine: Historical Perspectives and Contemporary Concerns.* Cambridge, Mass.: MIT Press, 1977.

Shannon, Thomas A., ed. *Bioethics: Basic Writings on the Key Ethical Questions That Surround the Major Modern Biological Possibilities and Problems.* New York: Paulist Press, 1976.

Veatch, Robert and Branson, Roy, eds. *Ethics and Health Policy.* Cambridge, Mass.: Ballinger Publishing Co., 1976.

Reference Works:

Reich, Warren T., ed. *Encyclopedia of Bioethics.* New York: Macmillan and Free Press, 1978. Vols. 1–4.

Sollitto, Sharmon and Veatch, Robert M., comps. *Bibliography of Society, Ethics and the Life Sciences.* Hastings-on-Hudson, N.Y.: Institute of Society, Ethics, and the Life Sciences. Updated periodically.

Veatch, Robert M. *Case Studies in Medical Ethics.* Cambridge, Mass.: Harvard University Press, 1977.

Walters, LeRoy, ed. *Bibliography of Bioethics.* Vols. 1–   Detroit: Gale Research Co. Issued annually.

Journals:

We here offer a list only of some of the more significant journals, arranged according to their various emphases.

There are a few journals which deal primarily, if not exclusively, with issues of biomedical ethics. Among these are *Ethics in Science and Medicine, The Hastings Center Report,* and *The Journal of Medical Ethics.* Other journals deal both with the history and philosophy of medicine and biomedical ethics. Journals such as *The Bulletin of the History of Medicine, The Journal of Medicine and Philosophy, Man and Medicine,* and *Perspectives in Biology and Medicine* are representative.

Some journals with a more general ethical orientation frequently include articles that apply basic ethical principles to problems raised by contemporary biology and medicine. Such journals include *Ethics, The Journal of Religious Ethics,* and *Philosophy and Public Affairs.* In addition, several medical and legal journals routinely publish articles dealing with biomedical ethics. Representative are *The American Journal of Law and Medicine, The Journal of Legal Medicine, The Journal of Thanatology, The Journal of the American Medical Association, Lancet, The New England Journal of Medicine,* and *Obstetrics and Gynecology.*

U.S. Government Documents:

HEW Secretary's Task Force on the Compensation of Injured Research Subjects. DHEW Publication No. (OS) 77–003 (1977).

The National Commission for the Protection of Human Subjects of Biomedical and Behavioral Research:

Report and Recommendations: Research on the Fetus. DHEW Publication No. (OS) 76–127 (1976). *Appendix to Report and Recommendations: Research on the Fetus.* DHEW Publication No. (OS) 76–128 (1976).

Report and Recommendations: Research Involving Prisoners. DHEW Publication No. (OS) 76–131 (1976). *Appendix to Report and Recommendations: Research Involving Prisoners.* DHEW Publication No. (OS) 76–132 (1976).

Report and Recommendations: Psychosurgery. DHEW Publication No. (OS) 77–0001 (1977). *Appendix to Report and Recommendations: Psychosurgery.* DHEW Publication No. (OS) 77–0002 (1977).

Disclosure of Research Information Under the Freedom of Information Act. DHEW Publication No. (OS) 77–0003 (1977).

Report and Recommendations: Research Involving Children. DHEW Publication No. (OS) 77–0004 (1977). *Appendix to Report and Recommendations: Research Involving Children.* DHEW Publication No. (OS) 77–0005 (1977).

Report and Recommendations: Research Involving Those Institutionalized as Mentally Infirm. DHEW Publication No. (OS) 78–0006 (1978). *Appendix to Report and Recommendations: Research Involving Those Institutionalized as Mentally Infirm.* DHEW Publication No. (OS) 78–0007 (1978).

Report and Recommendations: Institutional Review Boards. DHEW Publication No. (OS) 78–0008 (1978). *Appendix to Report and Recommendations: Institutional Review Boards.* DHEW Publication No. (OS) 78–0009 (1978).

Report and Recommendations: Ethical Guidelines for the Delivery of Health Services by DHEW. DHEW Publication No. (OS) 78–0010 (1978). *Appendix to Report and Recommendations: Ethical Guidelines for the Delivery of Health Services by DHEW.* DHEW Publication No. (OS) 78–0011 (1978).

The Belmont Report: Ethical Guidelines for the Protection of Human Subjects of Research. DHEW Publication No. (OS) 78–0012 (1978). *Appendices A and B to The Belmont Report: Ethical Guidelines for the Protection of Human Subjects of Research.* DHEW Publication Nos. (OS) 78–0013–14 (1978).

Report of the President's Biomedical Research Panel. DHEW Publication No. (OS) 76–500 (1976).

Index